REHABILITATION OF PERSONS WITH RHEUMATOID ARTHRITIS

THE REHABILITATION INSTITUTE OF CHICAGO PUBLICATION SERIES

Don A. Olson, PhD, Series Coordinator

Spinal Cord Injury: A Guide to Functional Outcomes in Physical Therapy Management

Lower Extremity Amputation: A Guide to Functional Outcomes in Physical Therapy Management, Second Edition

Stroke/Head Injury: A Guide to Functional Outcomes in Physical Therapy Management

Clinical Management of Right Hemisphere Dysfunction, Second Edition

Spinal Cord Injury: A Guide to Functional Outcomes in Occupational Therapy

Spinal Cord Injury: A Guide to Rehabilitation Nursing

Head Injury: A Guide to Functional Outcomes in Occupational Therapy Management

Speech/Language Treatment of the Aphasias: Treatment Materials for Auditory Comprehension and Reading Comprehension

Speech/Language Treatment of the Aphasias: Treatment Materials for Oral Expression and Written Expression

Rehabilitation Nursing Procedures Manual

Psychological Management of Traumatic Brain Injuries in Children and Adolescents

Medical Management of Long-Term Disability

Psychological Aspects of Geriatric Rehabilitation

Clinical Management of Dysphagia in Adults and Children, Second Edition

Cognition and Perception in the Stroke Patient: A Guide to Functional Outcomes in Occupational Therapy

Spinal Cord Injury: Medical Management and Rehabilitation

Clinical Management of Communication Problems in Adults with Traumatic Brain Injury

Rehabilitation
Institute of
Chicago

REHABILITATION OF PERSONS WITH RHEUMATOID ARTHRITIS

Edited by

Rowland W. Chang, MD, MPH

Associate Professor
Departments of Preventive Medicine and Physical Medicine and Rehabilitation
Northwestern University Medical School

Co-Director
Arthritis Center
Rehabilitation Institute of Chicago
Chicago, Illinois

with

Patricia A. Lee

Consulting Editor and Writer
Past President
American Medical Writers Association, Chicago Chapter
Chicago, Illinois

AN ASPEN PUBLICATION®
Aspen Publishers, Inc.
Gaithersburg, Maryland
1996

Library of Congress Cataloging-in-Publication Data

Rehabilitation of persons with rheumatoid arthritis / edited by Rowland W. Chang.
p. cm. — (Rehabilitation Institute of Chicago procedure manual) (The Rehabilitation Institute of Chicago publication series)
ISBN 0-8342-0679-X
1. Rheumatoid arthritis—Patients—Rehabilitation. 2. Rheumatoid arthritis—Treatment. I. Chang, Rowland W. II. Series. III. Series: The Rehabilitation Institute of Chicago publication series.
[DNLM: 1. Arthritis, Rheumatoid—rehabilitation. WE 346 R345 1996]
RC933.R365 1996
616.7′22706—dc20
DNLM/DLC
for Library of Congress
96-21624
CIP

The authors have made every effort to ensure the accuracy of the information herein. However, appropriate information sources should be consulted, especially for new or unfamiliar procedures. It is the responsibility of every practitioner to evaluate the appropriateness of a particular opinion in the context of actual clinical situations and with due considerations to new developments. Authors, editors, and the publisher cannot be held responsible for any typographical or other errors found in this book.

Editorial Resources: Ruth Bloom
Library of Congress Catalog Card Number: 96-21624
ISBN: 0-8342-0679-X

Printed in the United States of America

1 2 3 4 5

We dedicate this book
in memory of
Susan G. Perlman, MD

Table of Contents

Contributors

Victoria A. Brander, MD
Medical Director, Subacute Services and Co-Director, Arthritis Center
Rehabilitation Institute of Chicago
Assistant Clinical Professor
Departments of Orthopaedic Surgery and Physical Medicine and Rehabilitation
Northwestern University Medical School
Chicago, Illinois

Rowland W. Chang, MD, MPH
Associate Professor
Departments of Preventive Medicine and Physical Medicine and Rehabilitation
Northwestern University Medical School
Co-Director
Arthritis Center
Rehabilitation Institute of Chicago
Chicago, Illinois

Karen J. Connell, MS
Director, Educational Development
Department of Family Medicine
University of Illinois at Chicago
Chicago, Illinois

Judith A. Falconer, PhD, MPH, OTR/L
Associate Professor of Physical Therapy and Medicine
Programs in Physical Therapy
Northwestern University Medical School
Chicago, Illinois

Sharon V. Feldmann, MS, PT
Senior Physical Therapist
Physical Therapy Department
Rehabilitation Institute of Chicago
Chicago, Illinois

Karen W. Hayes, PhD, PT
Curriculum Coordinator
Assistant Professor of Physical Therapy
Programs in Physical Therapy
Northwestern University Medical School
Chicago, Illinois

Richard T. Katz, MD
Vice President of Medical Affairs
SSM Rehabilitation Institute
St. Louis, Missouri

Lynn Westerman Kirkbride, MS
Project Specialist
Wyoming Institute for Disability
University of Wyoming
Laramie, Wyoming

Mary C. Kozy, MSW, LCSW, ACSW
Social Work Consultant
Dupage Center for Independent Living
Chicago, Illinois

Kenneth A. Lefebvre, PhD
Senior Psychologist
Spinal Cord Injury, Amputee, and Orthopaedic Clinical Operating Group
Rehabilitation Institute of Chicago
Assistant Professor
Department of Rehabilitation Medicine
Northwestern University Medical School
Chicago, Illinois

Holly Yvonne Lusa, MOT, OTR/L
Supervisor, Hand Rehabilitation
Mercy Hospital and Medical Center
Chicago, Illinois

Christina Marciniak, MD
Assistant Professor
Departments of Physical Medicine and Rehabilitation
Northwestern University Medical School
Attending Physician
Rehabilitation Institute of Chicago
Chicago, Illinois

Jane E. Marlor, CO, CPED, LPTA
formerly, Senior Orthotist
Prosthetic Orthotic Clinical Services
Rehabilitation Institute of Chicago
Chicago, Illinois

Marion Jackson Mito, MA, CCC-SLP
Senior Speech/Language Pathologist
Lutheran General Hospital
Park Ridge, Illinois

Karen Freeman Ortmann, MM, PT
Director, Physical Therapy Department
Rehabilitation Institute of Chicago
Chicago, Illinois

Caroline K. Ross, ScD
formerly, Research Health Scientist
Department of Veterans Affairs
West Side Veterans Administration Medical Center
formerly, Assistant Professor
Division of Health Policy and Administration
School of Public Health
University of Illinois at Chicago
Chicago, Illinois

Anne V. Sasso, MA, CCC-SLP
Senior Speech/Language Pathologist
Department of Speech Pathology and Audiology
Marianjoy Rehabilitation Hospital & Clinics
Wheaton, Illinois

John T. Schousboe, MD
Consulting Rheumatologist
Rheumatology Treatment and Resource Center
Park Nicollet Clinic, Health System Minnesota
Minneapolis, Minnesota

Pamela A. Semanik, BSN, MS
Rheumatologic Nurse Practitioner
Rehabilitation Institute of Chicago
Chicago, Illinois

Dale C. Strasser, MD
Assistant Professor of Rehabilitation Medicine
Emory University School of Medicine
Chief of Rehabilitation Medicine
Wesley Woods Geriatric Hospital
Medical Co-Director
Atlanta Veterans Administration Research and Development Center
Atlanta Veterans Administration Medical Center
Decatur, Georgia

Judith A. Sutin, MD
Clinical Assistant Professor
Department of Rehabilitation Medicine
State University of New York at Buffalo
Buffalo, New York

Foreword

Despite remarkable advances in the treatment of rheumatoid arthritis it remains a disease of unknown etiology for which we have no cures. It is a chronic illness that reduces life expectancy; it also profoundly affects patients' ability to function and their quality of life. Advances in the basic understanding of function and rehabilitation techniques have made it possible for most patients to adapt and adjust, and to participate in normal activities even with the impairments and functional limitations resulting from rheumatoid synovitis.

This book, edited by an outstanding practitioner of the art and a very capable medical editor/writer, presents a multidisciplinary, authoritative, and practical guide to the rehabilitation management of rheumatoid arthritis. Rehabilitation follows a paradigm different from that of curative medicine, which is based on the medical model, and focuses on ways to reduce or prevent the functional consequences of rheumatoid synovitis. It is dependent on an accurate description of functional status and knowledge of the mechanisms of functional limitation rather than that of the mechanism of disease. The formulation of a functional (in addition to medical) diagnosis and treatment and an active therapeutic partnership with the client are essential features. Rehabilitation is a venerable specialty and its ethos has been "discovered" by those formulating and changing health policy. This discovery has occurred because of society's desire for more outcomes assessment, something in which rehabilitation professionals are expert. The bottom line for patients is their ability to function, to be productive members of society, and to participate fully in their family life. This book is an important contribution toward these goals.

Matthew H. Liang, MD, MPH
Professor of Medicine, Harvard Medical School
Professor of Health Policy and Management,
Harvard School of Public Health
Medical Director, Rehabilitation Services Director,
Robert B. Brigham Multipurpose
Arthritis Center
Brigham and Women's Hospital
Boston, Massachusetts

Preface

This book is the result of the cumulative expertise of the past and present members of the Arthritis Center at the Rehabilitation Institute of Chicago (RIC) and the Multipurpose Arthritis and Musculoskeletal Disease Center at the Northwestern University Medical School (NUMS). The RIC Arthritis Center was first established in the 1970s by Dr Henry Betts, CEO of the RIC and immediate past Chairman of Rehabilitation Medicine at RIC and NUMS, and Dr Frank Schmid, Northwestern's Chief of the Arthritis-Connective Tissue Diseases Section. This book project began during the time when Dr Rowland Chang and Dr Judith Sutin were the leaders of the program. Now Dr Chang and Dr Victoria Brander co-direct the program.

There has been considerable growth in the clinical activities of the RIC Arthritis Center in the past 10 years. As a result, there has been a growing cadre of health professionals who have committed much time and energy toward exploring the strengths and weaknesses of arthritis rehabilitation care and developing experience with significantly disabled arthritis patients. This has led to a clinically successful program.

The role of rehabilitation in arthritis care, training, and research traditionally has been undervalued. However, several factors, including the renaissance of rehabilitation in general, the increased societal and medical consciousness of the benefits of physical activity, the disinclination to rely totally on pharmacotherapy, and the burgeoning field of total joint replacement, have thrust rehabilitation into the forefront of arthritis care.

Our program has undergone a progressive evolution with respect to content and philosophy. We believe this was due to the realization that (1) the issues in the rehabilitation of the arthritis patient are different from those of the patient with other impairments and that (2) the "medical model" that continues to push the frontiers of scientific knowledge forward in rheumatology and its allied basic sciences of immunology, biochemistry, and molecular biology often is not useful in solving rehabilitation problems. All participating professionals have had to deal with complex problems stemming from the increasing age of the total joint replacement population to the unknown prognosis of newly diagnosed patients with rheumatoid arthritis (RA). Other problems relate to the established and maladaptive coping behaviors of long-term patients with RA. We have tried to coalesce the established literature that serves as a basis for rational decision making. Where literature is lacking, we believe our extensive experience may benefit others struggling with similar problems.

The selection of the chapter titles and authors parallels the philosophy of our arthritis rehabilitation program. Our team is multidisciplinary, with representatives from rheumatology, physiatrics, orthopaedic surgery, nursing, social work, clinical psychology, occupational therapy, physical therapy, communicative disorders, vocational rehabilitation, and therapeutic recreation. The interdisciplinary nature of the team is exemplified by the cooperation among physicians, nurses, and therapists to form a unique team with expertise in various rehabilitation topics. For example, one team member, an occupational therapist, runs a daily aerobic-like upper extremity exercise class for arthritis and orthopaedic surgery patients.

While there are chapters that are specific to a particular area of expertise (eg, vocational rehabilitation and speech therapy), we have attempted to maintain an interdisciplinary stance for as many chapters as possible. Unlike those of other multiauthored books on arthritis rehabilitation, all authors of this book are team members or past team members in the RIC-NUMS arthritis rehabilitation clinical and/or research program.

We hope that all health care professionals interested in the care of persons with RA will benefit from reading each chapter, since we intend the chapters to be useful for those in all disciplines.

SCOPE OF THIS BOOK

There was a conscious decision to restrict the scope of this book to rehabilitation problems of those with adult RA. Arthritis rehabilitation programs generally are modeled around the care of the RA patient. While many of the topics discussed could be applied to patients with other musculoskeletal and connective tissue diseases, we thought it best for clarity and parsimony of thought that our authors restrict discussion to a single disease. It is left to the reader to decide not only who should provide the therapy but also which patients might benefit from any particular rehabilitation strategy.*

Given this purpose, we have consciously attempted to emphasize the principles underpinning rehabilitation practice for persons with RA rather than protocols of rehabilitation care. We have taken this stance to emphasize that much practitioner decision making is necessary for the optimal use of the vast panoply of rehabilitation services, particularly for those with RA, a disease that leads to a myriad of possible consequences of varying severity. For instance, the use of methotrexate is appropriate for a person with recent-onset, active inflammatory joint disease but useless or even harmful for a person with longstanding, destructive disease with no evidence of acute inflammation. Similarly, strengthening and aerobic exercises are encouraged for most persons with RA, but these need to be modified during disease flares of acute inflammation. Also, when considering the use of splints, the particular type of hand splint prescribed and fabricated for a person with RA depends on the disease activity and the purpose for the splint.

A person's RA is ever changing. Individuals at any given time in their natural history will present with different challenges and rehabilitation opportunities. We expect that future outcome studies, such as those ongoing at our university, will define more accurately which specific rehabilitation strategies are most effective and which patients are most likely to benefit.

RESEARCH AND RHEUMATOID ARTHRITIS

Finally, we wish to emphasize the importance of research. Arthritis rehabilitation is a relatively young field. There are few investigators whose primary job or passion it is to broaden and deepen the scientific and empirical basis of rehabilitation practice for the arthritis patient. Several members of our program are involved in research. Some have studied the effect of ultrasound in improving treatment for soft tissue contractures. Others have assessed the effect of a computer-assisted management technique on the efficiency of inpatient rehabilitation care. Still others have merged an educational program with an aerobic exercise training program (Educize) and assessed its effect on health behaviors and functional status. Much needs to be done to understand further which are the most effective and efficient rehabilitation services for persons with RA and also what patient characteristics (related and unrelated to RA) are associated with improved outcome after rehabilitation. Whenever possible, we have attempted to clarify the rationale for these and other ongoing and contemplated studies and provide a stimulus for others to be creative in thinking about and solving arthritis rehabilitation problems.

This book was written for health care professionals interested in the clinical management of RA. Its purpose is to focus on the application of team care concepts in the rehabilitation of those with RA. Most chapters provide some theoretical and research under-

*Note that this book does not address rehabilitation after hand surgery. This area has become very specialized and typically is performed outside the team care setting.

pinnings so that intelligent, practical, clinical applications can be achieved.

Chapter 1 discusses the rationale for team care and the evidence for its efficacy in patients with RA. Both the theoretical and practical aspects of team care are addressed.

Chapter 2 is a broad overview of assessment issues in RA. Rather than presenting the traditional discipline-specific approach to this topic, assessment is discussed from a more global perspective to encourage interdisciplinary communication. The author believes that interdisciplinary assessment is important for providing optimal care for the RA patient. The chapter's conceptual framework is centered around the disability model created by the Institute of Medicine. By use of a fictionalized case history for illustration, the rationales, context, and paradigms of RA assessment are reviewed. Assessment forms for immediate use or adaptation are also included in Appendix A.

Chapter 3, "Tissue and Joint Impairments in Rheumatoid Arthritis," begins with a review of the structure and function of normal tissue and joints and progresses to tissue impairments, such as synovitis, and joint impairments, such as flexor tenosynovitis. Later, the pattern and course of RA are described for the upper and lower extremities and the cervical spine. This chapter will be particularly useful for those who wish to understand the relationship between RA's pathology and deformity.

Chapter 4, "Functional Limitations Associated with Rheumatoid Arthritis: A Guide to Rehabilitation Prescription," reviews some of the most common functional limitations in RA, such as early nondestructive RA, RA with active inflammation and modest joint destruction, and RA with severe deformities and extra-articular manifestation. Selected detailed case presentations give insights into the types of problems the rehabilitation professional faces regularly. This chapter also provides a structured approach to prescription writing for rehabilitation treatment referencing the Institute of Medicine's disability model. Those needing a theoretically based approach for deciding which rehabilitation approach to prescribe for any given patient will especially appreciate this chapter.

Electrodiagnostic testing is the topic of Chapter 5. This chapter presents an overview of electrodiagnostic methods and then proceeds to discuss the diagnosis of several neuromuscular disorders associated with RA in some detail.

Chapter 6, "Current Medical Treatment of Rheumatoid Arthritis," comprehensively reviews the general approach and rationale for using medication when treating patients with RA. Details about which drugs have proven effective for RA patients in specific disease stages are given. Efficacy of aspirin, nonsteroidal anti-inflammatory drugs, corticosteroids, and the more toxic disease-modifying drugs is weighed. Typical dosages, expected effects, and contraindications are also discussed. A distinctive feature of this chapter is that medication decisions are discussed in the context of the patient's functional status.

Chapter 7 focuses on the use of heat and cold treatments for relieving some of the predominant symptoms of RA. Both the theoretical rationale and empirical support for modality use are discussed.

Chapter 8, "Exercise for the Person with Rheumatoid Arthritis," provides practical instruction about which exercises are useful for maintaining or increasing daily level of function and also decreasing pain. Historically exercise was thought to be detrimental to patients with RA, but recent studies suggest that carefully prescribed and monitored exercise can be beneficial. Flexibility training, strength training, and cardiovascular conditioning for RA patients are reviewed.

Chapter 9, "Hand Splinting in Rheumatoid Arthritis: A Perspective on Current Knowledge and Directions for Research," provides principles that are useful for the rational prescription of the many varieties of hand splints available for persons with RA.

Chapter 10, "Orthotic Management of Rheumatoid Arthritis in the Foot and Ankle," discusses which orthotics are appropriate and why they are appropriate for a variety of foot and ankle problems related to RA. This chapter also provides information about some of the techniques used by orthotists and advises the reader about issues of concern when working with the orthotist and the RA patient.

"Psychological Components in the Understanding and Treatment of Patients with Rheumatoid Arthritis," Chapter 11, describes the psychological reactions of many RA patients to this chronic disease. The author also presents a comprehensive review of the current psychology literature that relates to RA patient treatments and outcomes.

Chapter 12, "Nutrition and Rheumatoid Arthritis," presents what is known about the relationship between RA and diet. The process of nutritional assessment, the nutritional status of RA patients, and possible nutritional interventions are explored. This topic is not commonly addressed in the context of RA management; it is an important one, however, so this chapter is especially welcome.

Chapter 13, "Speech, Language, and Swallowing Disorders in Rheumatoid Arthritis," reviews the symptoms of RA related to speech and considers appropriate patient treatment. Particular conditions, such as rheumatoid involvement of the cricoarytenoid joint, rheumatoid nodules, and atlantoaxial subluxation in the cervical spine, are addressed, as are conditions that may co-occur with RA, such as Sjögren syndrome.

Chapter 14, "Rehabilitation Following Hip, Knee, and Shoulder Arthroplasty," discusses in detail what these types of surgeries entail for the RA patient. Appropriate rehabilitation exercises are given, as are expectations about rate of recovery. Total joint replacement surgery has led to substantial improvements in function and reduction in pain for thousands of patients with RA. Although much of what is done for other patients can be adapted to patients with RA, there are specific modifications of postoperative rehabilitation procedures that should be considered.

Chapter 15, "Adaptive Equipment and Assistive Devices," highlights the equipment and devices available for improving mobility and making the activities of daily life easier for those coping with RA.

Chapter 16, "Insights from Problem-Solving Theory for Arthritis Patients Education," tells what has been learned about how to educate successfully the RA patient about this chronic disease so that achievement of a high quality of life is a realizable goal.

Chapter 17, "Vocational Rehabilitation for Persons with Rheumatoid Arthritis," explains in detail what is involved in the process of vocational counseling, an underutilized resource for persons with RA.

The final chapter, "Social Supports and Community Resources for Persons with Rheumatoid Arthritis," provides an overview of the range of resources available to those with RA. Related government services and not-for-profit organizations' services, such as those offered by the Arthritis Foundation, are listed and explained.

Acknowledgments

The editors thank all the contributing authors for both their contributions and their patience. Special thanks to Dr Don Olson, who believes in the rehabilitation team care concept and thought that what we'd learned through our work at the Arthritis Center was worth sharing with a wider audience. We also thank Aspen Publishers for patience and suggestions. Thanks too to Mary Keen, MD, and Lillian Anaya for their work when this project was in its infancy. Finally, thanks to Julie Mack for her many skills and good humor as she works each day with all of us!

CHAPTER 1

Process and Outcomes of Team Care in Rheumatoid Arthritis

Dale C. Strasser, MD, and Rowland W. Chang, MD, MPH

Persons suffering from rheumatoid arthritis (RA) present complex problems to rehabilitation professionals. The uncertainty of etiology, the variable natural history of the disease, and the need for an array of toxic medications and complicated orthopaedic procedures are challenging. This serious disease has profound ramifications on the physical, psychological, social, and economic well-being of the patient. According to a review of the subject by McDuffie (1985), persons afflicted with RA have a divorce rate 70% above that of the general population. He found that a person with destructive RA is likely to experience a 60% decline in earnings during the first 6 years of the disease. When the consequences of RA begin to have a serious impact on a person's life, the rehabilitation care is best handled by a specialized health care team.

A health care rehabilitation team consists of two or more professionals from different disciplines who share common values and goals (Halstead, 1976). Team care should be a comprehensive, coordinated, and integrated approach to patient management. Furthermore, teamwork surpasses the sum of the work of the individual members (Ducanis & Golin, 1979; Horwitz, 1970; Rothberg, 1985) as expressed in the distinction between multidisciplinary and interdisciplinary activities (Fordyce, 1981; Melvin, 1980).

Special thanks to Ann VanSlyke, MA, Judith A. Falconer, PhD, MPH, OTR/L and Meyer S. Gunther, MD, for their insightful comments.

While practitioners applaud the "team approach," many have only vague notions of how such a team should function. This chapter explores the nature of team care rehabilitation as it relates to RA patients and offers suggestions on how team management can be provided effectively.

PSYCHOSOCIAL ADAPTATION, PAIN MANAGEMENT, AND THE REHABILITATION TEAM

Individuals with RA suffer psychological difficulties as their disease progresses. These difficulties profoundly affect and are affected by the rehabilitation process. The interdisciplinary team makes a concerted effort to optimize functional abilities by addressing the multidimensional medical, surgical, physical, and social-psychological consequences of RA. The strength of this comprehensive approach is evident when addressing the complicated issues of psychosocial independence and pain.

Psychological states influence adaptation for individuals with RA. Depression, dependency, anxiety, sexual dysfunction, and family discord are common with advanced disease (Baum, 1982; Rogers, Liang, & Partridge, 1982), and psychological factors influence functional adaptation to the disease. Nosek, Parker, and Larsen (1987) studied the relationship between psychosocial independence and functional abilities in adults with severe musculoskeletal impairments, including RA. They found no significant relationship between physical impairments and functional abilities on the one hand and psychological and social independence on the other. Similarly, McDuffie (1985) discovered that job-related factors influenced continued employment at least as much as course of the disease or success of medical intervention.

The perception of pain is influenced by one's psychological state. In addition, pain has a unique meaning and influence in the care of RA patients. In a study comparing pain, physical disability, and psychological disability in arthritis patients, Kazis, Meenan, and Anderson (1983) found that current pain was the best predictor of subsequent pain, functional limitation, and disability. They also reported that pain was the most important component in explaining medication usage in a study of patients with rheumatic diseases. Clinically, pain or fatigue affects medication use, exercise prescription, activity level, and vocational considerations. The psychological environment of both patient and staff alters the interpretation of these subjective feelings. For example, does the pain or fatigue represent a disease flare-up, a worsening of a depression, a poor relationship with staff, a reinforcement of a secondary gain, or a combination of all four? The well-integrated team is better equipped to treat these elusive, but crucial issues.

The psychological state of the patient may also affect the team by countertransference. Team members may identify emotionally with the patient. A physician may be reminded of his or her father's hip replacement and become overly cautious about activity tolerance. A physical therapist may associate a patient's depression with that of a close relative and become inappropriately anxious around the patient. The countertransference that staff members experience frequently is anxiety provoking and alters the rehabilitation environment (Gunther, 1987).

Team dynamics and the patient's own psychodynamics influence each other. Commonly, patients with depression will drain the team of energy. A patient who does not participate in the rehabilitation activities may evoke staff feelings of frustration and inadequacy. Typically, a patient with a borderline personality splits the team into "good guys" and "bad guys." A team conflict may be initiated or augmented by the internal conflict of the patient (Nason, 1981).

TEAM CARE OUTCOMES IN RHEUMATOID ARTHRITIS

An arthritis team typically consists of a physician, a nurse, a physical therapist, an occupational therapist, a psychologist, and a social worker. For selected patients an orthotist and a vocational counselor will also become involved. This diversity of professional perspectives allows the team to treat the interrelated consequences of RA, namely impairments, functional limitations, and disabilities.

Team members usually concentrate on different consequences of RA. For example, an occupational therapist focuses primarily on functional limitations when he or she helps the patient acquire a greater functional ability with hand activity. The relative importance of acquiring a specific skill (eg, the disability) is usually influenced by the assessment of the social worker, psychologist, and vocational counselor. Likewise, the progress made with the occupational therapist will probably affect the work of the social worker, psychologist, and vocational counselor.

While the benefits of team care are difficult to prove, this approach appears to benefit patients with RA. Katz, Vignos, Moskowitz, Thompson, and Svec (1968) compared one group of RA outpatients treated by a team with a control group treated in a more traditional medical clinic setting. Patients in the treatment groups did better in terms of activities of daily living, economic independence, and clinical manifestations of disease activity. Duff, Carpenter, and Neukom (1974) also studied the effects of comprehensive management of patients with RA in an outpatient setting for 1 year. Similar to Katz et al. (1968), they examined five indices of disease activity and found that the experimental group did relatively better than the control group. In a smaller study lasting 2 years, Feinberg and Brandt (1984) found improvements in disease activity, grip strength, range of motion, and attitude of patients treated by an experimental team compared with those in a control group.

A primary benefit of team care may be in the area of psychosocial adaptation. Vignos et al. (1972) found that RA patients treated by a team approach showed improved psychosocial adjustment and functional activities of daily living. In a randomized, prospective study, Ahlmen, Sullivan, and Bjelle (1988) compared team versus non–team outpatient care for individuals with RA. Individuals managed by a treatment team had increased mental well-being and improved health as measured by the Sickness Impact Profile, without any differences in pharmacological treatment, orthopaedic evaluations, disease activity, specific joint dysfunction, or self-rated physical discomfort. These two studies suggest that team care enhances global functioning and adaptation without necessarily decreasing disease activity.

The value of team care remains to be proven conclusively (Keith, 1991). Methodological issues are numerous and complex and include patient mix, organizational context, and specific team characteristics (Schmidt, Farrell, & Heinemann, 1988).

Many would agree with Diller (1990) that rehabilitation professionals have yet to develop an adequate understanding or theoretical framework of rehabilitation teams. On the one hand, psychological factors are underemphasized in rehabilitation (Rintala et al., 1986). On the other hand, team care is an expensive process with limited, rigorously proven, benefit. Several commonly cited problems, including professionalization (eg, "turf"), leadership, and economic considerations, are discussed.

PROFESSIONALIZATION

The professional background of each team member encompasses a specific and particular body of values, skills, and knowledge. As reviewed by Kane (1975), individual health care professionals have poor understanding of the activities of other team members. Rehabilitation staff perceive difficulties in interprofessional boundaries (Strasser, Falconer, & Martino-Saltzman, 1994). Conflicts can arise when team members are asked to share concerns with team members of another profession, to soften the definition of their own professional roles, and—perhaps most importantly—to accept that the agenda of a different professional may be more appropriate in a particular situation.

The inherent tension of professionalization can be helped by taking the perspective of the patient and focusing on the particular needs of the individual. This change in focus corresponds to a shift from professional roles and toward specific tasks (Horwitz, 1970; Kane, 1975; Levinson, 1977). Emphasis is placed on tasks such as ambulation, activities of daily living, and psychosocial adaptations to the illness instead of the professional roles of each team member.

Professional departments and hospital administration contribute to the fragmentation of teams in subtle and inadvertent ways. Prestige, salary, scheduling, and employment are usually made at the departmental level with guidelines from the hospital administration. Decisions on team membership and staffing are made at the convenience of the department. When a conflict arises between what is best for the team and what is best for the department, the interests of the team can be slighted. The allegiance to the team as a "reference group" (Horwitz, 1970) characteristically lags behind the allegiance to the department and to the hospital administration.

Offered below are several suggestions to improve the inherent tension among professionals on teams. First, team activities must be focused on the patient's well-being. Second, individual team members need to be recognized for their particular insight and work. Third, a congenial atmosphere that highlights the need for collaborative work should be cultivated. And fourth, hospital administrators and department heads must be reminded of the importance of teamwork. Administration decisions should be judged not only by their effects on the department but also by their effects on the team and their patients.

TEAM LEADERSHIP AND THE PHYSICIAN

Team leadership encompasses a set of both subtle and complex issues that are often ignored by health professionals. First, there is the issue of who is versus who should be in charge. Second, the style of effective leadership is talked about extensively, but no preferred style has emerged. Third, leadership performs a variety of functions essential to interdisciplinary team care. And finally, the patient's experience of leadership provides interesting insights into the rehabilitation process.

Formal Leadership

Typically, team leadership is bestowed upon the physician by the administration. Many blame the woes of rehabilitation teams on this professional dominance

(Noren, 1977; Peake, 1971; Sawner, 1971; Siller, 1971). Physician dominance in team leadership reflects physician dominance in health care. While no particular profession in arthritis or rehabilitation care has much formal training in team management, the principles of good team leadership apply to any team leader. Leadership involves more than who the leader is.

A sense of mission should emanate from the leader. He or she needs special skills to negotiate the goals of rehabilitation. The ground rules for team decisions and activities should be clearly stated at the beginning. While it is important that all relevant considerations be weighed, decisions should be timely. When staff conflicts arise, the perceptive leader chooses the appropriate forum for airing these concerns. The team should feel secure in disagreeing but should acknowledge the importance of consistent activity after a decision has been made.

Leadership Styles

Leadership styles have been classified in different ways. Some have found the concepts of promotor, supporter, controller, and analyzer to be useful (Daresh, 1988). Another classification characterizes leadership styles as autocratic, democratic, and laissez faire (Browne & Bishop, 1980). Most ideas of leadership styles emphasize that there is no "right" or "wrong" style. For example, the strong leader who establishes clear delineation of authority and responsibility may be quite effective in directing the care of a complex technical problem, while the same leader may have difficulty with staff relations when there is a demanding patient. This could hamper the work of the team. Individuals with chronic diseases such as RA have rehabilitation issues combining "technical" and "psychological" concerns. No leadership style appears to have an advantage in meeting these multidimensional issues.

Leadership Functions

Leadership encompasses several functions inherent in effective team management. These functions include the coordination of activities for task accomplishment, the maintenance of the team's ability to accomplish these tasks, and the communication with the patient about the rehabilitation process (Parker, 1972). A designated leader usually excels in certain areas. Commonly, the physician will direct task accomplishment and medical management, while a social worker or psychologist may perform leadership functions associated with team development and team maintenance. A nurse, a physical therapist, or an occupational therapist may maintain the primary patient relationship or be the de facto case manager. Any team member may be a "spiritual" leader, providing some of the "glue" that holds the team together. These leadership functions do not lessen the importance of the designated leader, but they add to the complexity of the team process.

In a sense, the patient experiences different "leadership" through the rehabilitation process. Initial concerns may be primarily medical and nursing, whereas occupational and physical therapies dominate the process later. Frequently, the concerns of vocational counselors and social workers may dominate toward the end of an inpatient stay. This evolution of leadership highlights the process of team activities for a given patient.

Staff members should acknowledge the importance (eg, the leadership) of certain team members at particular times in the patient's rehabilitation course. A physician's emphasis on the importance of the goals of the occupational therapist may enhance the patient's participation in therapy. Likewise, a physical therapist's endorsement of the work of the vocational counselors may help the patient understand the connection between therapy tasks and work-related issues.

Finally, the role of the patient should be considered. While the patient does not have the technical knowledge or objectivity to be the administrative leader, he or she should have an active role in the formulation of goals and participation in therapy. Often a patient is steamrolled through therapy and retains limited knowledge for use away from the rehabilitation setting.

ECONOMICS OF TEAM CARE

Team care is expensive. If specialists in arthritis are unable to understand, justify, and improve team care, the ability to continue such a comprehensive approach will be forfeited. Although it seems obvious that team care provides the most comprehensive approach to the multifaceted problems encountered in arthritis rehabilitation, rehabilitation professionals must undertake the arduous task of understanding the nature of the team approach.

Continuous quality improvement and critical path methodologies may offer insights on how to make team care rehabilitation more cost effective. Researchers at Northwestern University (Falconer, Roth, Sutin, Strasser, & Chang, 1993) recently completed an ambitious experiment on adapting critical path methods to inpatient rehabilitation. In this study a critical path of rehabilitation activity was determined after specific goals had been established. With the identification of a critical path, team meetings were devoted to efficient allocation of staff resources to achieve more cost-effective rehabilitation.

Although this study failed to demonstrate improved cost effectiveness with a critical path methodology, insights into the complexities and subtleties of team care emerged. The researchers concluded that external regulations may influence practice dramatically and that the relationships between service delivery and patient outcome are not clear. Additionally, potential sources of problems on treatment teams include professional boundaries, team leadership and trust, and less favorable perception of the rehabilitation environment among older patients (Strasser, Falconer, & Martino-Saltzman, 1992, 1994).

TEAM DEVELOPMENT AND TEAM MAINTENANCE

While team care is promoted in the management of complex disabling conditions, most rehabilitation professionals have limited time or skill to devote to team development. The American Congress of Rehabilitation Medicine has produced valuable curriculum to promote team development and foster team cohesion among rehabilitation professionals (American Congress of Rehabilitation Medicine, 1992). Outside professionals can be helpful in facilitating team development (Banta & Fox, 1972; Gunther, 1987).

Techniques devised to enhance team process are proving increasingly difficult to implement because of time, finances, and lack of trained personnel. Nevertheless, devoting staff time and energy to team development can improve staff morale and patient outcome. The importance of staff's articulating a philosophy of team care and patient service should not be underestimated.

Additionally, regular meetings devoted to such issues as staff conflicts, organization of services, and the management of difficult patients can, in the long run, enhance the delivery of effective rehabilitation services. Paradoxically, in this era of limited health care dollars, understanding and promoting optimal team function is even more pressing.

CONCLUSION

The rehabilitation issues of patients with RA ideally are managed by an interdisciplinary team. Patients with RA present a unique constellation of physical and psychological issues that cut across several professional disciplines. The particular significance of pain and fatigue for these patients highlights the need for integrated, coordinated care. Issues of leadership, professionalization, economics, and the psychological environment influence the rehabilitation process. Effective management of patients with RA requires that professionals be well versed in the specifics of arthritis rehabilitation and have an understanding of the benefits and difficulties inherent in a team approach.

Interdisciplinary teams require a delicate balance of structure and flexibility. Whether it be issues of leadership or boundaries, the professional roles of each member should have flexibility. Rigid professional perceptions must be adapted to accomplish the integrated work necessary for effective rehabilitation.

Finally, the health of the interdisciplinary team also must be considered. Appropriate forums are needed to deal with team development and maintenance. Developing effective strategies to deal with issues surrounding interdisciplinary health care teams is one of the most challenging and important issues facing arthritis rehabilitation.

REFERENCES

Ahlmen, M., Sullivan, M., & Bjelle, A. (1988). Team versus nonteam outpatient care in rheumatoid arthritis. *Arthritis and Rheumatism*, 31, 471–479.

American Congress of Rehabilitation Medicine. (1992). *Guide to interdisciplinary practice in rehabilitation settings.* Skokie, IL: Author.

Banta, H.D., & Fox, R.C. (1972). Role strains of a health care team in a poverty community: The Columbia Point experience. *Social Science and Medicine*, *6*, 697–722.

Baum, J. (1982). A review of the psychological aspects of rheumatic diseases. *Seminars in Arthritis and Rheumatism*, *11*, 352–361.

Browne, J.A., & Bishop, D.S. (1980). Team functioning: A professional versus lay perspective. In D.S. Bishkop (Ed.), *Behavioral problems and the disabled: Assessment and management* (pp. 378–400). Baltimore: Williams & Wilkins.

Daresh, J.C. (1988). Applying leadership skills in conflict management. *American Journal of Physical Medicine and Rehabilitation*, *67*, 34–36.

Diller, R. (1990). Fostering the interdisciplinary team, fostering research in a society in transition. *Archives of Physical Medicine and Rehabilitation*, *71*, 275–278.

Ducanis, A.J., and Golin, A.K. (1979). *The interdisciplinary health care team: A handbook.* Gaithersburg, MD: Aspen Publishers Inc.

Duff, I.F., Carpenter, J.O., & Neukom, J.E. (1974). Comprehensive management of patients with rheumatoid arthritis. *Arthritis and Rheumatism*, *17*, 635–645.

Falconer, J.A., Roth, E.J., Sutin, J.A., Strasser, D.C., & Chang, R.W. (1993). The critical path method in stroke rehabilitation: Lessons from an experiment in cost containment and outcome improvement. *Quality Review Bulletin*, *19* (1), 8–16.

Feinberg, J.R., Brandt, K.D. (1984). Allied health team management of rheumatoid arthritis patients. *American Journal of Occupational Therapy*, *38*, 613–620.

Fordyce, W.E. (1981). Interdisciplinary peers. *Archives of Physical Medicine and Rehabilitation*, *62*, 51–53.

Gunther, M.S. (1987). Catastrophic illness and the caregivers: Burdens and solutions. In B. Caplan (Ed.), *Rehabilitation psychology desk reference* (pp. 219–244). Gaithersburg, MD: Aspen Publishers Inc.

Halstead, L.S. (1976). Team care in chronic illness: A critical review of the literature of the past 25 years. *Archives of Physical Medicine and Rehabilitation*, *57*, 507–511.

Horwitz, J.J. (1970). *Team practice and the specialist: An introduction to interdisciplinary teamwork.* Springfield, IL: Charles C Thomas.

Kane, R.A. (1975). *Interprofessional teamwork* (Manpower Monograph No. 8). Syracuse, NY: Division of Continuing Education and Manpower Development, Syracuse University School of Social Work.

Katz, S., Vignos, P.J., Moskowitz, R.W., Thompson, H.M., & Svec, K.H. (1968). Comprehensive outpatient care in rheumatoid arthritis: A controlled study. *Journal of the American Medical Association*, *206*, 1249–1254.

Kazis, L.E., Meenan, R.F., & Anderson, J.J. (1983). Pain in the rheumatic diseases: Investigation of a key health status component. *Arthritis and Rheumatism*, *26*, 1017–1022.

Keith, R.A. (1991). The comprehensive treatment team in rehabilitation. *Archives of Physical Medicine and Rehabilitation*, *72*, 269–274.

Levinson, D. (1977). Roles, tasks and practitioners. *New England Journal of Medicine*, *296*, 1291–1293.

McDuffie, F.C. (1985). Morbidity impact of rheumatoid arthritis on society. *American Journal of Medicine*, *78* (Suppl. 1A), 1–5.

Melvin, J.L. (1980). Interdisciplinary and multidisciplinary activities and the ACRM. *Archives of Physical Medicine and Rehabilitation*, *61*, 379–380.

Nason, F. (1981). Team tension as a vital sign. *General Hospital Psychiatry*, *3*, 32–36.

Noren, R.L.R. (1977, Spring). The team approach. *American Archives of Rehabilitation Therapy (AART)*, 1–6.

Nosek, M.A., Parker, R.M., & Larsen, S. (1987). Psychosocial independence and functional arthritis: Their relationship in adults with severe musculoskeletal impairment. *Archives of Physical Medicine and Rehabilitation*, *68*, 840–845.

Parker, A.W. (1972). *The team approach to primary health care.* (Neighborhood Health Center Seminar Program Monograph Series No. 3). The Regents of the University of California.

Peake, L.N. (1971). Occupational therapy, nursing, and physical therapy. *Archives of Physical Medicine and Rehabilitation*, *52*, 406–408.

Rintala, D.H., Hanover, D., Alexander, J.L., Sanson-Fisher, R.W., Willems, E.P., & Halstead, L.S. (1986). Team care: An analysis of verbal behavior during patient rounds on a rehabilitation hospital. *Archives of Physical Medicine and Rehabilitation*, *67*, 118–122.

Rogers, M.P., Liang, M.H., & Partridge, A.J. (1982). Psychological care of adults with rheumatoid arthritis. *Annals of Internal Medicine*, *96*, 344–348.

Rothberg, J.S. (1985). Rehabilitation team practice. In P.J. Lecca & J.S. McNeil (Eds.), *Interdisciplinary team practice: Issues and trends* (pp. 19–41). New York: Praeger.

Sawner, K.A. (1971). Physical therapy, medicine, and occupational therapy. *Archives of Physical Medicine and Rehabilitation*, *52*, 408–410.

Schmidt, M.H., Farrell, M.P., & Heinemann, G.D. (1988). Conceptual and methodological problems in studying the effects of interdisciplinary geriatric teams. *Gerontologist*, *28*, 753–764.

Siller, J. (1971). A summary: On the delineation of boundaries of professional practice in rehabilitation. *Archives of Physical Medicine and Rehabilitation*, *52*, 410–412.

Strasser, D.C., Falconer, J.A., & Martino-Saltzman, D. (1992). The relationship of patient's age to the perceptions of the rehabilitation environment. *Journal of the American Geriatrics Society*, *40*, 445–448.

Strasser, D.C., Falconer, J.A., & Martino-Saltzman, D. (1994). The rehabilitation team: Staff perceptions of the hospital environment, the interdisciplinary team environment, and interprofessional relations. *Archives of Physical Medicine and Rehabilitation*, *75*, 177–182.

Vignos, P.J., Thompson, H.M., Katz, S., Moskowitz, R.W., Fink, S., & Svec, K.H. (1972). Comprehensive care and psycho-social factors in rehabilitation in chronic rheumatoid arthritis: A controlled study. *Journal of Chronic Diseases*, *25* (8), 457–467.

SUGGESTED READING

Bishop, D., Green, A., Cantor, W., & Torresin, W. (1987). Depression, anxiety, and rheumatoid arthritis activity. *Clinical and Experimental Rheumatology, 5*, 147–150.

Figley, B.A. (1983, January/February). The roles of allied health professionals in the management of arthritis. *Clinical Rheumatology in Practice,* pp. 43–46.

Karlen, I., Lee, M., & McEwen, C. (1973). Rheumatoid arthritis: Five-year study of rehabilitation. *Archives of Physical Medicine and Rehabilitation*, *54*, 120–128.

Swezy, R.L. (1986) Arthritis rehabilitation: Staff, facilities, and evaluation. In G.E. Ehrlich (Ed.) *Rehabilitation management of rheumatic conditions* (pp. 1–23). Baltimore: Williams & Wilkins.

CHAPTER 2

Assessment of Rheumatoid Arthritis and Its Consequences

Rowland W. Chang, MD, MPH

The objectives of this chapter are to define the goals of assessment, to present a model of disability as a context for assessment, and to discuss certain concepts and paradigms of assessment that are useful in the management of rheumatoid arthritis (RA) within this context. The premise of this chapter is that interdisciplinary assessment is important to providing optimal care for the patient with RA. Assessment relevant to specific rehabilitation approaches is addressed in many of the following chapters.

RATIONALES FOR ASSESSMENT

Assessment is vital to both research and clinical evaluation. Research assessment for RA has been the subject of at least two symposia that address its complex conceptual and measurement issues (Proceedings of Current Research, 1987; Proceedings of the Symposium, 1982). We concentrate here on clinical assessment, using many lessons learned in research and then applying them to clinical care.

Two important reasons to use assessment during clinical encounters are (1) to identify problems and strengths that would influence treatment plan content and strategy and (2) to monitor progress or deterioration over time. Consider this abbreviated case history: "Ms J.H. is a 35-year-old female who presents with a progressive 1-year history of pain, stiffness, and swelling of her hands and knees." What should we find out about Ms J.H.? Each health professional managing arthritis patients probably has a set of questions, observations, and strategies that he or she routinely uses to assess the state of people like J.H. A physician would be concerned with J.H.'s diagnosis initially. The history and physical examination would be directed toward an understanding of which anatomical structure was involved and whether the symptoms were caused by an inflammatory or noninflammatory process. A physical therapist would be interested in J.H.'s mobility and physical function, given her knee symptoms. Thus a physical therapist's assessment would include the quality and quantity of ambulation and stair climbing as well as bed mobility and transfer (eg, sit to stand) status. An occupational therapist would be concerned with the ability of the patient to perform activities of daily living (eg, dressing, grooming, feeding, toileting, and homemaking), while a social worker would ask about the patient's family and social environment and try to understand what stresses the patient's symptoms are placing on the family's social functioning. A clinical psychologist would be most concerned about the patient's coping abilities and interpersonal relationships. Assessing the patient's work requirements and environment and determining what effect RA is having on the patient's work performance would be the responsibility of a vocational counselor.

Typically, the patient does not have the time or the inclination to pursue all of these issues even though each is important and relevant to a future treatment plan. Generally, the patient seeks the help of health professionals and presents a set of problems, and it is these that guide the referral and subsequently direct the assessment. For instance, if J.H. stated that she could not climb stairs because of her knee symptoms despite anti-inflammatory drugs and a steroid injection, it is probable that a physical therapist would be consulted and a mobility and physical function assessment undertaken. However, if J.H. does not mention that she cannot do her secretarial work because of her hand symptoms, it is unlikely a vocational counselor would ever be consulted.

The patient-directed assessment has the advantage of increased patient acceptance of the assessment process because he or she accepts that an important issue (eg, mobility or physical function) is being monitored. If one were to assess only those parameters explicitly identified by the patient as being problems, however, potentially remediable conditions would be overlooked and future preventable problems neglected. The challenge is to determine how to assess a patient efficiently and choose the correct parameters to guide comprehensive and effective management. There is no controversy about the use of assessment parameters. As stated, they should direct treatment and monitor progress or deterioration.

CONTEXT OF ASSESSMENT IN RHEUMATOID ARTHRITIS

Given that the universe of potential assessment parameters is too great for any health professional to evaluate or any single patient to endure, how can we reorganize our thinking to devise efficient assessment strategies for individual patients? The World Health Organization's definitions of disease, impairment, disability, and handicap provided a framework for assessment (Wood, 1980). This was modified by the Institute of Medicine (IOM) in 1991. The definitions of common terms given below are from the IOM's report, *Disability in America* (IOM, 1991).

Pathology: Measurable cellular and tissue changes caused by disease, infection, trauma, congenital conditions, or other agents.

Impairment: Discrete loss or abnormality of mental, physiological, or biochemical function at the organ level. All pathologies are accompanied by impairments in either the specific functioning of an organ or organ system.

Functional Limitation: Effects of impairments which are manifested in the performance or performance capacity of the person as a whole and restrict an individual's ability to perform.

Disability: Any restriction or lack of ability to perform an activity in the manner or within the range considered normal for a human being, which is chronic or permanent in nature, and/or which is judged to be a cultural, social, economic, and/or environmental disadvantage.

Handicap: A condition, barrier or disadvantage imposed by society, the environment, or by one's self (eg, stairs are a handicap for a person in a wheelchair) that limits or prevents fulfillment of a role that is "normal" (depending on age, sex, and social and cultural factors) for an individual. Traditionally, "handicap" has been used synonymously with "disability" to mean limitations in performance, placing an individual at a disadvantage. Because of its negative connotation, this term is being replaced in common usage by the term "disadvantage" (IOM, 1991, pp. 76–83).

Since RA presently has no cure, its management is directed at treating or preventing the adverse consequences of disease. Treatment can be approached by attempting to alter disease activity (or pathology), joint impairments, functional limitations, disabilities, and handicaps associated with RA. Thus one way of considering the variety of assessment options for RA is to classify conceptually each parameter within the presented conceptual model (Figure 2–1).

The advantages of this perspective of assessment in RA are especially relevant to the interdisciplinary team. First, the model defines the breadth of knowledge and perspective of the collective group. Second, although no health professional is capable of being expert in all aspects of arthritis assessment and care, each has a particular leadership role to play in its management, depending on where the patient problems fall within the model. Thus the rheumatologist is well suited to assess and treat pathology. The orthopaedic surgeon via joint surgery can affect profoundly a consequence of pathology, joint impairment (ie, a destroyed hip or knee joint).

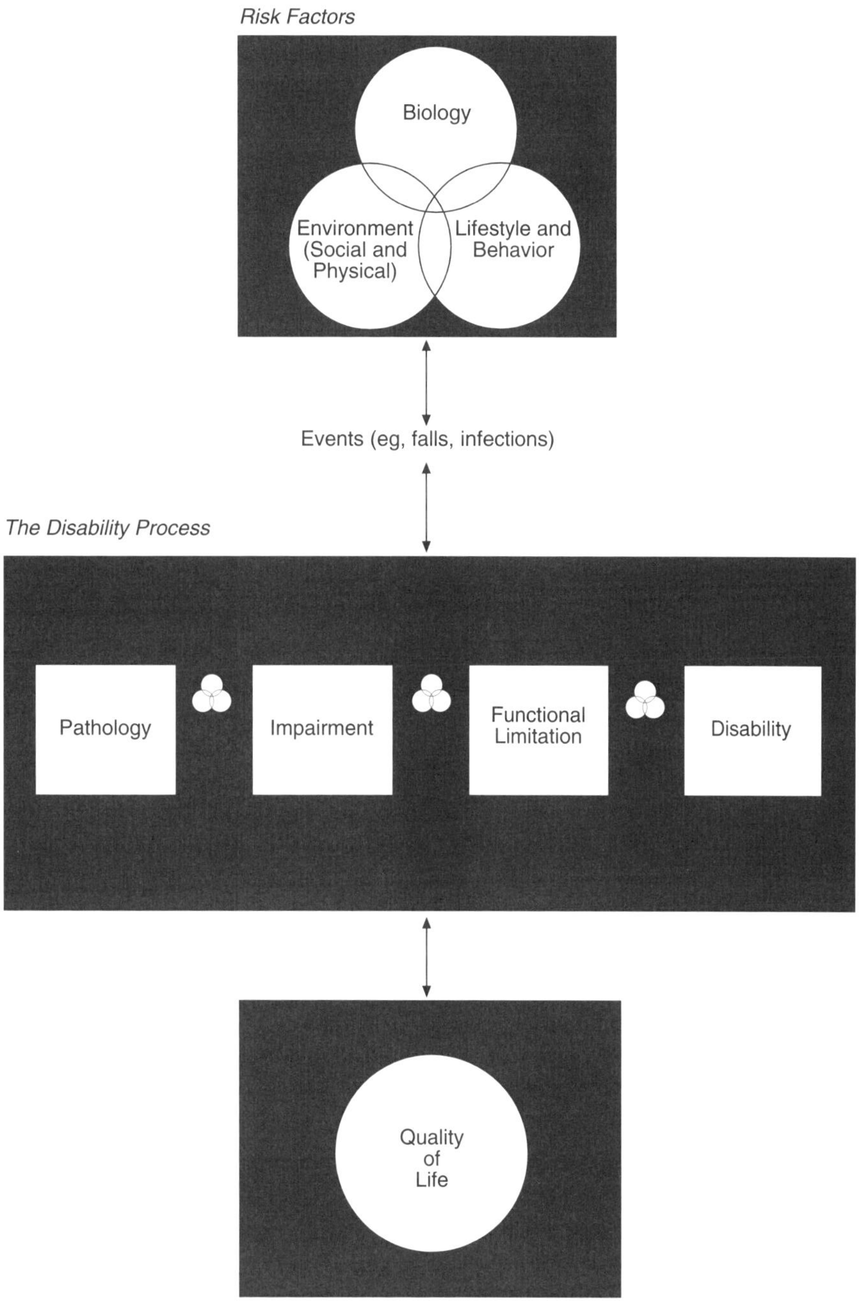

Figure 2–1 Model of disability showing the interaction of the disabling process, quality of life, and risk factors. Three types of risk factors are included: biological (eg, Rh type); environmental (eg, lead pain [physical environment], access to care [social environment]); and lifestyle and behavior (eg, tobacco consumption). Bidirectional arrows indicate the potential for "feedback." The potential for additional risk factors to affect the progression toward disability is shown between the stages of the model. These additional risk factors might include, depending on the stage of the model, diagnosis, treatment, therapy, adequacy of rehabilitation, age of onset, financial resources, expectations, and environmental barriers. *Source:* Adapted with permission from *Disability in America.* Copyright 1991 by the National Academy of Sciences. Courtesy of the National Academy Press, Washington, D.C.

Rehabilitation professionals such as physiatrists, physical therapists, occupational therapists, social workers, clinical psychologists, speech pathologists, orthotists, and vocational counselors experienced in arthritis care are expert in assessing and treating the functional limitations, disabilities, and handicaps associated with RA. Nurses often span a spectrum of experience, which makes them ideal for being a coordinator of care for persons with RA. Third, the model explicitly acknowledges the interrelations among professionals in the management of RA. The way a physical therapist assesses and treats a patient with RA should be influenced by an understanding of the unique nature of the pathology and its consequent effect on joint impairment and functional limitation. Similarly, a rheumatologist's understanding of RA's consequences beyond the pathology level will lead to a perspective that will maximize his or her ability to help RA patients manage their lives. Indeed, this conceptual framework can be a useful model for any group of health professionals committed to the care of RA patients, but it is especially useful to the interdisciplinary team.

PARADIGMS OF ASSESSMENT IN RHEUMATOID ARTHRITIS

Using the J.H. case as the example, specific assessment parameters in the context of the presented conceptual model are discussed.

Disease Activity

Disease activity is a synonym for pathology in the context of RA. The measurement of disease activity involves the synthesis of many clinical and laboratory parameters. The concept of interest is inflammatory synovitis, although another major concept that has been difficult to assess is synovial joint destruction potential. Inflammatory synovitis would be suspected if J.H. reported joint swelling, warmth, and stiffness, and generalized morning stiffness. If J.H.'s physical examination revealed soft tissue swelling of joints, joint effusion, warmth, redness, and loss of motion, one would conclude that the inflammatory process is active. Laboratory parameters thought to parallel the activity of the inflammation include the erythrocyte sedimentation rate.

Impairments Directly Related to Rheumatoid Arthritis

Joint impairment affects the mechanical state of the joint and can be measured in several ways. The integrity of articular cartilage can be assessed by X-ray or arthroscopically. Other commonly assessed parameters of joint impairment include the range of motion of a joint, the strength of muscles surrounding a joint, and the stability and/or deformity of a joint. Most health professionals assume that RA disease activity is primarily responsible for the assessed joint impairment, but other concomitant disease processes are possible etiologies as well. J.H.'s surgical and rehabilitation prescriptions would depend on the mechanical state of the joint as determined by physical examination and perhaps other imaging tests (eg, X-ray, computed tomography scan, magnetic resonance imaging scan) or procedures (arthroscopy).

Functional Limitation

Parameters that fit into this category include ambulation ability, stair climbing, transfer ability, and the ability to perform personal care such as feeding, dressing, bathing, and toileting. Several summary measures of function are available for research and clinical purposes (Fries, Spitz, Kraines, & Holman, 1980; Meenan, Gertman, & Mason, 1980; Pincus, Summey, Soraci, Wallston, & Hummon, 1983). Rehabilitation personnel, however, tend to use more detailed assessment protocols to identify problems and to monitor progress. This is primarily due to the self-report nature of the research measures and their lack of ability to detect small individual changes.

The measurement of functional limitation is not disease specific. While RA disease activity leading to joint destruction is often the reason for functional limitation, many other processes such as impaired cognition or psychological impairments may also influence function. Recognition of these other impairments that may coexist with RA is an important part of the assessment process and again argues for an interdisciplinary approach to RA management. Furthermore, the RA disease process can cause different joint impairments that may have different effects on functional activities. For instance, ambulation can be affected adversely by joint stiffness, swelling, and/or instability as well as muscle weakness or generalized deconditioning, all a consequence of RA disease activity. Successful treatment requires a clear understanding of what specific impairments are responsible for the functional limitation.

If J.H. were found to have significant functional limitations, interventions aimed at decreasing disease activity and/or specific joint impairments could be prescribed, but functional training could also be considered.

Disabilities and Handicaps

These more socially-oriented parameters include the abilities of a patient to be physically independent, to travel in the community, to work, to socialize, and to be economically viable. Again, the disabilities and handicaps confronting J.H. may not be attributed directly to the RA disease process, and the assessment level needs to appraise other etiologies as well as family and community support.

In the context of a multidisciplinary team, J.H.'s assessment could be quite complex and time consuming (see assessment forms in Appendix A). Prioritizing the challenges needs to be accomplished with the patient to create an efficient rehabilitation prescription. Communication among team members is also crucial in choosing appropriate therapies and minimizing conflicting therapy goals and approaches.

CONCLUSION

The primary rationales for assessment are (1) to identify problems and strengths that would influence treatment plan content and strategy and (2) to monitor progress or deterioration over time. A useful context in which to consider the assessment of a patient with RA are the Institute of Medicine's definitions of pathology, impairment, functional limitation, disability, and handicap (IOM, 1991). If viewed in this context, the paradigms of arthritis assessment represent powerful stimuli for a professional team approach to RA management.

REFERENCES

Fries, J.F., Spitz, P., Kraines, R.G., & Holman, H.R. (1980). Measurement of patient outcome in arthritis. *Arthritis and Rheumatism, 23*, 137–145.

Institute of Medicine. (1991). *Disability in America: A national agenda for prevention*, A.M. Pope & A.R. Tarlov (Eds.). Washington, DC: National Academy of Sciences.

Meenan, R.F., Gertman, P.M., & Mason, J.M. (1980). Measuring health status in arthritis: The arthritis impact measurement scales. *Arthritis and Rheumatism, 23*, 146–152.

Pincus, T., Summey, J.A., Soraci, S.A., Wallston, K.A., & Hummon, N.P. (1983). Assessment of patient satisfaction in activities of daily living using a modified Stanford Health Assessment Questionnaire. *Arthritis and Rheumatism, 26*, 1346–1353.

Proceedings of Current Research and Future Directions in Rehabilitation. (1987). *Journal of Rheumatology, 14* (Suppl. 15), 1–91.

Proceedings of the Symposium on Outcome Measures in Rheumatology Clinical Trials. (1982.) *Journal of Rheumatology, 9*, 749–806.

Wood, P.N.H. (1980). Appreciating the consequences of disease: The international classification of impairments, disabilities, and handicaps. *World Health Organization Chronicle, 34*, 376–380.

SUGGESTED READING

Meenan, R.F., Mason, J.H., Anderson, J.J., Guccione, A.A., & Kazis, L.E. (1992). AIMS II: The content and properties of a revised and expanded Arthritis Impact Measurement Scales. *Arthritis and Rheumatism, 35*, 1–10.

Chapter 3

Tissue and Joint Impairments in Rheumatoid Arthritis

Judith A. Sutin, MD

Patients with rheumatoid arthritis (RA) face more than pain and clinical joint deformity. There are multiple systemic, visceral, neurological, and secondary disease complications that can lead to significant functional deficits. This chapter describes the consequences of the underlying disease process by reviewing functionally significant local or regional tissue impairments.

STRUCTURE AND FUNCTION OF THE NORMAL JOINT

Synovium

The synovial or diarthrodial joint is characterized by bones united through a tough fibrous capsule and ligaments. The interposed cavity is lined by a synovial membrane, a vascular connective tissue, characterized by a capillary network and a relatively smooth surface from which a variable number of villi project. The function of this membrane is to secrete synovial fluid, a lubricating fluid that also provides nutrition for chondrocytes in articular cartilage. Normally, the synovial lining does not cover articular cartilage, but rather reflects off the capsule and inserts into the periosteum of subchondral bone, where it forms a vascularized fold. It is here that rheumatoid synovitis is initiated, potentially causing the typical rheumatoid marginal erosion.

The synovial membrane is relatively aneural compared with articular ligaments or bone, and much of its nerve supply is autonomic. Deliberate crushing and pulling in most areas results in little sensation, and even when pain is produced, it remains poorly localized (Kellgren & Samuel, 1950). Clinical observation reveals that synovitis is often painless, whereas ligamentous sprains or bone injuries are extremely painful.

Articular Cartilage

The articular surface is covered by hyaline cartilage, which also is devoid of innervation and has no sensation when stimulated (Kellgren & Samuel, 1950). This specialized connective tissue, with its abundant extracellular substance and relatively few cells, substantially loses reparative power when growth ceases (Gardner, 1963).

The viscoelastic behavior of cartilage accounts for its immediate deformation when stress is applied. Loading conditions produce observable indentations, which increase joint contact and conformity, thereby enhancing stability. The compliance of normal cartilage and subchondral bone promotes maximal congruence, with optimal pressure distribution under full-load conditions. Subchondral bone, in fact, substantially contributes to shock absorption, and its compliance under physiologic load is comparable to the give of soft wood (Radin, 1975). Joint motion combined with muscle lengthening under tension is suggested as another shock-absorption mechanism. Accordingly, Simon, Friedenberg, and Richardson (1973) observed thicker cartilage in joints of lesser congruence (such as hip and knee), a finding postulated to minimize load per unit area. These incongruent joints also show a high frequency of degenerative disease associated with cartilage attrition.

Tendons and Tendon Sheaths

Tendons transmit muscle tension to a mobile part, and also diminish muscle length, thereby decreasing distal extremity bulk. In general, direction of pull is altered by fibrous sheaths, pulleys, and retention bands, so that excessive bowstringing is avoided during muscle contraction. A delicate surrounding connective tissue meshwork transmits nerves, blood vessels, and lymphatics to tendon. Tendons also are richly innervated both by region nerves and by nerves emanating from attached muscles. Additionally, at the dorsal and volar wrist and along the flexor surface of digits, tendons are surrounded by synovial lined sheaths; and while few nerve receptors are found intrasheath, the synovial lining is replete with free nerve terminals. Also, tendons receive blood supply from adjacent bone, muscle, and intermediate vessels. As tendon metabolic rate is low, the preservation solely of intermediate vessels allows for continued flow throughout the length. With flexor tendon sheaths, however, the vascular arrangement is altered, with the volar surface devoid of arteries, and nourishment is provided by synovial fluid. Hypovascular areas are known to occur in several tendons, which are presumed to be subject to degeneration and rupture.

Tendons possess great mechanical strength parallel to fiber axis, as observed with other highly organized collagen structures (deep fascia and ligaments). Initial stress application (Canoso, 1981) straightens and lengthens the helically twisted collagen fibers, thereby increasing closeness of molecular packing and enhancing interchain forces. The property of elasticity is demonstrated by a small load resulting in appreciable lengthening. Progressively larger loads, however, do not affect length as much, and beyond a 4% length increase, tendon is less perfectly elastic. Resistance to elongation markedly decreases as interchain bonds are destroyed, and permanent elongation is commensurate with irreversible structural change. Eventually the tendon yields and rupture ensues (Benedict, Walker, & Harris, 1968).

Synovial tendon sheaths are considered a special class of deep bursae located in specific sites within the fibrous tunnels of digital flexors. Deep and superficial synovial layers reflect along an interrupted or continuous connective tissue septum (the mesotendon), carrying vascular channels and nerves. These tendon sheaths promote gliding of tendon and provide nutrition to the intrasheath region.

Ligaments

Structurally, ligaments resemble tendons, although less is known about their vascular supply (Canoso, 1981). Fibrous articular ligaments are richly endowed with somatic nerves, and numerous areas cause pain when mechanically stimulated. Hence, unlike the synovium, fibrous ligaments play a pivotal role in joint sensation and are a major source of joint pain (Kellgren & Samuel, 1950).

Immobilization affects the mechanical properties of ligament, much as it affects tendon (Noyes, Torvik, Hyde, & DeLucas, 1974). Following 9 weeks of immobilizing rabbit limb, for example, energy-absorbing potential of collateral ligament and ultimate load to failure diminished by one third when compared with the contralateral side (Woo, Gomez, Woo, & Akesou, 1982). Furthermore, recovery of mechanical parameters after immobilization is frequently highly protracted (Canoso, 1981), incomplete, and uneven. The threshold of activity required to maintain normal mechanical properties also remains largely undefined (Noyes et al., 1974).

Deep and Superficial Bursae

Bursae are closed sacs with synovial lining comparable to that of diarthrodial joints. By light microscopy this lining typically is one cell layer thick and supported by connective tissue and fat. The mechanism of lubrication is speculative but probably involves hyaluronic acid. Bursae are poorly vascularized, and information about terminal nerve endings is lacking (Canoso, 1981).

Bursal functions include facilitation of gliding by one musculoskeletal structure over another, or the creation of a potential reservoir for excess synovial fluid. For instance, deep bursae (such as the iliopsoas or gastrocnemius semimembranosus bursa) frequently communicate directly with the underlying synovial joint. Conversely, repetitive pressure and friction seem necessary to develop superficial or subcutaneous bursae, which do not communicate directly with the joint. Similarly, adventitious bursae appear later in life over bony prominences (such as a gibbus or hallus valgus) or a rheumatoid nodule.

Superficial bursae react less to disease stimuli than do diarthrodial joints, despite the similarity between their membranes. In particular, bursal leukocyte counts remain low in septic bursitis (Canoso & Yood, 1979). This lesser inflammatory response of bursae and infrequent involvement by hematogenous infection (Canoso, 1981) may reflect the lesser degree of vascularization when compared with synovial joints. Furthermore, traumatic bursitis contrasts with traumatic arthritis in its poor fluid viscosity and inadequate mucin clot, suggesting less differentiation.

Muscles

Muscle has an expansive blood supply, as increased activity demands this adaptation. Although the nerves to muscles are frequently considered only motor, they contain some 40% to 60% afferent fibers (Hollinshead, 1969). The disparity in tensile strength between muscle and tendon is enormous. Thus a large muscle acts through an extremely small tendon, and likewise, muscle belly, musculotendinous junction, or periosteal tendinous junction give way to stress long before tendon. Muscle strength is proportional to cross-sectional area and to the degree of motor unit synchrony. Velocity of contraction also contributes to muscle tension, with a fast, eccentric (lengthening) contraction developing greatest tension, and a rapid concentric (shortening) contraction developing the least.

TISSUE IMPAIRMENTS IN RHEUMATOID ARTHRITIS

Synovitis

Rheumatoid synovitis is characterized by proliferation, enlargement, and disarray of synovial cells and inflammation of the synovial tissue. Inflammatory cells, particularly lymphocytes, collect in the synovium, whereas polymorphonuclear cells are found in synovial fluid. Because joints are closed spaces with limited drainage capabilities (particularly for more viscous or particulate fluids), inflammatory/necrotic products are retained and inflammation is perpetuated.

Perhaps most damaging is the formation of pannus, a sprawling vascular granulated synovial tissue, which extends over articular cartilage, into and about capsuloligamentous attachments and tendons (Swanson & DeGroot Swanson, 1973). Alternatively, granulation may originate in subchondral bone and penetrate the cartilage from below (Hamerman, Rosenberg, & Schubert, 1970). The consequence of pannus formation is cartilage and subchondral bone erosion, cartilage destruction, and laxity of joint capsule and periarticular structures.

Tendinitis

Long flexors are affected by tendinitis most often, and to a lesser extent the long digit extensors, tendons about the ankle, and the Achilles tendon. Tendon surface dulling is noted as the earliest change. Later, tendons appear thickened, yellowed, and streaked with gray gelatinous material. Tendon nodularity is seen, at times to the extent that it appears as a large cauliflower mass seeming to burst from the tendon center. Peritendon and mesotendon sometimes are replaced by a thick layer of granulation tissue.

Histologically, tendon involvement is irregular and varied in severity. Some tendon centers contain necrotic fibrinoid granular mass, or in some cases the peritendon or mesotendon is entangled in fibroid necrosis. Notably, there is absence of inflammatory cellular infiltration related to necrotic degenerated areas. Also observed is considerable lack of uniformity in the microscopic fields. Tendon sheaths reveal scattered, nonspecific synovitis, with lymphocytes and plasma cells in edematous areas (Kellgren & Ball, 1950).

Myositis

Focal myositis is well established in RA muscles, and is more intense in peripheral muscles than in proximal muscle groups (Swezey, 1971–1972). Also described, however, is proximal weakness, not necessarily related to myositis or regional synovitis, and possibly due to disuse, pain response, or extra-articular RA manifestation.

Focal myositis is one potential source of proximal muscle weakness not related to inflammation of contiguous joints and resulting disuse atrophy. Histologically this myositis is characterized as bland, with small round cell infiltration, little muscle fiber destruction, and often the absence of serum enzyme elevation (Swezey, 1971–1972). Electromyography reveals the anticipated short duration, polyphasic motor units. Although rheumatoid myositis typically does not progress to diffuse, severe, muscle necrosis, the clinical myositis picture may occasionally become dramatic enough to resemble muscular dystrophy. Selective weakness of cervical extensors has been attributed to focal, concentrated myositis in the context of RA (Wiederholt & Ehrlich, 1985).

One study clearly confirms the occurrence of myositis in some individuals with RA, often as a mild patchy process associated with active joint disease, and either elevated creatine phosphokinase or a sedimentation rate elevated disproportionately to peripheral synovitis (Halla, Koopman, Fallatti, Oh, & Gay, 1984). Those rheumatoid patients with systemic (constitutional) features without vasculitis may have rheumatoid myositis. In addition, myositis secondary to D-penicillamine treatment of RA has been described (Swartz & Silver, 1984).

Rheumatoid Nodules

Nodules are a salient indication of seropositive disease. Cosmesis and interference with forearm resting are obvious problems. Although pulp space nodules are infrequent, they can thwart activities requiring fine manipulation skills. Nodules sometimes adhere to tendon sheath or surface, or occupy the tendon center and penetrate. The flexor mechanism may become handicapped by triggering or rupture.

Synovial Effusion and Intra-articular Pressure

Unphysiological strains have an impact on rheumatoid synovium and articular cartilage surfaces given that higher synovial fluid pressures are encountered (Jayson & Dixon, 1970a). Synovial effusions may impede cartilage nutrition by reversing the normal flow gradient, which depends on higher pressure in bone marrow than the joint space (Genovese, Jayson, & Dixon, 1972). Clinically, joint positions corresponding to least intra-articular pressure are spontaneously chosen by patients (Jayson, 1981), although they are not positions of optimal function (Gerser, 1985). For example, 30° to 40° of knee flexion is the position of least intra-articular pressure (Favreau & Laurin, 1963).

Classic studies by Jayson and Dixon (1970a) examined the relationship between joint effusion and intra-articular pressure. Joints were drained and progressively distended, with pressures recorded at increasing volumes using a pressure transducer. Rheumatoid knees developed higher pressures than the knees of control subjects with the most marked and statistically significant values at higher volumes (40 to 80 mL). Then, using initial effusion volumes as baseline, results were even more striking.

A later study monitored intra-articular pressure under dynamic conditions (Jayson & Dixon, 1970b). Similarly, at each successive volume and with movement, rheumatoid knees developed statistically significant higher mean intra-articular pressures, whereas the empty knees of control subjects demonstrated subatmospheric pressures upon quadriceps contraction or stance. The authors conjecture that quadriceps contraction distracts a lax capsule, tending to enlarge the joint space, and creating a negative (subatmospheric) pressure. No negative pressure phase, however, was recorded for the rheumatoid knees.

Of particular interest is the higher pressure developed by RA patients, insofar as they were typically female, older, and more frail, and had weaker quadriceps than the healthy young males of the control group (Jayson & Dixon, 1970a). The higher rheumatoid pressures were attributed to inflammatory alteration of the joint lining (Rask, 1978), along with synovial hypertrophy. In a complementary study, both age and disease are blamed for the low capsular compliance (distensibility) observed in those with RA over age 40 (Myers & Palmer, 1972).

Quadriceps inhibition occurs at larger volumes of simulated effusion, and although no pain occurs, subjects become unable to sustain contraction. This is seen at volumes where pressures plateau or actually decrease (about 60 to 80 mL) and is attributed to afferent intracapsular receptors sensing joint capsule stretch, rather than to the level of intra-articular pressure achieved. Quadriceps exercises therefore are fruitless with a knee effusion, and quadriceps wasting may reflect muscle inhibition (Jayson, 1981; Jayson & Dixon, 1970b).

Secondary Osteoarthritis

Since all weight-bearing cartilage is subject to variable loading, normal alignment is necessary to transmit force uniformly and to minimize trauma. Although cartilage deteriorates with age, even in non–weight-bearing areas, any malalignment or instability (which imposes chronically increased impact loading) acts to incite osteoarthritis (Swanson & DeGroot Swanson, 1973). When invasion by rheumatoid pannus and distention by effusion stretch periarticular tissues and joint capsules, any unstable area is particularly vulnerable.

Hypermobility correlates with premature osteoarthritis and traumatic synovitis even in nonrheumatic clinical settings (Bird, Trise, & Bacon, 1978). Also, unanticipated (impulse) loading, or that too rapid for timely neuromuscular response, poses potential threat even to cartilage of normal joints, but particularly to that of diseased joints. Impulse loading causes subchondral microfractures, which heal by stiffening and further encourage cartilage damage. Bone changes therefore can be a major determinant in the amount of cartilage destruction.

Further degenerative changes result from subtle anatomical hip distortion or from angular knee deformity (Radin, 1975). Kostuik, Schmidt, Harris, and Wooldridge (1975) report that a 3° shift in tibial femoral alignment in normal subjects under static conditions transforms equal weight bearing to unicompartmental weight bearing. Thus small changes in alignment effect marked shifts in relative weight bearing between different areas. It is estimated that 20% of patients with early RA and 48% of those having RA for more than 10 years show later osteoarthritis change (Fletcher & Rowley, 1952).

Osteoporosis

Osteoporosis is a frequent, early occurrence in RA, and the two patterns seen are juxta-articular and shaft. Juxta-articular osteoporosis is usually widespread in a region (Fletcher & Rowley, 1952), whereas true, generalized osteoporosis is seen only in longstanding, diffuse cases.

Clinically, stress fractures occur either from abnormal stress to bone that has normal elastic resistance or from normal stress to bone that has less than normal elastic resistance (Schneider & Kaye, 1975). In particular, the onset of new lower extremity pain in an RA patient should signal a stress fracture. Coexistent angular limb deformity, osteoporosis, or unaccustomed exercise after reconstructive surgery are predisposing factors. Flexion contractures also contribute, with deformity enhancing stress contiguous to a joint.

PATTERNS AND COURSE OF RHEUMATOID ARTHRITIS

Natural History of Rheumatoid Arthritis

Multiple authors (Duthie, Brown, Truelove, Barajar, & Laurie, 1964; Fleming, Benn, Corbett, & Wood, 1976; Jacoby, Jayson, & Cosh, 1973; Mitchell et al., 1986) address patterns of disease onset or involvement, relating these to functional outcome or disease course. Frequently comparisons are obscured by variance in study design (ie, patient numbers, demographics, length of time studied, stage at which study entry or treatment initiated, and outcome measures). Obviously, the course of any individual case is unpredictable, although some generalizations can be made.

Duthie et al. (1964) followed 247 RA patients for approximately 6 years and broadly concluded that 65% either were unimpaired or were able to carry out most ordinary activities at follow-up. Nearly half their cases showed inactive disease at final evaluation. Many patients with mild symptoms probably escape medical attention.

Jacoby and colleagues (1973) described 100 patients within 3.7 months of onset and found that the majority showed functional deterioration over 11 years, although relatively few showed considerable deterioration. Many patients have a level of disease activity that fluctuates within small limits.

Fleming, Benn, Corbett, and Wood (1976) followed 102 patients seen within the first year of disease for up to 4 or 5 years. As noted in other studies, older patients or those having early progression to symmetrical disease tended to fare worse in terms of disease progression (especially with regard to deformity), and those having severe acute onset tended to respond to treatment more favorably (Duthie et al., 1964; Fleming, Benn, Corbett, & Wood, 1976; Krane & Simon, 1986). Shoulder, elbow, wrist, and knee involvement was more prevalent in older age groups, and was associated with seropositivity and a worse prognosis. In addition, Fleming, Benn, Corbett, & Wood (1976) noted that involvement of metatarsophalangeal joints 2 to 5 was associated with younger patients and a better outcome, whereas involvement of metatarsophalangeal joints 1 and 2 was associated with seropositivity, worse disease, and erosions. Duthie et al. (1964) found that nodules, high rheumatoid factor titers, and high sedimentation rates tend to be associated with more severe forms of disease.

In contrast, some studies assert a lack of influence of type and site of disease onset, pattern of joint involvement, and presence or absence of prodrome in predicting disease outcome (Duthie, Brown, Knox, & Thompson, 1957; Duthie et al., 1964; Jacoby et al., 1973).

Patterns of RA in the Upper Extremity

Synovitis in the Hand

The joint apparatus of each digit (Figures 3–1 and 3–2) consists of a capsule plus strong lateral collateral ligaments, which continue onto the palmar aspect to fuse with sides of the accessory palmar plate. The resulting tough fibrous plate (volar plate, volar ligament) on the palmar joint surface is not present dorsally. Thus proliferating synovium expands much more readily in a dorsal direction. The hands and wrists are early salient targets for synovitis, with the dorsal wrist, metacarpophalangeal joint, and proximal interphalangeal joint being frequent sites of swelling. Erosion and subluxation of the first carpometacarpal joint may impair opposition and lateral pinch.

Flexor tenosynovitis occurs in 38% to 55% of patients with RA and may be even more prevalent, but it is difficult to detect with early involvement beneath the flexor retinaculum (Macauley, Evans, & Ansell, 1981). Synovial proliferation of the tendon sheath potentially thwarts active digit flexion or results in fibrosis, with concomitant limitation of passive digit flexion or tendon rupture. Surprisingly, there is little correlation between tenosynovial bulk and the extent of tendon damage (Backhouse, Kay, Coomes, & Kates, 1971) although synovial sheaths may be prominently distended by excess fluid (Kellgren & Ball, 1950) or the tendon itself may be markedly enlarged.

On examination, firm, tender swellings are palpated at the metacarpal heads, which move with the tendons as digits are passively manipulated. Flexor tenosynovitis variously presents as blocking or catching, or as digital stiffness, diffuse digital pain (although this is not obligatory) as crepitant flexion, painless diffuse digital swelling, compromised active range, or as pain referred to the dorsal proximal interphalangeal joint. A

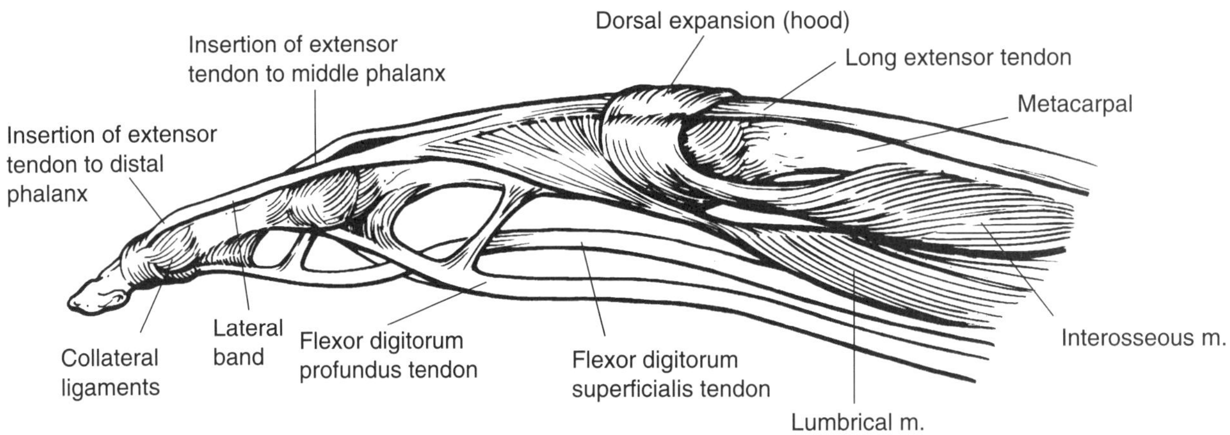

Figure 3–1 Lateral view of joint apparatus of a digit.

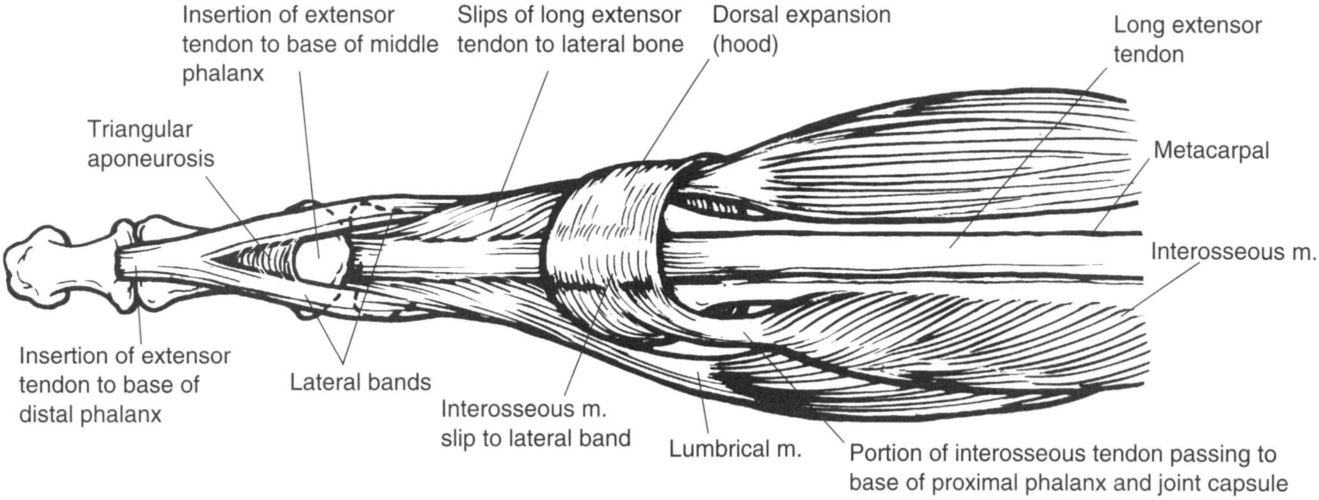

Figure 3–2 Anterior view of joint apparatus of a digit.

secondary loss of passive range commonly develops as joints are moved infrequently (Millis, Millender, & Nalebuff, 1976), and the subsequent joint stiffening and passive range impairment are easily confused with joint destruction.

In actuality, tendon involvement often coexists with underlying joint inflammation and damage, and it is difficult to determine the proportionate contribution of each to the impairment (Kellgren & Ball, 1950). In other words, the extent of flexor tenosynovitis has no necessary relationship to the amount of underlying synovitis in the joints of the same digits. Triggering, locking, or complete inhibition of active flexion at all but the metacarpophalangeal (MCP) joint suggests flexor tendon nodules. Passive motion at interphalangeal joints is preserved, and neither joint ranging nor palpation is uncomfortable. The localized pain of a tendon under load indicates tendon damage (Backhouse et al., 1971.)

Extensor Tendon Rupture

Extensor tendon ruptures are more frequent than flexor ruptures (Burke, 1984), and ulnar extensors particularly tend to rupture because of their greater degree of directional change plus loading (Backhouse et al., 1971). Although often painless, dorsal synovitis is readily apparent through distention of the extensor retinaculum on the dorsal aspect of the wrist. (Extensor tendon sheaths begin shortly above the proximal extensor retinaculum and continue proportionately a greater distance into the hand below the retinaculum.)

As a result of metacarpophalangeal synovitis, extensor tendons slip ulnarward into valleys between the metacarpal heads, where they act as lateral deviators, increasing ulnar drift. Severe subluxation is distinguished from tendon rupture by the palpable or visible tension developed during attempted active extension. Additionally, inflamed extensor tendon sheaths become compressed between the extensor retinaculum and the jagged, posteriorly subluxating ulnar edge. Sequential drop of the ulnar three digits results from rupture of their tendons over this ulnar contour. The extensor pollicis longus also ruptures due to attrition at Lister's tubercle (Millender & Nalebuff, 1975).

Ulnar Deviation

The MCP joints are characterized by potential instability. Because of metacarpal head asymmetry, the proximal phalangeal base tends to rotate in an ulnar direction as the finger flexes (Kay, 1979). The normal hand also has metacarpophalangeal collateral ligaments of dissimilar size and strength. Specifically, the radial collateral of the long and index digits is longer, thinner, and more distally attached than the ulnar collateral. This anatomical distinction accounts for the small amount of ulnar drift established in the normal hand during firm grip (Flatt, 1983). As collateral ligaments are disrupted and grip instability occurs, progressive compensatory flexion power is applied, which results in increasing ligamentous disruption. Once palmar subluxation and ulnar deviation have occurred, muscle pull and gravity aggravate the deformity. Normal forces are potentially deforming, but are restrained by intact ligaments and soft tissues in the nonpathological state.

In the normal hand, bowstringing of flexor tendons is prevented by an intact collateral ligament sling arrangement, with collateral ligaments attaching to the volar plate. Additionally, common flexor tendons enter their fibrous sheath at an angle, such that their forces have both an ulnar and a palmar component. In the rheumatoid hand, however, joint distention occurs along with capsular and ligamentous spread, and the tenosynovial stretch of the fibrous flexor sheaths at the digit bases. As the volar MCP flexor tendon support becomes lax, resistance to deformity is lost, and the full extent of ulnar and palmar deviation is realized. As anticipated, a higher frequency and severity of MCP synovitis is found in joints developing subluxation and ulnar drift (Kay, 1979).

Intrinsic muscles also contribute to deformity once restraining forces are lost at the MCP joints. For example, ulnarly located intrinsics have a mechanical advantage, which is enhanced by MCP subluxation (Swanson & DeGroot Swanson, 1973). The inflamed MCP capsule purportedly induces an increase in intrinsic muscle tension, painful stretch, and protective contracture. An exaggeration of intrinsic action contributes to swan-neck deformity, or intrinsic muscle tension plus deformities (Flatt, 1983).

Also conducive to deformity is the extensor hood, which is thinner in its radial expansion. Therefore, hypertrophied synovium typically herniates radially, stretching the MCP horizontal fibers between the long extensor tendon and radial wing tendon of the interosseous muscle (Swezey, 1971–1972). The radial interosseous fibers are weakened, permitting ulnar slippage of the extensor tendons (Burke, 1984). Long extensor tendons then drift ulnarly into the subjacent sulci, with further extensor tendon bowstringing and digital pull into flexion.

Wrist Deformities

Proper wrist balance depends on intact bony configuration, with integrity and tension of ligaments. Ligamentous loosening is common on the radial aspect of the wrist, allowing for ulnar displacement of the proximal row of carpi, with secondary radial deviation of the hand on the forearm (Swanson & DeGroot Swanson, 1973). The resultant radial rotation of distal carpi and metacarpals (due to relatively unopposed radial wrist extensors) is noted, along with compensatory ulnar phalangeal drift (Swezey, 1971–1972). Shapiro (1970) contends that ulnar drift thus originates at the wrist, with radial rotation and radial metacarpal deviation preceding zigzag, compensatory ulnar phalangeal drift. He also highlights the radial bias of normal functional wrist movements. Radial deviation, palmar subluxation, and pronation are associated with decreased capability for positioning and adaptation of the hand to the environment (Swanson & DeGroot Swanson, 1973).

An early manifestation of wrist disease is synovitis at the distal radioulnar joint, which stretches the capsule, disrupts the triangular disc and ulnar collateral ligament, and results in dorsal subluxation of the distal ulna (Millender & Nalebuff, 1975). This dorsal ulnar prominence generally is associated with decreased rotatory and dorsiflexion function, and pain on movement. Also seen with dorsal ulnar subluxation is dysfunction of the extensor carpi ulnaris, which slips ulnar and palmarward, and may act as a flexor. Increased mobility of the fourth and fifth metacarpals widens the hand's transverse arch and acts as a source of ulnar extensor tendon displacement (Swanson & DeGroot Swanson, 1973).

Swan-Neck Deformity

Swanson and DeGroot Swanson (1973) attribute swan-neck deformity to synovitis of the flexor tendon sheath, which restricts interphalangeal flexion. For example, the major long flexor function is to flex the distal interphalangeal (DIP) joint during early bending movement. Patients with flexor synovitis have difficulty initiating this action, and flexor power becomes more concentrated on the MCP joint. This then facilitates pull on the intrinsics across the extensor apparatus. Beyond this, proximal interphalangeal (PIP) synovitis causes loosening of the palmar plate and collaterals, allowing PIP hyperextension to occur. Swan-neck deformity also is attributed to tightened interossei coupled with lax PIP joints, with consequent undue tension on the long extensor at the PIP, and DIP flexion generated by the overtight profundus (Swezey, 1971–1972). As the lateral tendons sublux dorsally, transverse fibers of the retinacular (Landsmeer's) ligaments are stretched out.

Boutonniere Deformity

In boutonniere deformity, hyperplastic synovial tissue lengthens or disrupts the central tendon or its insertion onto the base of the middle phalanx, and transverse fibers connecting the lateral to the central tendon dislocate palmarward (Swanson & DeGroot Swanson, 1973; Swezey, 1971–1972). The PIP joint protrudes between the lateral bands of the extensor tendon, and the digit may stiffen in this position owing to soft tissue contracture. The lateral bands then act as PIP flexors, and as they are shortened relatively by displacement there is distal insertional pull, causing hyperextension at the DIP (Swanson & DeGroot Swanson, 1973). This follows the generalization regarding collapse of a three-joint system, where, for example, hyperextension is surrounded by reciprocal flexion.

The Shoulder

Shoulder motion encompasses four discrete components—sternoclavicular, acromioclavicular, scapulothoracic, and glenohumeral. The glenohumeral component permits more motion than any other joint in the body, and itself sometimes is referred to as "the shoulder joint" (Figure 3–3). The rotator cuff muscles promote stability during movement.

Passively, the humerus can be abducted to 120° while the scapula is restrained from moving (Lucas, 1973). The glenohumeral joint is oriented upward, laterally and posteriorly (Rothman, Marvel, & Heppenstall, 1975). Radiologically, therefore, the joint is best examined by an oblique view. Anteroposterior views of the shoulder in internal and external rotation

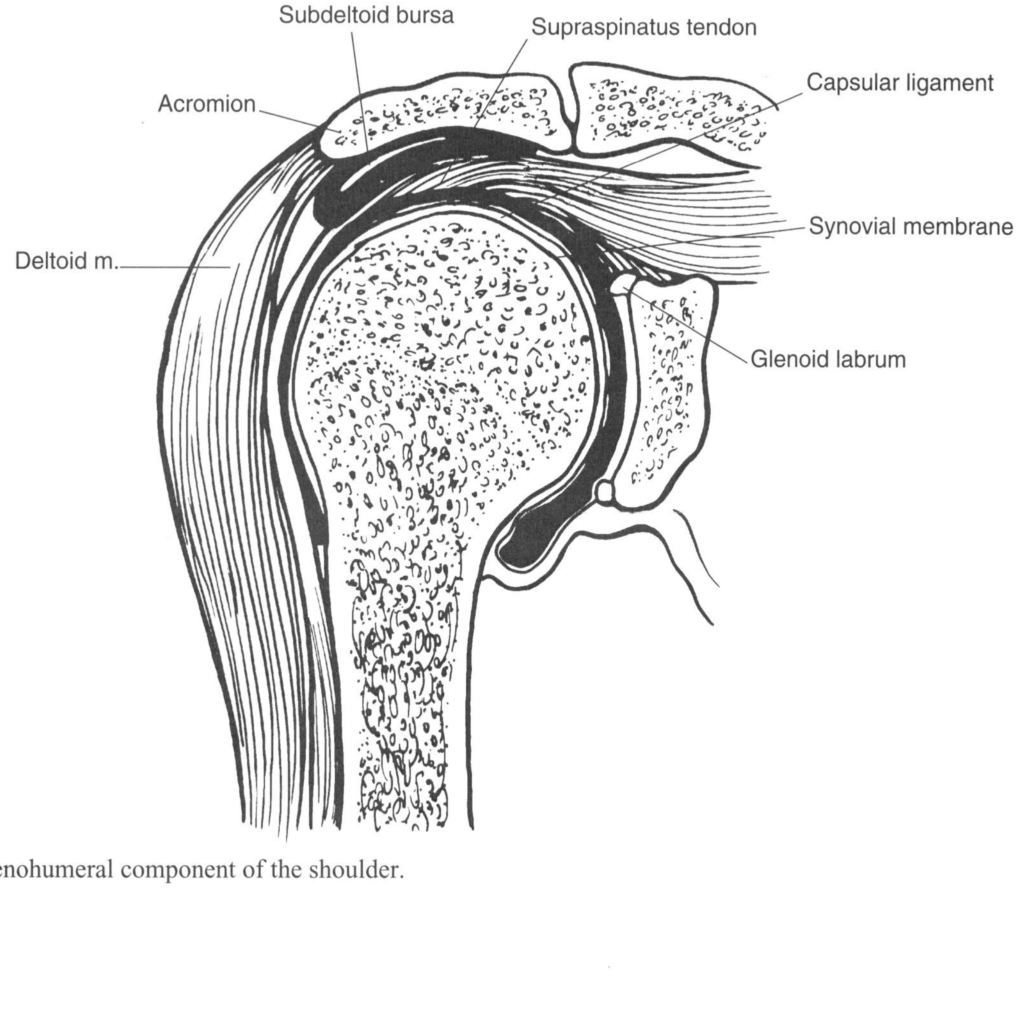

Figure 3–3 Glenohumeral component of the shoulder.

are useful to identify subjacent soft tissue calcifications, marginal erosions, and periarticular spurs (Curran, Ellman, & Brown, 1982).

The fibrous capsule of the shoulder is adapted for mobility, as it occupies approximately twice the volume of the humeral head (Rothman et al., 1975). The joint's synovial capsule is prolonged distally to line the bicipital groove and is reflected over the biceps tendon. Normally, the rotator cuff separates the subdeltoid bursa from the glenohumeral joint. There is no communication between the shoulder (glenohumeral) joint cavity and the subdeltoid bursa—except in the pathological state, with attendant rotator cuff tear (Weiss, Thompson, Doust, & Burgener, 1975).

Normally the rotator cuff muscles contribute the vertical force, which tethers the humerus downward such that the humeral head can pivot effectively in the glenoid when the deltoid contracts. In particular, the supraspinatus reaches peak activity at 100° of abduction and acts throughout the range with the deltoid; the other cuff muscles then act as depressors during abduction (Rothman et al., 1975). Hence, vertical forces provided by the deltoid and cuff muscles render balance and stabilization to the head of the humerus in the glenoid. When rotator cuff function is absent, the unopposed deltoid lacks a fulcrum and subluxes the humeral head against the overhanging acromial process (Lucas, 1973; Schneck, 1977–1980).

Functionally, the shoulder acts in concert with the elbow and wrist in placing the hand, and also in grosser power tasks such as throwing, pushing, lifting, and carrying. Consequently, inability to abduct and rotate at the shoulder serves to enhance the importance of more distal deformities of the elbow, wrist, and digits. Bilateral painful, restricted shoulders, in particular, may severely threaten ability for independent hygiene after toileting.

Subacromial (Subdeltoid) Bursitis and Rotator Cuff Dysfunction

Under normal circumstances, the bursa provides a mechanism for smooth, gliding movement between the rotator cuff tendons and the coracoacromial arch, and cushions the greater tuberosity of the humerus against the overhanging arch. Yet, roughening of the tuberosity or underlying cuff serves as an irritant, with eventual thickening and redundancy of the bursa. Tears or calcium deposits in cuff tendons evoke a bursal inflammatory response. Rarely, the bursa becomes chronically distended, with accommodation of up to several hundred milliliters of fluid (Sbarbaro, 1975). The bursa, therefore, is comparable to the abdominal peritoneum, as underlying cuff disturbances frequently are discovered as the result of bursal symptomatology (Bateman, 1978).

The screw home mechanism that shoves the humeral head directly against the bursa and overhanging arch unfortunately is utilized in the performance of many routine tasks. Subacromial bursitis presents as an obstacle to smooth, unrestricted, or resisted abduction and external rotation.

Rotator cuff atrophy and attrition are visualized radiographically as progressive cephalad migration of the humeral head with respect to the glenoid cavity. The space between the superior humerus and the undersurface of the acromion is narrowed, with the humeral head articulating with acromion as a secondary socket (Chand & Potter, 1972). The coracoacromial arch limits the cuff tendons during abduction, and a painful arc develops. Cuff degeneration, tears, bursal inflammation, and impingement follow, sometimes relieved by acromioplasty. Another mechanism proposed for rotator cuff tear is erosion of the supraspinatus tendon undersurface by adjacent synovium (Weiss et al., 1975). Alternatively, the undervascularized region immediately proximal to the supraspinatus tendon insertion is vulnerable to tearing (Rothman et al., 1975). A torn cuff is almost always sensitive (Bateman, 1978) and the rent may be palpable with the arm extended, as more of the cuff is exposed. Therefore, the sudden onset of increased unilateral shoulder pain during active motion should not be mistaken for flare or new joint infection in the patient with chronic RA (Weiss et al., 1975). Active range (especially abduction or rotation) decreased out of proportion to pain and limitation of other joints suggests a rotator cuff tear. Cuff tear may result in complete loss of active abduction, 30° of active abduction, or full active abduction that is overcome by minuscule resistance. Full passive range of motion may be preserved. Cuff rupture is common in the patient with RA, described as a manifestation of ongoing synovial activity, and usually associated with minor trauma (Sbarbaro, 1975). A cuff tear is further corroborated when subacromial anesthesia eliminates pain but fails to affect weakness (Bateman, 1978). During arthrography, dye moves from the shoulder joint into the bursa via the abnormal passage created by a tear (Weiss et al., 1975).

Glenohumeral Articular Cartilage Destruction

In addition to soft tissue involvement, RA causes progressive destruction of the glenohumeral articular surfaces. Glenohumeral cartilage destruction, with associated joint narrowing, incongruity, periarticular muscle attrition, and intractable pain on movement, contributes to the marked restriction of motion. Some such shoulders retain no more than 30° of flexion, extension, and abduction, and virtually no rotation (Sbarbaro, 1975).

The Elbow

Elbow and shoulder involvements occur most frequently with established disease. Nonetheless, an ankylosed shoulder or wrist is much more readily tolerated than an immobile elbow. Inability to supinate is typically the earlier, more severe impairment (Sturge, 1984), and results in problems with hygiene and toileting. Likewise, loss of pronation compromises writing and most household tasks and further necessitates shoulder abduction and truncal/shoulder rotation in compensation. In contrast, an extension lack can be tolerated as long as active flexion range exists. Reasonable elbow stability is an important requirement for the adequate use of an assistive device.

Patterns of Rheumatoid Arthritis in the Lower Extremity

The Hip and Protrusio Acetabuli

Protrusio acetabuli, an intrapelvic protrusion of the acetabulum, is the typical end stage of rheumatoid hip involvement. Protrusio also is considered a pressure type erosion, with bone-on-bone contact and exacerbation by weight bearing (Monsees and Murphy, 1985). Rheumatoid hip disease is relatively infrequent and usually is described in cases of greater disease chronicity and severity (Bossingham, Schorn, & Morgan, 1975; Hastings & Parker, 1975). Appearance and acceleration of protrusio has been associated with steroid use (Bossingham et al., 1975; Hastings & Parker, 1975), and a high incidence of coexistent avascular necrosis (uncorrelated to drug therapy) also has been reported.

With progressive deformity, subchondral acetabular bone and the adjacent femoral head develop cystic degeneration, presumably due to direct synovial invasion. Deformity accrues both with weight bearing and activity associated with medial wall fracture and femoral head flattening. The rate of acetabular collapse curiously is described as approximately twice that of femoral collapse, with deformity progression more closely parallel to acetabular collapse. The femoral head shifts inward, with direction of horizontal force application comparable to normal, which may account for the surprising mobility sometimes retained by these hips at advanced stages (Hastings & Parker, 1975). Typically, an antalgic or waddling gait is noted as abductor advantage is compromised. In some cases abutting of the greater trochanter against the lateral acetabular brim may decelerate the deforming process (Monsees & Murphy, 1985). Since force borne by the hip comprises body weight and abductor components, greater force is applied as abductors slacken and greater muscle effort is needed for control. As with other hip pathologies, treatment is aimed at force reduction per unit area, and a contralateral walking stick is helpful (Denham, 1959).

Popliteal Cysts and the Pseudothrombophlebitis Syndrome

The gastrocnemius semimembranosus bursa is a constant popliteal structure, which often acquires knee joint communication through a valvular opening (Figure 3–4). The bursa is defined by three sections: a deep, flat area between the gastrocnemius tendon and joint capsule; a neck between the gastrocnemius tendon and semimembranosus; and a superficial expanse beneath the deep fascia. In full extension, the gastrocnemius tendon eliminates passage to the joint between the muscle and medial femoral condyle. Furthermore, in extension, the semimembranosus occludes the connecting neck, and any fluid is driven posteriorly as egress from the joint is blocked. In the normal condition, probably only traces of fluid are found in the bursa, although exact bursal size is undetermined (Canoso, 1981). In contrast, cystic bursal enlargement is designated a Baker's or popliteal cyst.

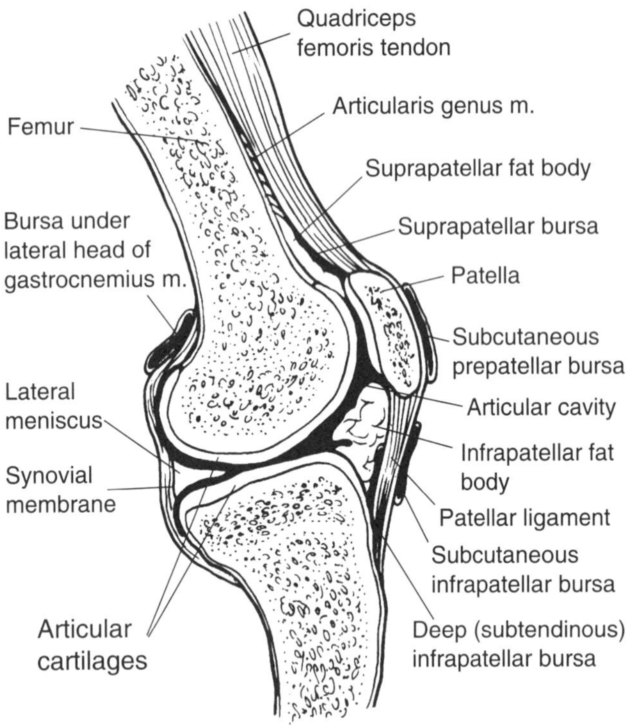

Figure 3–4 Anatomy of the knee.

Popliteal cysts arise either as posterior synovial herniation through the joint capsule wall or by distention and enlargement of the communicating gastrocnemio-semimembranous bursa (Genovese et al., 1972; Jayson, 1981). Again, the enlarged popliteal cyst is always joined to the knee by a valvular connection. This mechanism then serves as a reservoir to reduce intra-articular fluid and to minimize the potentially deleterious effects of joint effusion (Canoso, 1981). The valvular passage to the knee is typically narrow and tortuous, allowing passage of fluid from knee to cyst, but not the reverse. Given an intact valve mechanism, even in the absence of joint pathology, bursal fluid is as viscous as joint fluid; in those with RA, the cyst may actually contain fibrin clumps (Canoso, 1981). With simultaneous pressure measurements, the cyst pressure is characteristically higher than the joint space (Jayson, 1981), again suggesting a protective role for cyst expansion.

Popliteal cysts can occur without ostensible clinical symptomatology (Genovese et al., 1972) or they can amplify greatly and extend down the calf to the ankle. Large cysts at times obstruct venous return, or occasionally are mistaken for solid tumors (Jayson, 1981). A ruptured cyst is characterized by loss of the usual smooth contour and leakage of injected contrast material to fascial planes of the calf. Cystic consistency varies significantly with position, becoming softer in flexion and firmer in extension (Canoso, 1981). Characteristically, cysts develop to more tense, more painful structures after exercise, and to relatively flaccid configurations at rest (Jayson, 1981). Treatment is frequently unsatisfying because fluid recurs, the aspirating needle becomes blocked by fibrin debris, or attempts at excision are unsuccessful.

The pseudothrombophlebitis syndrome is characterized by acute calf inflammation masquerading as new deep vein thrombosis. Rupture of popliteal synovial cysts with synovial fluid extravasation and consequent calf dissection is responsible. Differentiation, starting with venography, has critical therapeutic implications.

Knee Deformities

Convery, Conaty, and Nickel (1971) assessed several forms of management for the rheumatoid knee in 82 patients having at last 10° of flexion contracture and duration of 6 months or more. The mild deformities of 15° or less were corrected in 50% of the patients by physical therapy alone, and remained corrected if the patient stayed ambulatory. Deformities of greater severity or in nonambulatory patients were refractory to physical therapy alone. Plaster casts corrected three fifths of any absolute deformity, regardless of extent, yet with predictable deterioration demonstrated at follow-up. Posterior surgical release resulted in a mean 78% correction, but with regular regression by 15° or 20° at the next visit.

As a generalization, hip or knee flexion contractures of more than 30° present considerable challenge, especially when longstanding and treated by nonoperative means (Hall, 1975). Nonetheless, surgical correction may compromise the neurovascular bundle or require sacrifice of bone and limb length.

Functionally, knees with 10° to 20° of lateral instability are painful (Hall, 1975), and may give way and contribute to falls. Inability to flex the knee beyond 90° requires augmented upper-extremity thrust for rising from a chair, and is greatly complicated by upper limb pain and instability. Weight-bearing function superimposed on affected upper extremities may hasten joint damage and deterioration.

The Foot and Ankle

Rheumatoid arthritis first attacks the foot in 16% of cases, with the ankle and metatarsophalangeal (MTP) joints affected the earliest (Benson & Johnson, 1971). Major deformities include hallux valgus, dropped metatarsals, hammer or claw toes, calcaneovalgus, pronation, and tendocalcaneal bursitis. All contribute to multiple gait deviations, including decreased heel-to-toe pattern, decreased cadence, diminished stride length, abnormal weight bearing, and decreased knee range of motion (Dimonte & Light, 1982; Marshall, Myers, & Palmer, 1980). Frequently pain is mechanical in origin.

As elsewhere, synovial assault compromises joint integrity, with correlative damage to capsule, ligaments, tendons, and cartilage. Weight bearing serves to enhance the inflammation and strain. Imbalance of long muscles ensues, with hammer or claw toe deformities, and new areas of potential skin pressure. Patients having MTP subluxation feel that they are "walking on tacks," and pain evoked by lateral metatarsal head compression suggests involvement of these joints. Widening of the forefoot, tenderness, or puffiness may be associated. Exquisite pain at the plantar metatarsal heads and gross subluxation are often demonstrable.

Hallux valgus begins with MTP inflammation, followed by ligamentous laxity and lateral phalangeal deviation. A painful medial bunion often results, which becomes aggravated or ulcerates. Weight-bearing capacity is diminished at the first MTP, and the burden is unnaturally shifted to the lateral border of the foot.

The hindfoot sometimes instigates other deformities contributing to instability. Typically the calcaneus is subluxed into valgus, the talar head is displaced inferomedially, and the forefoot is abducted due to loss of subtalar inversion. Normal locking mechanisms at the subtalar and midtarsal joints are overcome. With subtalar involvement, walking on uneven ground, inversion, and eversion are extraordinarily painful. A painful, flexible hindfoot will respond to orthotic intervention, whereas inflexible valgus with painful metatarsals often will require surgery. With subcutaneous plantar nodules, discomfort is caused by weight bearing and shoe pressure. Calcaneal erosion sometimes develops at the site of the plantar fascial attachment.

Rheumatoid feet commonly develop tendon and bursal lesions. Usual sites of tenosynovitis include tendons of the tibialis posterior and peronaei, less often extensor tendons on the dorsum of the foot, or rarely any tendon (Benson & Johnson, 1971; Calabro, 1962). The constant synovially lined bursa beneath the achilles tendon participates in the rheumatoid process and becomes inflamed. Achilles tendon rupture has been reported in this circumstance (Rask, 1978).

The Cervical Spine

Cervical spine disease frequently is linked to widespread, even mutilating peripheral joint disease (Matthews, 1974; Nakano, 1975; Pellicci, Ranawat, Tsairis, & Bryan, 1981), peripheral laxity, seropositivity, and nodule formation. Bland (1974), however, has suggested a less common variety of cervical rheumatoid disease with little peripheral joint involvement.

Unexplained strength loss (with quiescent arthritis) should suggest the possibility of cervical myelopathy. Furthermore, muscle power, tone, and plantar responses are obscured by severe structural changes, and these changes delay myelopathy recognition.

Bone and ligament in proximity to the 32 cervical synovial joints are prone to synovial destruction. Synovial inflammation occurs around the anterior and posterior dens, and about its anchoring apical and alar ligaments. Stability is compromised through bony erosion, granulomatous disc invasion (Bland, 1974), and altered ligamentous support. Granulation tissue solely, rather than canal narrowing by subluxation, can account for cord compression (Whaley, 1968). Although canal width is greatest at C-1 to C-2, ultimately compression reflects absolute width (such that patients with intrinsically wider canals tolerate more atlantoaxial subluxation; Nakano, 1975). Between C-3 and C-7, canal depth averages 17 mm, with a scatter of 5 mm (Ehni, 1984).

Laxity of the transverse ligament (or odontoid erosion) allows the atlas and skull to move forward en bloc during neck flexion, trapping the cord between the odontoid and the posterior rim of C-1. Torsion of the vertebral artery may occur concomitantly. Also, transverse ligament loosening and severe atlantoaxial subluxation potentially compress the medullary respiratory center.

Vertical subluxation of the ondontoid and C-2 body follows bone loss variously in the occipital condyles, basilar skull, and atlantoaxial joints. In 1948 McGregor determined that the uppermost odontoid tip should rest no more than 4.5 mm cephalad to the line connecting the caudal occiput and posterior hard palate (Cabot & Becker, 1978). Furthermore, as the odontoid is wider at its base, gradual upward translocation progressively fills the canal. The illusion of improved atlantoaxial subluxation is created, as the upwardly migrating odontoid presents its larger circumference to a fixed bony outlet (Cabot & Becker, 1978; Matthews, 1974). The proximity of the dens to critical brain stem structures suggests that upward migration is more ominous than atlantoaxial subluxation (Rana, Hancock, Taylor, & Hill, 1973).

Multiple staircase, subaxial subluxations may occur in relationship to apophyseal disease. At times, lesser degrees of midcervical displacement produce symptomatic compression, as the cord more completely fills the canal at this level (Cabot & Becker, 1978; Marks & Sharp, 1981). Postural signs occasionally reveal serious underlying cervical processes. Suboccipital prominence of the axis spinous process (as observed with the neck flexed) suggests that skull and atlas are subluxing on the axis (Bland, 1974; Robinson, 1966). Rotation and slight tilting of the head imply asymmetrical erosion of atlanto-occipital or atlantoaxial joints. Some situations, such as general anesthesia, unwittingly expose the patient to serious risk.

Clinical expression of cervical spine disease varies dramatically. Deep, aching, upper cervical and occipital pain is frequent with high cervical involvement or otherwise stiffness, or occipital headache triggered by flexing the head forward is noted. With increasing severity, pain is referred temporally or retro-orbitally. Crepitus and instability may be prominent, or Lhermitte's sign readily elicited. Patients sometimes complain that the head seems heavy and difficult to support, or that vertigo, nausea, vomiting, or visual symptoms are evoked by rotatory neck movement. Pain commonly is worsened by secondary muscle spasm.

Onset of cord compression can be insidious. Sensory myelopathic symptoms are easily mistaken for entrapment or peripheral neuropathies. More subtle degrees of spastic quadriparesis are easily overshadowed by extensive joint deformities, although acute and severe quadriparesis/quadriplegia occasionally is seen. Also reported is late advanced quadriparesis/plegia, spastic paraparesis, Brown-Séquard syndrome, drop attacks (Christophidis & Huskisson, 1982), flexor spasms of the lower extremities, bowel/bladder disturbance (incontinence or retention), marble sensation of the trunk and limbs, impairment in the trigeminal sensory distribution, giddiness on neck extension, or (rarely) dysphagia due to brain stem compression (Davidson, Horn, Herndon, & Grin, 1977). Neurological manifestations at times regress, only to return.

On examination, deep tendon reflexes may be disproportionately brisk, and superficial abdominal or cremasteric reflexes sometimes are absent. Trigeminal abnormalities derive from the descending tract of that nerve, which reaches as low as the second cervical segment. The upper level of sensory loss is described as seldom relating to the level of presumed compression (Marks & Sharp, 1981). Spastic weakness is perhaps the most easily identified finding.

Not surprisingly, a dichotomy exists between clinical and radiological findings, though initial appearance of either may be delayed over years. One series reports that 106 patients with RA who had cervical spine complaints were followed for 5 years. At final evaluation, 36% had progressed neurologically, whereas 80% had progressed radiologically (Pellicci et al., 1981). Indeed, even serial radiological examinations, in isolation, disclose a varied natural history (Smith, Benn, & Sharp, 1972).

CONCLUSION

Patients with RA require intensive resources and frequently reach the rehabilitation setting in the later disease stages (Karlen, Lee, & McEwen, 1973). While functional gains are possible, they remain tempered by consequences of advanced structural change. The guiding principle of care is early diagnosis, recognition of primary and secondary complications, and the judicious and timely choice of interventions to prevent, mitigate, or contain functional compromise. Despite incomplete ability to control inflammation, well-chosen interventions can minimize effusion, supplement ligamentous or muscular support, protect weight bearing, circumvent use of painful or damaged structures, and overall enhance function. To these ends, rehabilitation provides an avenue to maximize activity performance and quality of life in the patient with RA.

REFERENCES

Backhouse, K.M., Kay, A.G., Coomes, E.N., & Kates, E. (1971). Tendon involvement in the rheumatoid hand. *Annals of the Rheumatic Diseases*, *30*, 236–242.

Bateman, J.E. (1978). *The shoulder and neck*. New York: Saunders.

Benedict, J.V., Walker, L.B., & Harris, E.H. (1968). Stress strain characteristics and tensile strength of unenbalmed human tendon. *Journal of Biomechanics*, *1*, 53–63.

Benson, G., & Johnson, E.W. (1971). Management of the foot in rheumatoid arthritis. *Orthopaedic Clinics of North America*, *2* (3), 733–744.

Bird, A., Trise, C.R., Bacon, P.A. (1978). Joint hypermobility leading to osteoarthrosis and chondrocalcanosos. *Annals of the Rheumatic Diseases*, *37*, 203–211.

Bland, J. (1974). Rheumatoid arthritis of the cervical spine. *Journal of Rheumatology*, *1*, 319–342.

Bossingham, D.H., Schorn, D., & Morgan, G. (1975). Patterns of hip involvement in rheumatoid arthritis. *Annals of the Rheumatic Diseases*, *37*, 293.

Burke, F. (1984). The effects of rheumatoid diseases of the hand. *Clinical Rheumatology Diseases*, *10* (3), 435–448.

Cabot, A., & Becker, A. (1978). The cervical spine in rheumatoid arthritis. *Clinical Orthopaedics and Related Research*, *131*, 130–140.

Calabro, J.J. (1962). A critical evaluation of the diagnostic features of the feet in rheumatoid arthritis. *Arthritis and Rheumatism*, *5*, 19–29.

Canoso, J. (1981). Bursae, tendons, and ligaments. *Clinics in Rheumatic Diseases*, *7* (1), 189–221.

Canoso, J., & Yood, R. (1979). Reaction of superficial bursae in response to specific disease stimuli. *Arthritis and Rheumatism*, *22*, 1361–1364.

Chand, K., & Potter, J.A. (1972). Rheumatoid arthritis and the shoulder joint. *International Surgery*, *57*, 969–973.

Christophidis, N., & Huskisson, E.C. (1982). Misleading symptoms and signs of cervical spine subluxation in rheumatoid arthritis. *British Medical Journal*, *285*, 364–365.

Convery, F.R., Conaty, J.P., & Nickel, V.L. (1971). Flexion deformities of the knee in rheumatoid arthritis. *Clinical Orthopaedics and Related Research*, *74*, 90–93.

Curran, J.F., Ellman, M.H., & Brown, N.L. (1982). Rheumatologic aspects of painful conditions affecting the shoulder. *Clinical Orthopaedics and Related Research*, *173*, 27–37.

Davidson, R.C., Horn, J.R., Herndon, J.H., & Grin, O.D. (1977). Brain stem compression in rheumatoid arthritis. *Journal of the American Medical Association*, *238*, 2633–2634.

Denham, R.A. (1959). Hip mechanics. *Journal of Bone and Joint Surgery [Br]*, *41*, 550–557.

Dimonte, P., & Light, H. (1982). Pathomechanics: Gait deviations and treatment of the rheumatoid foot. *Physical Therapy*, *62*, 1148–1156.

Duthie, J.J., Brown, P.E., Knox, J.D., & Thompson, M. (1957). Course and prognosis in rheumatoid arthritis. *Annals of the Rheumatic Diseases*, *16*, 411–424.

Duthie, J.J., Brown, P.E., Truelove, L.H., Barajar, F.D., & Laurie, A.J. (1964). Course and prognosis in rheumatoid arthritis: A further report. *Annals of the Rheumatic Diseases*, *23*, 193–202.

Ehni, G. (1984). *Cervical arthrosis*. Chicago: Year Book.

Favreau, J.C., & Laurin, C.A. (1963). Joint effusions and flexion deformities. *Canadian Medical Association Journal*, *88*, 575.

Flatt, A.E. (1983). *Care of the arthritic hand* (4th ed.). St. Louis: Mosby.

Fleming, A., Benn, R.T., Corbett, M., & Wood, P.N. (1976). Early rheumatoid disease, II: Patterns of joint involvement. *Annals of the Rheumatic Diseases*, *35*, 361–364.

Fletcher, D.E., & Rowley, K.A. (1952). The radiological features of rheumatoid arthritis. *British Journal of Radiology*, *25*, 282–295.

Gardner, E.D. (1963). Physiology of joints. *Journal of Bone and Joint Surgery [Am]*, *45*, 1061–1066.

Genovese, G.R., Jayson, M.I., & Dixon, A.S. (1972). Protective value of synovial cysts in rheumatoid knees. *Annals of the Rheumatic Diseases*, *31*, 179–182.

Gerser, L.H. (1985). Rehabilitation of patients with rheumatic diseases. In W.N. Kelley, E.D. Harris, S. Ruddy, & C.B. Sledge (Eds.), *Textbook of rheumatology* (Vol. II, 2nd ed.). Philadelphia: Saunders.

Hall, A. (1975). The decision to operate in rheumatoid arthritis. *Orthopaedic Clinics of North America*, *6*, 675–684.

Halla, J.T., Koopman, W.J., Fallatti, S., Oh, S.J., & Gay, R.E. (1984). Rheumatoid myositis: Clinical and histological features and possible pathogenesis. *Arthritis and Rheumatism*, *27*, 737–743.

Hamerman, D., Rosenberg, L.C., & Schubert, M. (1970). Diarthrodial joints revisited. *Journal of Bone and Joint Surgery [Am]*, 52, 725–774.

Hastings, D.E., & Parker, S.M. (1975). Protrusio acetabuli in rheumatoid arthritis. *Clinical Orthopaedics and Related Research*, *108*, 76–83.

Hollinshead, W.H. (1969). *Anatomy for surgeons: The back and limbs* (Vol. 3). New York: Harper & Row.

Jacoby, R.K., Jayson, M.I., & Cosh, J.A. (1973). Onset, early stages, and prognosis of rheumatoid arthritis: A clinical study of 100 patients with 11 year follow-up. *British Medical Journal*, *2*, 96–100.

Jayson, M.I. (1981). Intra-articular pressure. *Clinics in the Rheumatic Diseases*, *7*, 149–166.

Jayson, M.I., & Dixon, A. (1970a). Intra-articular pressure in rheumatoid arthritis of the knee: Pressure changes during passive joint distention. *Annals of Rheumatic Diseases*, *29*, 261–265.

Jayson, M.I., & Dixon, A. (1970b). Intra-articular pressure in rheumatoid arthritis of the knee. *Annals of the Rheumatic Diseases*, *29*, 401–408.

Karlen, I., Lee, M., & McEwen, C. (1973). Rheumatoid arthritis: A five-year study of rehabilitation. *Archives of Physical Medicine and Rehabilitation*, *54*, 120–128.

Kay, A.G. (1979). Management of the rheumatoid hand. *Rheumatology Rehabilitation* (Suppl.), 76–81.

Kellgren, J.H., & Ball, J. (1950). Tendon lesions in rheumatoid arthritis: A clinico-pathological study. *Annals of the Rheumatic Diseases*, *9*, 48–65.

Kellgren, J.H., & Samuel, E.P. (1950). The sensitivity and innervation of the articular capsule. *Journal of Bone and Joint Surgery [Br]*, *32*, 84–92.

Kostuik, J.P., Schmidt, O., Harris, W.R., & Wooldridge, C. (1975). A study of weight transmission throughout the knee joint with applied varus and valgus loads. *Clinical Orthopaedics and Related Research*, *108*, 95–98.

Krane, S.M., & Simon, L.S. (1986). Rheumatoid arthritis: Clinical features and pathogenetic mechanisms. *Medical Clinics of North America*, *70* (2), 263–283.

Lucas, D.B. (1973). Biomechanics of the shoulder joint. *Archives of Surgery*, *107*, 425–432.

Macauley, D.I., Evans, D.M., & Ansell, B.M. (1981). Assessment of flexor tenosynovitis in rheumatoid arthritis. *Rheumatology Rehabilitation*, *20*, 25–30.

Marks, J.S., & Sharp, J. (1981). Rheumatoid cervical myelopathy. *Quarterly Journal of Medicine*, *199*, 307–319.

Marshall, R., Myers, O., & Palmer, D. (1980). Disturbance of gait due to rheumatoid disease. *Journal of Rheumatology*, *7*, 617–623.

Matthews, J.A. (1974). Atlantoaxial subluxation in rheumatoid arthritis: A five year follow-up study. *Annals of the Rheumatic Diseases*, *33*, 526–531.

Millender, L.H., & Nalebuff, E.A. (1975). Evaluation and treatment of early rheumatoid hand involvement. *Orthopaedic Clinics of North America*, *6*, 697–708.

Millis, M.B., Millender, L.H., & Nalebuff, E.A. (1976). Stiffness of the protioral interphalangeal joints in rheumatoid arthritis. *Journal of Bone and Joint Surgery [Am]*, *58*, 801–805.

Mitchell, D.M., Spitz, P.W., Young, D.Y., Bloch, D.A., McShane, D.J., & Fries, J.F. (1986). Survival, prognosis and causes of death in rheumatoid arthritis. *Arthritis and Rheumatism*, *29*, 706–714.

Monsees, B., & Murphy, W. (1985). Pressure erosions: A pattern of bone resorption in rheumatoid arthritis. *Arthritis and Rheumatism*, *28*, 820–824.

Myers, D.B., & Palmer, D.G. (1972). Capsular compliance and pressure volume relationships in normal and arthritic knees. *Journal of Bone and Joint Surgery [Br]*, *54*, 710–716.

Nakano, K.K. (1975). Neurologic complications of rheumatoid arthritis. *Orthopaedic Clinics of North America*, *6* (3), 861–880.

Noyes, F., Torvik, P., Hyde, W., & DeLucas, J. (1974). Biomechanics of ligament failure. *Journal of Bone and Joint Surgery [Am]*, *56*, 1406–1418.

Pellicci, P.M., Ranawat, C.S., Tsairis, P., & Bryan, W.J. (1981). A prospective study of the progression of rheumatoid arthritis of the cervical spine. *Journal of Bone and Joint Surgery [Am]*, 63, 342–350.

Radin, E.L. (1975). Mechanical aspects of osteoarthrosis. *Bulletin of Rheumatic Diseases*, *26*, 862–864.

Rana, N.A., Hancock, D.O., Taylor, A.R., & Hill, A.G. (1973). Upward translocation of the dens in rheumatoid arthritis. *Journal of Bone and Joint Surgery [Br]*, *55*, 471–477.

Rask, M.R. (1978). Achilles tendon rupture secondary to rheumatoid disease. *Journal of the American Medical Association*, *239*, 435–436.

Robinson, H.S. (1966). Rheumatoid arthritis: Atlanto-axial subluxation and its clinical presentation. *Canadian Medical Association Journal*, *94*, 470–477.

Rothman, R.H., Marvel, J.P., & Heppenstall, R.B. (1975). Anatomic lorsidextions in the glenohumeral joint. *Orthopaedic Clinics of North America*, *6*, 341–352.

Sbarbaro, J.L. (1975). The rheumatoid shoulder. *Orthopaedic Clinics of North America*, *6*, 593–596.

Schneck, C. (1977–1980). Instructional anatomy courses. Philadelphia: Temple University.

Schneider, R., & Kaye, J.J. (1975). Insufficiency and stress fractures of the long bones occurring in patients with rheumatoid arthritis. *Radiology*, *116*, 595–599.

Shapiro, J.S. (1970). A new factor in the etiology of ulnar drift. *Clinical Orthopaedics and Related Research*, *68*, 32–43.

Simon, W.H., Friedenberg, S., & Richardson, S. (1973). Joint congruence: A correlation of joint congruence and thickness of articular cartilage in dogs. *Journal of Bone and Joint Surgery [Am]*, *55*, 1614–1620.

Smith, P.H., Benn, R.T., & Sharp, J. (1972). Natural history of rheumatoid cervical luxations. *Annals of the Rheumatic Diseases*, *31*, 431–439.

Sturge, R.A. (1984). The remote effects of rheumatic diseases on the hand and their management. *Clinics in Rheumatic Diseases*, *10* (3), 449–477.

Swanson, A.B., & DeGroot Swanson, G. (1973). Pathogenesis and pathomechanics of rheumatoid deformities in the hand and wrist. *Orthopaedic Clinics of North America*, *4* (4), 1039–1056.

Swartz, M.O., & Silver, R.M. (1984). D penicillamine induces polymyositis in juvenile chronic arthritis: Report of a case. *Journal of Rheumatology*, *11*, 251–252.

Swezey, R.L. (1971–1972). Dynamic factors in deformity of the rheumatoid arthritis hand. *Bulletin of Rheumatic Diseases*, *22* (1&2), 649–656.

Weiss, J.J., Thompson, G.R., Doust, V., & Burgener, F. (1975). Rotator cuff tears in rheumatoid arthritis. *Archives of Internal Medicine*, *135*, 521–525.

Whaley, K. (1968). Fatal subaxial dislocation of the cervical spine in rheumatoid arthritis. *British Medical Journal*, *2*, 31.

Wiederholt, W.C., & Ehrlich, G.E. (1985). Responses to K.A. Weinberger: Rheumatoid arthritis and floppy head syndrome. *Journal of the American Medical Association*, *253*, 93.

Woo, S., Gomez, M.A., Woo, Y.K., & Akesou, W. (1982). Mechanical properties of tendons and ligaments. *Biorheology*, *19*, 397–408.

SUGGESTED READING

Bombardier, C., Tugwell, P., Sinclair, A., Dok, C., Anderson, G., & Buchanan, W. (1982). Preference for endpoint measures in clinical trials: Results of Structured Workshops. *Journal of Rheumatology*, *9*, 798–806.

Canoso, J. (1955). Effect of ultrasound on tendon extensibility. *American Journal of Physical Medicine, 34*, 362–369.

Freyberg, R. (1968). A study of the time of onset of structural joint damages in rheumatoid arthritis. *Arthritis and Rheumatism, 11*, 481.

Hall, J.T., Koopman, W.J., Fallatti, S., Oh, S.J., Gray, R.E., & Schrohenloher, R.E. (1984). Rheumatoid myositis: Clinical and histological features and possible pathogenesis. *Arthritis and Rheumatism*, *27*, 737–743.

Henderson, P.R., Jayson, M.I., & Tribse, C.R. (1975). Lack of correlation of synovial histology with joint damage in rheumatoid arthritis. *Annals of the Rheumatic Diseases*, *34*, 7–11.

Jacobs, J.C., Dick, H.M., & Downey, J.A., Edgar, A., Sternstein, R., & Berdon, W.E. (1981). Weightbearing as a treatment for damaged hips in juvenile rheumatoid arthritis [Letter to the editor]. *New England Journal of Medicine*, *305*, 409.

Meijers, K.A., Van Beusekom, G.T., Luyendijk, W., & Duijfjes, F. (1974). Dislocation of cervical spine with cord compression in rheumatoid arthritis. *Journal of Bone and Joint Surgery [Br], 56*, 668–680.

CHAPTER 4

Functional Limitations Associated with Rheumatoid Arthritis: A Guide to Rehabilitation Prescription

Victoria A. Brander, MD

The rehabilitation prescription aims to minimize or eliminate disability through maximizing the medical management of rheumatoid arthritis (RA), optimizing the patient's physical and functional capacity, modifying the environment, and eliminating societal handicaps.

It is helpful to refer to a global scheme for conceptualizing impairment and disability when considering the rehabilitation prescription. As described in Chapter 2, the Institute of Medicine and the National Council on Disability have proposed specific definitions for terms used in a model of disability in the *Prevention of Disability Working Paper*, which was published in 1991.

REHABILITATION HISTORY AND PHYSICAL EXAMINATION

In addition to a comprehensive neurological and musculoskeletal examination, the rehabilitation history and physical examination must include a detailed social history. This would include addressing the accessibility of the patient's home environment. Are there many stairs? Are bathrooms wheelchair accessible? Are there handrails in the bathtub and near the toilet? Also important is identifying the primary caregivers and issues related to their services. Is the spouse in good health? A comprehensive vocational history should determine whether or not the patient is having work difficulties related to disability. Homemakers should be asked about their ability to perform household activities. Are they relying more on family members? Has this caused family strife? Avocational activities add quality to life. Patients should be asked whether they have hobbies and whether their impairments interfere with them.

The patient's ability to perform functional tasks should be ascertained by interview and/or direct observation. Functional skills are commonly described as activities of daily living (ADLs), such as feeding, toileting, oral facial hygiene, bathing, and upper extremity and lower extremity dressing; instrumental ADLs, such as laundry, shopping, cooking, and homemaking; and mobility skills, such as bed mobility, transfers, and ambulation.

Function is rated by using a simple scale to determine the amount of assistance an individual needs with a task. The ratings commonly used are as follows:

- Independent
- Modified independent (with a device); set up, supervised (hands-off guarding)
- Minimal assistance (the patient performs about 75% of the task, and the helper needs to perform only about 25%)
- Moderate assistance (the patient performs 50% of the task)
- Maximal assistance (the patient performs 25% of the task or is dependent but able to direct self care)
- Total assistance (dependent)

If the patient needs equipment, such as a walker, the term *with equipment* is added to the rating (eg, independent with equipment ambulating 150 ft). If the patient needs ongoing instruction or reminders from someone, the term *with cues* is added.

In general, when addressing a case of RA, synovitis/ inflammation must be eliminated; medical co-morbidities treated; physical impairments minimized through specifically prescribed exercise or rest; functional impairments improved through practice with use of altered techniques and equipment; and disability limited by minimizing societal barriers.

To illustrate the process of rehabilitation prescription, five case studies of patients with different severity levels of RA are presented and discussed.

CASE PRESENTATION 1: EARLY NONDESTRUCTIVE RHEUMATOID ARTHRITIS

The patient is a 45-year-old woman who has had RA for 5 years. She presents asking whether exercise will help her arthritis. Her RA primarily affects her hands, feet, and knees and is well managed with daily nonsteroidal anti-inflammatory drug use.

Minimize Physical and Functional Impairments

The overall benefits of exercise in the general population are well known, including improved longevity and quality of life. Inactivity is an independent predictor of morbidity and mortality, perhaps as significant as family history of heart disease or obesity. Patients with RA unfortunately have traditionally been precluded from exercise by their doctors and health care professionals who feared that exercise would accelerate joint damage. A few studies have documented that individuals with RA have poorer muscle strength and endurance than the normal population (Basmaijian, 1987; Ekblom, Lovgren, Alderin, Fridstrom, & Satterstrom, 1974; Minor, Hewett, Webel, Dreisinger, & Kay, 1988). Recent literature supports exercise (both aerobic and resistance training) as beneficial in individuals with RA.

Exercise improves aerobic capacity, speed and quality of gait, depression, anxiety, and function. There is some evidence that exercise alone may actually decrease active joint count and independently *improve* disease (Minor, Hewitt, Webel, Anderson, & Kay, 1989; Perlman et al., 1990). In a study of subjects with RA having symptomatic weight-bearing joints who participated in a 12-week course of graded aerobic exercise, significant improvements were made in aerobic capacity, abnormal involuntary movement scale (AIMS) scores on physical activity, anxiety and depression, 50-ft walk time, grip strength, and flexibility. The number of inflamed joints either remained the same or improved, without a change in drug treatment. Gains were maintained at 1 year (Minor, Hewett, Webel, Anderson, & Kay, 1989). In a study of the effectiveness of a dance-based aerobic exercise program combined with education on problem-solving skills for subjects with RA, improvements were noted in quality-of-life measures (depression, overall functioning, and increased vigor) as well as 50-ft walk time, without increases in disease activity (Perlman et al., 1990).

Muscle-strengthening exercises have been shown in a number of studies to increase muscle strength and endurance in individuals with arthritis. Ekblom, Lovgren, and Alderin (1975) showed increases in the ability to perform a series of physical fitness tests such as stair climbing, speed walking, and muscle strength. In a study of male subjects with knee osteoarthritis, Fisher et al. (1993) demonstrated improved muscle strength, endurance, and overall function without any exacerbation of joint pain after a program of resisted muscle strengthening and range of motion (ROM) exercises. A more comprehensive review of exercise in RA is presented in Chapter 8.

In summary, exercise is important for those with RA to manage inflammation, improve overall fitness, maintain mobility and vigor, counteract the muscle atrophy and debility that accompany joint inflammation, and perhaps to reduce long-term disability.

Exercise prescription should include a program of muscle strengthening and aerobic conditioning, with specifics about the duration of exercise, the intensity (based on target heart rate or perceived exertion), and the frequency (see Chapter 8). Assessment of the degree of joint instability is important to the prescription. If patients have full ROM of joints and good muscle strength, resistance training can begin immediately. When ROM and strength are limited, more care should be taken, using isometrics, active ROM (AROM) without resistance of weights, or exercise in water until maximal ROM without pain is obtained. Aquatic exercise is an excellent way for individuals with arthritis to exercise. The warmth and buoyancy of a heated pool allows maximal ROM, strengthening, and endurance training in a pain-free environment. Pool therapy improves both strength and conditioning (Danneskiold-Samsoe, Lyngberg, Risum, & Telling, 1987).

The typical instructions for this patient would be that she should begin an aerobic conditioning and strengthening program. Aerobic exercises should be performed at least three to four times weekly, for a minimum duration of 20 to 30 minutes. There is recent evidence that exercise performed throughout the day is cumulative, so that three exercise sessions of 10 minutes may be as effective as one 30-minute session. Aerobic exercise should be preceded by a 5-minute warm-up and 15-minute cool-down period of active ROM exercises, but even moderate-intensity exercise (at 40 to 60 degrees maximal heart rate, or 3 to 4 metabolic equivalents [METS]) is effective. Optimally she should try to reach her target heart rate (180 – age) 60% to 80%.

Older patients or those with cardiorespiratory impairments should focus on perceived exertion or attaining a safe heart rate (as determined by pre-exercise stress test). Aerobic conditioning in the pool or on a bike, or other low-impact exercises are the most prudent. Muscle strengthening should begin with low weights and higher repetitions, and then can be increased as tolerated. Novices to exercise may benefit from a session with a physical therapist or physical trainer to learn proper techniques and receive a complete program. It is certainly appropriate to refer patients with joint impairments to a physical therapist for one or two sessions to design a home exercise program. As described in Chapter 18, "Social Supports and Community Resources for Persons with Rheumatoid Arthritis," the Arthritis Foundation sponsors a number of land- and water-based aerobic exercise programs for patients with arthritis.

CASE PRESENTATION 2: ACTIVE INFLAMMATION, MODEST JOINT DESTRUCTION

A 65-year-old woman with a history of RA presents for evaluation of knee pain and lower leg swelling, which have bothered her for 1 week. On physical examination, she has a right knee joint effusion, a 15° flexion contracture, limited active flexion to 90°, and a painful, swollen calf. There is quadriceps atrophy. She reports that climbing stairs has been causing her mild knee pain for several months and is increasingly difficult. Radiographs obtained during her last visit revealed modest symmetrical knee joint narrowing.

Maximize Disease Management

The history and physical examination suggest a pseudothrombophlebitis secondary to a popliteal, or Baker's, cyst. Synovial effusion can create a communication between the knee joint and the semimembranosus-gastrocnemius bursa. If the cyst dissects into the calf, leg swelling and pain may occur, mimicking thrombophlebitis. Popliteal cysts may occur in individuals with RA, osteoarthritis, or other knee disorders. Ultrasound has become the diagnostic method of choice, confirming the presence of the cyst and excluding thrombophlebitis. The popliteal cyst in an individual with inflammatory arthropathy is treated with a corticosteroid (eg, 40 mg of triamcinolone acetonide or its equivalent) injection into the knee joint.

Minimize Physical and Functional Impairments

The physical impairments identified in this individual include a knee flexion contracture, limited active knee flexion, and quadriceps weakness and atrophy. Treating the popliteal cyst alone is not likely to reverse these impairments. A focused exercise regimen should be prescribed. An appropriate exercise program is as follows:

- Range of motion: active knee flexion and extension, 10 repetitions performed twice daily; stretching the knee in extension (on a flat surface) twice daily
- Strengthening: quadriceps sets; straight leg raises; terminal knee extension; progress to full ROM knee extension exercises with low weights (1 to 3 lb) as tolerated by pain within 2 weeks
- Endurance training: 30 minutes of accumulated aerobic exercise, maintaining the target heart rate or perceived exertion three to four times weekly

Whether or not physical modalities assist in the management of acute knee synovitis is not clear. Superficial cold application is a well-tolerated method of pain relief and can be safely added to the prescription (Kirk & Kersley, 1968). Cold packs are usually prescribed for use three to four times daily, for 15 minutes' duration. There is no good evidence of their effectiveness or data guiding prescription of duration or intensity. Deep-heating methods (eg, ultrasound, microwave, shortwave) likely increase intra-articular temperature. Whether or not this is beneficial in individuals with acute synovitis is debated (Hollander & Horvath, 1949; Weinberger et al., 1990; Weinberger, Fadilah, Lev, & Pinkhas, 1989). Ultrasound is a useful adjunct to ROM exercises in eliminating contractures secondary to soft tissue pathology. Ultrasound added to physical therapy, however, has not been shown to improve pain or AROM in patients with contractures from knee osteoarthritis (Falconer, Hayes, & Chang, 1992). In this patient, if the knee contracture is felt to be soft tissue–related, referral to physical therapy for modalities (such as ultrasound) is appropriate as an adjunct to the stretching and strengthening exercises.

Finally, the knee limitations in ROM and strength are likely the primary factors in impairing the patient's ability to climb stairs. Once the physical deficits are improved, the stair-climbing ability should be reassessed.

CASE PRESENTATION 3: ACTIVE INFLAMMATION, MINIMAL TO MILD JOINT DESTRUCTION, AND DEFORMITY

The patient is a 40-year-old man who has had RA primarily affecting his hands and feet for several years. He presents for evaluation of forefoot pain that is worse by the end of the day and during walking. He is also having increasing difficulty manipulating small objects and typing. He is employed as a data-entry computer operator. His medication is naproxen, 375 mg twice daily, for his arthritis. On physical examination, there is mild synovitis of the metacarpophalangeal joints (MCPs) and wrists. He has triggering of the right fourth digit during active extension, with a nodular thickening palpable at the base of the fourth MCP and decreased active finger flexion. There are ulnar deviations and swan-neck deformities in both hands. Examination of the foot reveals forefoot spread, cock-up and hammer toes, and hallux valgus. He has flexible but flat arches, tenderness over the metatarsal heads, and mild synovitis at the ankles.

Maximize Disease Management

The first step in this rehabilitation prescription is to improve drug management of the patient's synovitis. This patient has evidence of active synovitis, and he is taking only a small dose of nonsteroidal anti-inflammatory medication. Aggressive reduction of inflammation is warranted. Increasing the anti-inflammatory dose is appropriate, but a patient with structural deformities as a consequence of RA and active disease can be treated with a remittive agent, such as methotrexate (see Chapter 6).

Minimize Physical and Functional Impairments

This individual's hands exhibit many of the manifestations of RA described in Chapter 3. Tenderness on the dorsum of the hand, triggering of the fingers, decreased flexion, and a palpable nodule along the flexor tendon are characteristic of flexor tenosynovitis, which may occur in more than 50% of individuals with the disease. Corticosteroid injection (triamicinalone acetonide 20 mg or its equivalent) into the tendon sheath at the level of the nodule may alleviate the pain and triggering, and should be followed by exercise and other methods described.

Occupational therapy should be considered for fabrication of proximal interphalangeal (PIP) splints, resting hand splints, adaptive equipment evaluation, ROM and strengthening exercises, and education about energy conservation and joint protection. Splinting the PIP joints may reduce PIP hyperextension in individuals with flexible swan-neck deformities. These splints may improve pain and increase functional use of the fingers. Resting hand splints immobilize the wrist in a position of slight extension and the MCPs of the fingers in slight flexion. They can be used to assist in limiting inflammation, reducing pain, and attempting to preserve functional range until the synovitis of the hand is resolved. Self-help aids, such as built-up utensils and buttonhooks, may be useful to maintain function (see Chapter 15). Range of motion and strengthening exercises help preserve hand integrity. Improving active finger flexion should be a primary goal for this patient with flexor tenosynovitis. Strengthening the finger extensors is important to counterbalance the chronic flexor pull of a hand with tenosynovitis and contractures. Intrinsic muscle strengthening may ultimately improve the capacity to grasp and manipulate objects. Stretching and strengthening exercises should be initiated once synovitis is resolved to prevent exacerbation of inflammation or tendon rupture.

The foot disorders described necessitate referral to an orthotist for fabrication of proper footwear. A wide, deep, toe box is prescribed to accommodate the hallux valgus, forefoot spread, and hammer and cock-up toes. The flexible, flat arches and painful metatarsal heads may be alleviated through a total-contact, custom-fabricated arch support with relief for the metatarsal heads. If metatarsal pain is severe, a rocker-bottom shoe can be prescribed. Regular treatment from a podiatrist will prevent callus formation and the consequent skin breakdown that occurs commonly in individuals with impaired feet. Finally, intrinsic foot muscle-strengthening (eg, grabbing a tissue off the floor with the toes) and ankle and foot ROM exercises help preserve the function of the feet.

Education about joint protection teaches the patient to perform daily tasks without exerting undue stress on the abnormal joints, to avoid overuse, and to maintain proper posture and joint alignment. Energy-conservation techniques focus on maximizing joint biomechanical function and on performing tasks in the most energy-efficient manner. This would include the use of an adapted typewriter to promote a longer capacity to type. In addition, rest periods and smart task planning will conserve energy and improve the individual's ability to perform throughout the day.

Finally, as described in case presentation 2, aerobic conditioning exercise will limit the physical impairments (generalized deconditioning, fatigue, decreased strength) that accompany RA. Daily exercise should become an integral part of this individual's routine.

Limit Disability

Because his employment requires repetitive use of his hands as he types, this patient is at high risk for developing a work disability. Many investigators have shown the extent of work disability associated with RA. A review of those studies is presented in Chapter 17.

Employers are obliged by the Americans with Disabilities Act to make "reasonable accommodations" to assist persons with disabilities in performing their jobs. Honest, proactive discussions with the employer to develop creative solutions may help prevent future problems related to declining job performance secondary to disease. For this individual, the simple modification of a typing stick can be used if he is no longer able to type on individual keys. Forearm rests may help prevent fatigue. Wrist immobilization may limit repetitive wrist flexion and extension with its consequent exacerbation of pain. As technology advances, voice-activated keyboards should become more prevalent and inexpensive. Vocational rehabilitation specialists can assist in more difficult cases (see Chapter 17).

CASE PRESENTATION 4: SEVERE DEFORMITY EXTRA-ARTICULAR MANIFESTATION

> The patient is a 70-year-old woman with RA who has been on remittive agents, including steroids, for several years. She presents for evaluation of her increasing fatigue (associated with dyspnea), shoulder pain, and generalized weakness. She has had increased difficulty managing her ADLs and homemaking duties during the past year. She has limited and painful AROM and passive ROM of both shoulders, with erythema and effusions. Deltoid atrophy and tenderness are present over the superior lateral shoulders. She has ulnar deviation and swan-neck deformities of the hands, without evidence of active synovitis. Cardiac examination reveals normal findings. There are diffuse crackles throughout both lung fields, without wheezing. Results of the remainder of the examination are unremarkable. A chest radiograph reveals interstitial fibrosis. Shoulder films reveal periarticular osteopenia, marginal erosions, and bony sclerosis with superior migration of the humeral heads bilaterally.

Maximize Disease Management

Of most immediate concern is the patient's history of increasing dyspnea with findings consistent with interstitial lung disease. Cardiac and pulmonary impairments can occur in individuals with RA and frequently manifest as fatigue. Cardiac lesions that occur include rheumatic heart disease, pericarditis, interstitial myocarditis, rheumatoid heart disease, aortic stenosis or insufficiency, hypertension, and myocardial infarction (Hough & Sokoloff, 1989).

Pulmonary manifestations include interstitial lung disease (either primary or as a consequence of medication), granulomatous lesions, pleuritis, and infections. Many patients with RA have vasculitis, and may develop pulmonary arteritis and pulmonary hypertension as a consequence of interstitial fibrosis. Lung impairment puts patients at risk for a variety of secondary complications, including heart disease and infection, anxiety and depression, cognitive problems secondary to hypoxemia (eg, irritability, decreased short-term memory, and poor new learning), malnutrition, muscle wasting, and social isolation. Thus, management of lung impairments is important. Chest radiograph and pulmonary function tests will confirm the diagnosis of interstitial fibrosis. Pulmonary function tests show decreased diffusion lung capacity, reduced lung volumes, and hypoxia worsened by exercise.

The patient's shoulder synovitis and restrictions in shoulder motion and strength must also be addressed. Shoulder impairment from RA may be a consequence of both articular and periarticular destruction (Table 4–1). Commonly, the rheumatoid shoulder displays multiple intermingled diagnoses, which are not easily separable as distinct clinical entities. In an attempt to limit pain, the patient splints the arm in adduction and internal rotation, which results in capsular and ligamentous adhesions. Joint effusions limit both strength and motion, and occasional capsular ruptures can occur. Destruction of cartilage and subchondral bone causes not only pain but weakness as a result of biomechanical disadvantage. Weakness is exacerbated by the muscle atrophy that accompanies disuse and inflammation. Glenohumeral synovitis often coexists with rotator cuff inflammation. Rotator cuff dysfunction (tendinitis, tears) may cause profound limitations and pain that is worse at night. Subdeltoid bursitis is a common companion of glenohumeral arthritis and cuff tendinitis, further exacerbating pain and impairment. The end result is a painful shoulder that cannot flex, abduct, or rotate, such as in this case. The patient complains of difficulty performing functional tasks, such as hair styling, upper body dressing, oral facial hygiene, placing or retrieving items from higher shelves or cabinets, and carrying heavy items.

Aspiration of the fluid from the shoulder joints may help relieve pain. Local injection of corticosteroid can provide relief of pain, when systemic management of inflammation has been maximized. This is particularly true if a subdeltoid bursitis is present, as in this case. Chronic rotator cuff tendinitis can lead to complete rotator cuff tears, and inflammation should be managed aggressively. Surgical repair of the rotator cuff is not warranted in individuals with severe RA because of the frailty of soft tissue structures.

Minimize Physical and Functional Impairments

Medications, rest, exercise, and education are the cornerstones of rehabilitation management. Local rest is appropriate until the shoulder pain and inflammation begin to subside. However, prolonged immobilization is not advisable because of the adhesions and muscle atrophy associated with immobility. The critical shoulder motion necessary for functional activities is 75° of flexion, 75° of abduction, 20° of external rotation, and 45° of internal rotation (Hicks, 1990). Thus, acutely inflamed joints should have ROM exercises performed daily to maintain at least these critical motions. Active ROM exercises should begin after pain and inflammation have been reasonably controlled. These exercises should focus on shoulder flexion, abduction, and rotation. Pendulum exercises (progressive arm circles performed with the patient seated on a table leaning forward with the arm dangling) should be prescribed as a gentle ROM and strengthening activity. When the joint is essentially quiet, strengthening exercises should begin.

Isometric exercise can be progressed to isotonic exercise with low weights (1 to 3 lb) as tolerated by pain, focusing again on the critical shoulder motions. Outpatient occupational therapy prescription is appropriate to attain the goals of increased shoulder strength and motion and improved status, including elimination of the household work disability.

Pulmonary rehabilitation referral is appropriate for this patient with restrictions secondary to lung disease. Pulmonary rehabilitation aims to improve exercise capacity and endurance in order to improve capacity to manage ADLs, reduce respiratory symptoms and recurrent hospitalizations from exacerbation of lung disease, and improve overall quality of life. Patients learn

Table 4–1 Common Shoulder Disorders

Conditions	*Clinical Features*
Glenohumeral joint disorders (including synovitis and degenerative joint disease)	Generalized shoulder pain; crepitation or inflammatory signs, limitation in all motions, particularly rotation; generalized atrophy may be present; radiographs or synovial fluid analysis
Acromioclavicular and sterno-clavicular joint disorder	Shoulder arch painful and limited in mid–late abduction; painful shrugging; tender joint
Cervical radiculopathy	Painless arc of shoulder motion; neck rotation or compression may trigger pain; dermatomal dyesthesia or weakness; electrodiagnostic testing may confirm the diagnosis
Bursitis/supraspinatus tendinitis	Painful arc from 60° to 120° abduction; tender subacromial region; painful resisted abduction; subacromial anesthetic injection may be diagnostic
Bicipital tendinitis	Tenderness at biceps insertion and along tendon sheath; localized pain at biceps insertion with resisted forearm flexion and supination (Yergason's sign); shoulder ROM is normal
Impingement syndrome	"Catch" is reported between 60° and 70° and is maximum at 100° to 120° abduction; recurrent pain from compression of subacrominal tissue occurs at 90° to 100° of forward flexion; abnormalities may be present on radiograph
Rotator cuff tear or rupture	Following trauma, abrupt pain, and weak active abduction; "drop-arm" sign; tears present as gradual increase in pain and weakness of active abduction in older person; shoulder ROM is normal; radiographs may reveal a superior-lying humeral head; ultrasound and magnetic resonance imaging are diagnostic, but arthrography is the gold standard, with the diagnostic extrusion contrast into the subacrominal space
Adhesive capsulitis	Gradual onset of diffusely painful shoulder; restriction in all planes of active and passive motion

to self-assess shortness of breath, nutrition, proper use of inhalers, energy-conservation techniques, and coping skills. Breathing retraining exercises taught include pursed-lip and diaphragmatic breathing techniques and inspiratory muscle training and pacing. Exercise training begins with a baseline stress test (electrocardiogram and oximetry) with subsequent incremental increases in workload. All exercise is monitored with oximetry, and target heart rates are prescribed from the baseline stress test. Bronchial hygiene is taught. The dietitian, physical or occupational therapist, psychologist, and social worker may be brought in to consult about the patient's care when appropriate.

Limit Disability

Household work disability adds to the burdens of individuals with RA. Allaire, Partridge, Andrew, and Liang (1993) reported that women with RA, particularly severe RA, performed a smaller proportion of the household work (except taking care of others) and that husbands and other family members spent more time doing work that at one point was the wife/mother's responsibility. These women with RA noted that their standards for cooking and cleaning lowered as their disability progressed. Ten percent of the women surveyed reported family discord related to their household work disability. Significantly more women with severe RA were separated or divorced compared with those with mild RA. Thus, household work disability is an important clinical issue to address in homemakers with RA.

Occupational therapy may be effective in improving the patient's capacity to perform necessary household chores. Occupational therapists not only work on improving upper extremity ROM and strength but teach adaptive techniques, incorporating joint protection and energy conservation and equipment for basic and instrumental ADLs. Six weeks of home occupational therapy was reported to improve functional capacity in subjects with RA (Helewa et al., 1991). The prescription should instruct the therapist to focus on higher level (or instrumental) ADLs, using adaptive equipment as necessary, and incorporating energy conservation and joint protection techniques.

CASE PRESENTATION 5: NO INFLAMMATION, SEVERE DEFORMITIES

The patient is a 58-year-old woman with long-standing severe RA. She has shoulder, elbow, knee, and hip contractures; substantial hand deformities; weakness and spasticity of the upper and lower extremities; urinary and fecal incontinence; and grade I sacral decubitus. There is no active synovitis. Radiographs reveal significant atlantoaxial subluxation and end-stage joint disease, with bone-on-bone changes at all the joints surveyed. She has a mild anemia, but otherwise laboratory findings are normal. Shc is taking acetaminophen for pain. She is cognitively intact, but her interaction with others is limited and her affect is blunted. She lives with her retired husband and her daughter, who is employed full-time. Her family feeds, bathes, and dresses her. She wears diapers. The patient uses a standard wheelchair, which she cannot propel. Her positioning in the chair is poor.

Maximize Disease Management

The first step in this rehabilitation prescription is evaluating disease activity. In this case there is no evidence of active synovitis. The quadriparesis, spasticity, and weakness are a consequence of the atlantoaxial subluxation and cord compression. Treatment in the earlier stages of cervical spine disease consists of a cervical collar for relief of pain and protection against sudden trauma. The timing of surgical stabilization is controversial. It is generally recommended for patients with intractable pain and progressive deterioration in neurological function. Some research suggests that about 10% of patients with radiographic evidence of disease may deteriorate and require surgery (Pellici, Ranawat, Tsairis, & Bryan, 1981). Return of neurological function after surgery cannot be guaranteed. Most patients are counseled that the purpose of surgery is to prevent further deterioration and that reversal of neurological abnormalities is not guaranteed. Considering that this patient has limited use of her extremities secondary to the severe joint disease, cervical decompression and fusion probably are not warranted.

Total joint arthroplasty should be considered when individuals have end-stage joint disease. Hip and knee replacements can be staged over a period of several weeks, and the patient can be rehabilitated in a comprehensive inpatient rehabilitation unit between and after surgeries. Because this patient has severe myelopathy and her pain is controlled with acetaminophen, how-

Table 4–2 Common Neurological Disorders, Bladder Dysfunction, and Potential Interventions

Neurological Disorder	*Usual Type of Bladder Dysfunction*	*Interventions*
Suprapontine lesions (eg, brain neoplasms)	Uninhibited bladder	Toileting at regular intervals
Lesions below the pons (eg, spinal cord injuries, myelopathy secondary to arthritis)	Small-capacity, spastic bladder; ± detrusor sphincter dyssynergia	Anticholinergic agents; regular toileting; α-blockers to reduce sphincter tone; intermittent catheterization
Conus lesions (eg, herniated intervertebral disk)	Reflexic bladder	Cholinergic agents; intermittent catheterization; Credé/Yalsalva maneuver; adrenergic agents to improve continence

ever, aggressive arthroplastic surgery is not indicated. Since there is no evidence of active synovitis, corticosteroids or remittive agents would be ineffective.

Minimize Physical and Functional Impairments

The neurogenic bowel and bladder are a consequence of the cervical myelopathy. The etiology of this patient's incontinence is most likely a disinhibited, small-capacity, spastic bladder (Table 4–2). Detrusor sphincter dyssynergia, causing urinary outlet obstruction, is not uncommon in individuals with spasticity. Longstanding urinary outlet obstruction can transform a small-capacity, spastic bladder into a hypotonic areflexic bladder, which may be associated with hydronephrosis. Thus a careful bladder evaluation is necessary. The amount of residual urine after a void revealed through use of a postvoid residual will ascertain whether or not the bladder is emptying completely. A cystometrogram (CMG) with a periurethral electromyogram (EMG) is necessary to determine the capacity of the detrusor muscle and the degree of dyssynergia. Because this patient is incontinent and has a myelopathy with spasticity, it is appropriate to obtain a CMG with EMG of the external sphincter. If the patient has a small-capacity, spastic bladder, anticholinergic medications (such as oxybutynin hydrochloride) may reduce bladder contractility and lead to continence.

Alternatively, cholinergic drugs (such as bethanechol chloride) increase detrusor contractions and may facilitate voiding in patients with hypotonic bladders. Antiadrenergic sympatholytic agents reduce bladder outlet pressures and are prescribed for patients with dyssynergia. Yearly evaluations of kidney function are necessary to prevent the secondary complications (hydronephrosis, chronic pyelonephritis, renal insufficiency) of neurogenic bladder. Measurements of electrolytes, blood urea nitrogen, and creatinine (kidney function tests) should be obtained yearly, and urinalyses should be performed when appropriate. Patients with chronic urinary retention will develop bacterial colonization of urine and should be treated with antibiotics *only* when actual infections develop (fever, chills, dysuria) to prevent colonization/superinfection with drug-resistant organisms.

Evacuation of the bowels is a reflex function, under voluntary central nervous system control. The patient's fecal incontinence is also a consequence of the cervical spinal cord pathology and can be regulated with bowel retraining. A specific time of day should be established for defecation, and the patient should be given a suppository (eg, bisacodyl) to stimulate reflex peristalsis. Preferably, this is done with the patient sitting on the commode. The patient's diet should be high in fiber, and stool softeners may be necessary. With this type of bowel program individuals with neurogenic bowels can reduce or eliminate incontinent episodes.

This patient exhibits features consistent with criteria of the fourth edition of *Diagnostic & Statistical Manual* (DSM-IV) for major depression, including anhedonia, fatigue, depressed mood, insomnia, and recurrent thoughts of death (without a specific plan). Severe depression is not uncommon in RA.

Depression as a side effect of drugs or coexistent medical comorbidity (eg, hypothyroidism) must be ruled out. There is a complex relationship between chronic pain and depression, and the presence of depression is associated with higher reported pain in RA patients. The treatment of clinical depression may be overlooked in patients with RA—particularly in substantially disabled patients such as this woman—for a host of reasons, including the overwhelming complexity of needs, the inexperience of physicians in treating depression, and a physician's pessimistic view of the outcome of treatment. The complexity of depression in this disabled patient with RA necessitates a multidimensional approach to treatment. For success, consideration must be given to ensuring adequate pain relief, improving functional impairments to increase feelings of self-worth, providing psychotherapy or counseling, using antidepressant medication, and providing therapeutic recreational and/or vocational rehabilitation services. A more comprehensive discussion of the psychological impairments in RA is presented in Chapter 11.

Limit Disability

The appropriate wheelchair prescription is critical for attaining optimal independence and minimizing secondary disability (such as pressure sores or contractures). A cognitively intact individual who cannot physically propel a manual wheelchair may need an externally powered chair if the individual's home is accessible. Those who use powered chairs also require special supportive lumbar cushions, thoracic pads, and limb supports to ensure proper positioning in the chair. Hand-operated controls, such as a joystick, can also be adapted to environmental control units if these are useful.

Alternatively, if the patient is not a candidate for a powered chair because the home is not accessible or the patient requires constant assistance or is not interested, a manual wheelchair is prescribed. Removable armrests will make transfers easier and should be specified in the prescription. The standard sling-back seat is not appropriate for a patient with profound weakness and spasticity because proper seated posture will not be maintained. A solid seat and back and lumbar support cushions assist in the maintenance of correct posture. Chair tires are prescribed according to the type of surface most often wheeled over. Solid, smooth tires are most commonly prescribed because they perform better on hard, indoor surfaces. If regular outdoor use is anticipated (eg, for individuals who are active in the community), treaded, pneumatic tires are more durable. A seat cushion is prescribed to prevent decubitus ulcers and maintain seated alignment. Cushions may be made of foam or air or may be custom fabricated. In this situation, physical therapy referral for wheelchair prescription is appropriate.

Adaptive equipment may be useful. A bedside commode is helpful for patients who must use the toilet in the middle of the night and cannot safely walk to the bathroom and for those whose bathrooms are inaccessible to wheelchairs or walkers. A bath bench with grab bars or shower seat will facilitate safe bathing. If the patient has some functional use of the upper extremities, adaptive equipment for the hands (eg, built-up utensils) may be useful. An occupational therapy referral is necessary for evaluation and ordering of appropriate equipment.

Finally, the patient should be referred to social services for evaluation and assistance in attaining necessary home resources, including attendant and/or respite care. The introduction of a department of rehabilitation services attendant to assist with care for this patient may unburden the family and help the patient attain some self-sufficiency. A thorough review of the social services available to patients is provided in Chapter 18.

CONCLUSION

Given the widespread effects of disability on individuals and societies, we must attempt to prevent and limit it. Traditionally the health of a population has always been measured in terms of mortality. We must begin to view our successes in public health in terms of quality of life. The National Council on Disability was created in 1978 by the US Congress and is responsible for coordinating a national strategy for disability prevention. In 1986 the organization published a landmark document entitled "Toward Independence" which set the stage for a national effort to prevent disability. With a congressional mandate, the Centers for Disease Control and Prevention and the Institute of Medicine published *Disability in America: A National Agenda for Prevention* as a foundation and strategy for disability prevention (Institute of Medicine, 1991). Recommendations address research, access to services, availability of services, professional education and training, family and public education, and coordination of services and advocacy. This publication is recommended reading for health care providers.

It is the fundamental premise of rehabilitation that intervention at various stages of the disability process can minimize or eradicate disability. If the framework of the Institute of Medicine is followed, as highlighted by the case presentations in this chapter, interventions to limit disability should be timed at all levels, from attempting to alter risk factors (research into the genetic basis of arthritis), to modifying the disease process (remittive agent prescription), to improving impairments (therapy to increase ROM), to minimizing functional limitations (adaptive dressing aids), to limiting societal disadvantages (lobby for uniform access).

REFERENCES

Allaire, S.H., Partridge, A.J., Andrew, H.F., & Liang, M.H. (1993). Management of work disability. *Arthritis and Rheumatism*, *36*, 1663–1670.

Basmaijian, J. (1987). Therapeutic exercise in the management of rheumatic diseases. *Journal of Rheumatology*, *14* (Suppl. 15), 78.

Danneskiold-Samsoe, B., Lyngberg, K., Risum, T., & Telling, M. (1987). The effect of water exercise therapy given to patients with rheumatoid arthritis. *Scandinavian Journal of Rehabilitation Medicine*, *19*, 31.

Ekblom, B., Lovgren, O., & Alderin, M. (1975). Effect of short term physical training in persons with rheumatoid arthritis. *Scandinavian Journal of Rheumatology*, *4*, 80.

Ekblom, B., Lovgren, O., Alderin, M., Fridstrom, M., & Satterstrom, G. (1974). Physical performance in patients with RA. *Scandinavian Journal of Rheumatology*, *3*, 121–125.

Falconer, J., Hayes, K.W., & Chang, R.W. (1992). Effect of ultrasound on mobility in osteoarthritis of the knee. *Arthritis Care and Research*, *5*, 29–35.

Fisher, N.M., Gresham, G.E., Abrams, M., Hicks, J., Horrigan, D., & Pendergast, D.R. (1993). Quantitative effects of physical therapy on muscular and functional performance in subjects with osteoarthritis of the knees. *Archives of Physical Medicine and Rehabilitation*, *74*, 840–847.

Helewa, A., Goldsmith, C.H., Lee, P., Bombardier, C., Hanes, B., Smythe, H.A., & Tugwell, P. (1991). Effects of occupational therapy home services on patients with rheumatoid arthritis. *Lancet*, *337*, 1453–1456.

Hicks, J.E. (1990). Exercise in the patient with inflammatory arthritis and connective tissue disease. *Rheumatic Disease Clinics of North America*, *16* (4), 845–869.

Hollander, J.R., & Horvath, S.M. (1949). The influence of physical therapy procedures on the intra-articular temperature of normal arthritis subjects. *American Journal of the Medical Sciences*, *218*, 543–548.

Hough, A.J., & Sokoloff, L. (1989). Pathology of rheumatoid arthritis and allied disorders. In D.V. McCarty (Ed.), *Arthritis and allied conditions* (11th ed., pp. 674–714). Philadelphia: Lea & Febiger.

Institute of Medicine. (1991). *Disability in America: A national agenda for prevention*, A.M. Pope & A.R. Tarlov (Eds.). Washington, DC: National Academy of Sciences.

Kirk, J.A., & Kersley, G.D. (1968). Heat and cold in the physical treatment of rheumatoid arthritis of the knee: A controlled clinical trial. *American Journal of Physical Medicine and Rehabilitation*, *9*, 270–274.

Minor, M.A., Hewitt, J.E., Webel, R.R., Anderson, S.K., & Kay, D.R. (1989). Efficacy of physical conditioning exercises in patients with rheumatoid arthritis and osteoarthritis. *Arthritis and Rheumatism*, *32*, 1396–1405.

Minor, M.A., Hewett, J.E., Webel, R.R., Dreisinger, T.E., & Kay, D.R. (1988). Exercise tolerance and disease related measures in patients with rheumatoid and osteoarthritis. *Journal of Rheumatology*, *15*, 905–911.

Pellici, P.M., Ranawat, C.S., Tsairis, P., & Bryan, W.J. (1981). A prospective study of the progression of rheumatoid arthritis of the cervical spine. *Journal of Bone and Joint Surgery [Br]*, *63*, 342–350.

Perlman, S.G., Connell, K.J., Clark, A., Robinson, M.S., Conlon, P., Gecht, M., Caldron, P., Sinacore, J.M. (1990). Dance-based aerobic exercise for rheumatoid arthritis. *Arthritis Care and Research*, *3*, 29–35.

Weinberger, A., Abramonrici, A., Fadila, R., Levy, A., Giler, S., & Lev, A. (1990). The effect of local deep microwave hyperthermia on experimental zymosan-induced arthritis in rabbits. *American Journal of Physical Medicine*, *89*, 239–444.

Weinberger, A., Fadilah, R., Lev, A., & Pinkhas, J. (1989). Intra-articular temperature measurements after superficial health. *Scandinavian Journal of Rheumatology*, *32*, 55–57.

SUGGESTED READING

Perkash, I. (1990). Management of neurogenic dysfunction of the bladder and bowel. In F.K. Kattke & J.F. Lehmann (Eds.), Krusen's handbook of physical medicine and rehabilitation (pp. 820–821). Philadelphia: Saunders.

Weinberger, A., Fadilah, R., Lev, A., Levy, A., & Pinkhas, J. (1988). Deep heat in the treatment of inflammatory joint disease. *Medical Hypothesis*, *25*, 231–233.

Yelin, E., Henke, C., & Epstein, W. (1987). The work dynamics of the person with rheumatoid arthritis. *Arthritis and Rheumatism*, *30*, 502–512.

CHAPTER 5

Role of Electrodiagnostic Testing in Rheumatoid Arthritis

Richard T. Katz, MD, and Christina Marciniak, MD

Neuromuscular disorders affecting the patient with rheumatoid arthritis can be produced by an abnormality anywhere in the motor unit complex, from the spinal cord to the muscle cell (Exhibit 5–1). This chapter is meant to be a detailed review of these disorders. In addition, we have included sufficient background on electrodiagnostic methods so that the clinician treating the patient with rheumatoid arthritis will have a reasonable understanding of the techniques used in making these diagnoses as well as some of the limitations. If more information on electrodiagnosis itself is desired, several excellent reviews and texts can be consulted (Aminoff, 1986a, 1986b, 1987; Brown & Bolton, 1993; Kimura, 1989; Oh, 1993).

Three components of electrodiagnosis are useful in the evaluation of the peripheral nervous system and spinal cord: (1) electromyography, (2) electroneurography (nerve conduction studies), and (3) somatosensory-evoked potentials. An overview of each electrodiagnostic method is presented and relevant pathological entities are discussed in greater depth.

Exhibit 5–1 Neuromuscular Disorders in the Patient with Rheumatoid Arthritis

- Peripheral neuropathy
  - Predominantly sensory, stocking-glove distribution
  - Sensorimotor, lower greater than upper extremity weakness
  - Autonomic neuropathy
  - Secondary to gold therapy
  - Secondary to penicillamine therapy
  - Secondary to chloroquine
- Mononeuritis multiplex
- Focal neuropathy
  - Median (carpal tunnel)
  - Posterior interosseous nerve (elbow)
  - Ulnar nerve (elbow, wrist)
  - Tibial (popliteal, tarsal tunnel)
  - Peroneal (popliteal)
- Myopathy
  - Myositis due to vasculitis
  - Steroid myopathy
  - Myopathy secondary to penicillamine therapy
  - Myopathy secondary to chloroquine
- Neuromuscular junction disorders
  - Penicillamine-induced myasthenia gravis
- Cervical myelopathy

ELECTROMYOGRAPHY

The electromyographic examination involves the introduction of a special recording needle into a muscle belly (Aminoff, 1986a, 1987; Daube, 1991; Ma, Pease, MacLean, Cassvan, & Johnson, 1987). Two types of needles are used by nearly all electromyographers: monopolar, composed of a steel wire insulated with Teflon, and concentric, a hollow needle through which runs a fine wire. Monopolar needles may be preferred because they cause less discomfort to the patient, but they require a surface reference electrode. Concentric needles have a more uniform exposed surface and thus may be more useful for quantification and comparison of motor unit potentials.

Electrical potentials located within a few millimeters of the needle radius are picked up by the electrode and then transmitted from the muscle to a preamplifier placed near the patient. These signals are further amplified and filtered, and displayed visually for examination by the electromyographer. The potentials are also transmitted over a loudspeaker, as auditory monitoring is a valuable adjunct to the visual inspection of the waveforms. The electromyographic examination consists of the analysis of waveforms of various muscles during relaxation, mild contraction, and vigorous contraction. The choice of muscles for study is dictated by the clinical problem and the history and physical examination.

Normally, when a needle is inserted into resting muscle, a brief spurt of electrical potentials (insertional activity) is produced, followed by silence. The electromyographer then moves the needle in several directions in search of spontancous activity, that is, electrical potentials that occur while the muscle is at rest. Although spontaneous activity may occur normally when the needle is in the vicinity of the neuromuscular junction, in other locations spontaneous activity generally is a pathological finding. Three particular types of spontaneous activity are of the greatest relevance to this discussion: positive sharp waves, fibrillation potentials, and fasciculations.

Positive sharp waves and fibrillations are small discharges that are the result of spontaneous depolarization of single muscle fiber membranes. Most often these potentials signify denervation. They are not synonymous with axonal loss, however, since they may be seen in a variety of disorders, including certain myopathies, periodic paralysis, botulism, and severe upper motor neuron injury. Fasciculations are the involuntary twitchings of a bundle of muscle fibers that are often obvious to the observer on visual inspection. Fasciculation potentials are noted to be irregular firing of a motor unit on the electromyographic (EMG) screen. They may or may not be a pathological finding, depending on the clinical and electromyographic scenario.

When the patient is asked to perform a mild muscle contraction, the electromyographer is able to analyze potentials from various motor units within the muscle. The motor unit—the anterior horn cell, nerve axons, and muscle fibers that they innervate—is the "final pathway" of motoric activity within the nervous system. Normally, motor units fire in characteristic recruitment patterns. Small motor neurons supplying fatigue-resistant (slow) muscle fibers are recruited first, and larger neurons supplying fatiguable high-tension (fast) muscle fibers are recruited later. The electromyographer can thereby study not only the characteristics (shape, amplitude, duration) of the first few recruited motor units but also their firing rate and pattern. Finally, the patient is asked to perform a vigorous contraction of the muscle. The screen normally is filled with motor unit potentials, also known as the interference pattern.

When studying the motor unit potentials during the electromyographic examination, several important characteristics are evaluated in distinguishing whether a neuropathic or myopathic process is present. Normally motor units range in size from 300 to 5000 μV and vary greatly (1 to 16 milliseconds) in duration. Motor units generally have two to four phases, whereas polyphasic motor unit potentials (greater than four phases) are noted no more than 15% of the time.

When a lower motor neuron insult has occurred, the inspection of the motor units may show waveforms of increased amplitude, phases, and duration. These changes are secondary to reinnervation of denervated muscle fibers by surviving neighboring axons. Also, as motor units are lost to the pathological process, those remaining need to compensate by firing faster than normal. On full recruitment, a dropout of motor units is seen on the oscilloscope interference pattern while low-pitched motor units are heard over the loudspeaker.

The most characteristic finding in a myopathic process is that of motor units of smaller amplitude and of shorter duration because loss of muscle fibers results in a smaller electrical potential. These motor units may also be polyphasic. As weakened muscles produce less desired force, more motor units must be recruited earlier to produce even a mild contraction. The interference pattern may be full until late in the disease, and characteristically high-pitched motor units are noted over the loudspeaker (Buchtal, 1985). In chronic inflammatory myopathies, long-duration polyphasic potentials may be seen. Satellic potentials, small motor unit action potentials firing at a time-locked interval from the main potential, are also seen in this setting (Uncini, Lange, Lovelace, Solomon, & Hays, 1990). The above findings may be spotty in location, with some areas of muscle normal while others show severe motor unit changes. Proximal muscles show the most marked changes, particularly paraspinals (Kimura, 1989).

ELECTRONEUROGRAPHY (NERVE CONDUCTION STUDIES)

Electromyography can help assess the status of nerve fibers indirectly, but the integrity of large myelinated sensory and motor neurons can be evaluated directly by nerve conduction studies (NCS), also known as electroneurography (Daube, 1986; MacLean, Pease, Ma, Cassvan, & Johnson, 1987; Oh, 1993). Nerve conduction studies involve the introduction of an electrical stimulus either by surface electrode or needle, and recording an evoked response, again using either a surface disc electrode or a needle electrode inserted through the skin. Nerve conduction studies can assess motor neurons, sensory neurons, or mixed nerve trunks depending on the strategy employed. Motor conduction studies are performed by applying an electrical shock via the stimulating electrode to a mixed nerve trunk, for example, the median nerve at the wrist (Figure 5–1). The nerve is usually stimulated at a fixed distance, often 8 or 10 cm, proximal to the recording electrodes. Recording electrodes, usually of the disc type, are taped to the skin over a muscle belly innervated by that mixed nerve, in this example the thenar eminence. Upon increasing the stimulus intensity just beyond the point at which the evoked muscle response (compound muscle action potential [CMAP]) is maximal, several useful parameters can be measured. The distal latency is a measure of the time from the onset of the stimulus until it reaches the muscle belly. Similarly, the amplitude of the CMAP is recorded, and sometimes its duration and shape. The nerve is then stimulated at a more proximal site and identical measurements are made. By using the value obtained by stimulating the nerve at two separate sites, measuring the distance between stimulating sites, and subtracting the difference in latencies, the motor conduction velocity can be calculated (see Figure 5–1). Although each electrodiagnostic laboratory may develop its own normal values for nerve conduction velocity and amplitude and duration of the CMAP, standardized values are readily obtained in the medical literature. An easy rule of thumb is that upper and lower extremity motor fibers generally conduct at or greater than 50 m/s and 40 m/s, respectively. Because of their anatomic availability, the most commonly performed motor conduction studies include median, ulnar, radial, tibial, and peroneal. Studies of the facial nerve are occasionally useful when cranial nerve function is to be assessed.

Sensory never fibers can be studied orthodromically or antidromically. Orthodromic and antidromic conductions imply that the electrical stimulus introduced by the examiner is traveling in the same direction (ortho-) or opposite direction (anti-) as the naturally occurring conduction of that nerve fiber. Stimulating purely sensory fibers and recording proximally over the mixed nerve trunk is orthodromic conduction, for example, placing ring electrodes around the index finger to stimulate the median digital nerves and recording with surface electrodes proximally. Antidromic conduction can be achieved by stimulating the mixed nerve at the wrist and recording from purely sensory fibers distally; using the median nerve as an example again, by stimulating at the wrist and recording from the index finger (Figure 5–2). Fourteen centimeters is a commonly used distance for distal sensory latencies; however, 10- and 12-cm distances are often used as well. Sensory nerve conduction velocity can be studied in a manner analogous to motor conduction velocity. Sensory fibers can be stimulated directly (eg, at the index finger), and the nerve evoked response can be measured at the wrist and elbow. The distance between recording sites divided by the difference between the latencies is the sensory conduction velocity. Nerves most routinely used for sensory conduction studies include median, ulnar, radial, sural, and peroneal.

Late responses (Cassvan, Pease, MacLean, Ma, & Johnson, 1987a; Fischer, 1992) are the third type of nerve conduction study frequently used. Late responses include F waves and the H reflex. The F wave is a small potential occurring after the CMAP during most motor conduction studies. Upon stimulating the mixed nerve trunk, the electrical volley travels not only distally toward the muscle belly but also antidromically toward the spinal cord. The F wave is believed to originate from electrical volleys that bounce back from the ante-

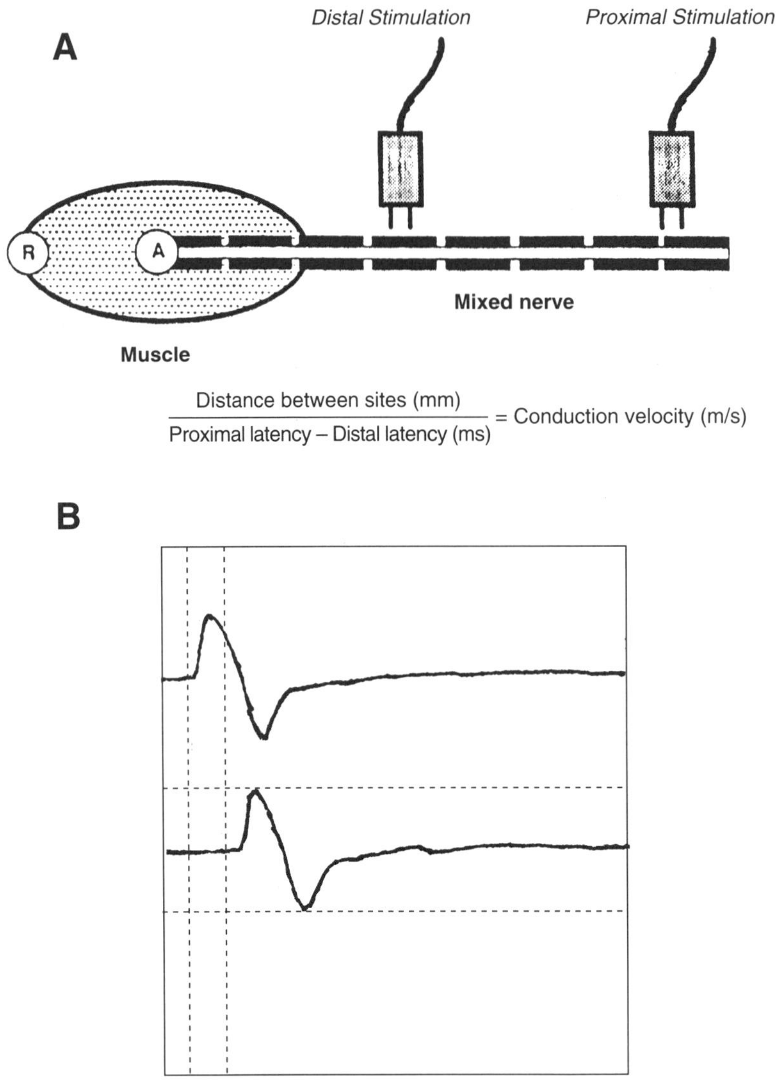

Figure 5–1 Motor conduction study. **A**, The mixed nerve is stimulated at a proximal site and a distal site. The distal site is often stimulated 8 cm from the active (*A*) electrode. The reference electrode (*R*) is placed more distally over the muscle tendon. **B**, The top tracing was obtained upon stimulation of the median nerve at the wrist and recording over the thenar eminence. Latency between stimulation and the onset of the compound muscle action potential is 3.12 milliseconds. The bottom tracing was obtained upon stimulation of the median nerve at the elbow and recording over the thenar eminence. Latency is 7.07 milliseconds. Both responses are approximately 38,000 μV. The motor nerve conduction velocity from the proximal to the distal site can be obtained according to the formula in this figure. The distance between sites is 245 mm, and the difference in the latencies is 3.95 milliseconds, resulting in a velocity of 62 m/s. *Source*: Reprinted with permission from *Orthopedics*, Vol. 12, No. 8, pp. 1098–1099, © 1989, Slack, Inc.

rior horn cell and then travel back down the nerve, orthodromically, to the muscle belly. Because the F wave has a substantially longer path than the orthodromically traveling motor latency, it occurs later and hence its descriptor as a "late" response.

The H reflex has a latency similar to that of the F wave, but it traverses different pathways. Upon stimulating the tibial nerve at the popliteal fossa (as this is the only site where the H reflex is readily elicited in normal subjects), the electrical volley travels ortho-

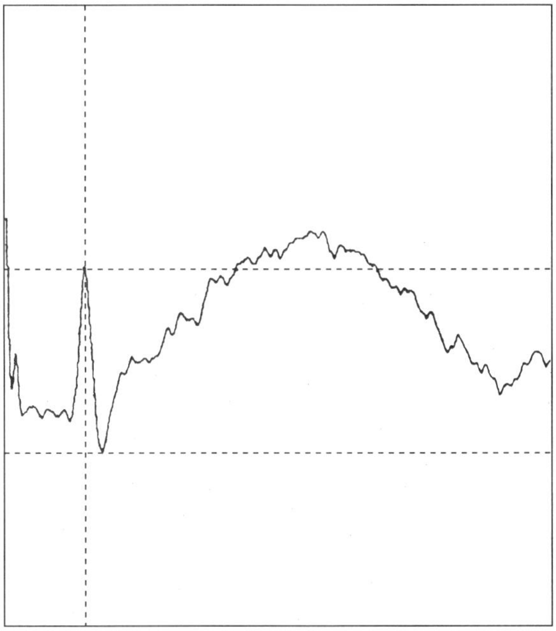

Figure 5–2 Sensory nerve action potential. The median nerve was stimulated 14 cm proximal to the metacarpal-phalangeal joint of the index finger. The latency to the peak of the sensory nerve action potential is 3.02 milliseconds with an amplitude of 40 μV. *Source*: Reprinted with permission from *Orthopedics*, Vol. 12, No. 8, pp. 1098–1099, © 1989, Slack, Inc.

dromically along Ia sensory afferent fibers, makes a primarily monosynaptic connection within the spinal cord, and continues orthodromically down motor fibers toward the muscle belly. Thus, the H reflex is similar to a muscle stretch reflex, except that it bypasses the mechanically induced stretch of the muscle belly. The H reflex can be reliably distinguished from the F wave by its shape and the stimulus intensity used. The H reflex is obtained with a submaximal stimulus (insufficient to generate a CMAP of maximal amplitude), whereas the F wave is elicited best by one that is supramaximal.

The F wave can be an extremely valuable adjunct to more distal nerve conduction studies because it can be used to evaluate the more proximal portions of the nerves. These sites are not as easily studied by usual nerve conductions because they require quite uncomfortable stimulus intensities to reach the nerves positioned more deeply within the limb. In patients with early stages of peripheral neuropathy, F waves may show abnormalities when conventional motor and sensory studies are unremarkable (Lachman, Shahani, & Young, 1980). H reflexes routinely are studied primarily for the evaluation of S-1 radiculopathy, but they may also be abnormal in polyneuropathies and plexopathies (Ackil, Shahani, Young, & Rubin, 1981; D'Amour, Shahani, Young, & Bird, 1979).

Autonomic pathways may be studied by a variety of methods to identify the presence and site of dysfunction (Ravits, 1990). In the electrodiagnostic laboratory, skin sympathetic nerve activity following an electrical stimulus can be easily measured (Shahani, Halperin, Bouly, & Cohen, 1984). Sympathetic skin potentials reflect changes in skin resistance to electrical conduction that are regulated by presecretory activity in the sweat glands. Abnormalities are an indication of disruption of unmyelinated axons. Most commonly, potentials are recorded from the palm of the hand and the plantar surface of the foot (Ravits, 1990).

Neuromuscular Junction Studies

Two techniques are especially useful for assessing disorders of the neuromuscular junction: repetitive stimulation, and single fiber electromyography (Jablecki, 1985). Repetitive stimulation studies are begun in the manner of a nerve conduction study (described above) with the exception that the nerve is not stimulated once, but rather many times. The examiner stimulates the mixed nerve and records the compound muscle action potential from a muscle innervated by that nerve. Before repetitive stimulation is attempted, the stimulation intensity is increased until a maximum CMAP is achieved. At that point the nerve is stimulated at a rate of two to three times per second until a total of 10 compound muscle action potentials are recorded. These potentials are then analyzed to determine whether a decrement in the amplitude of the CMAP has occurred. A loss in amplitude of greater than 8% to 10% is suggestive of a postsynaptic neuromuscular junction disorder, such as myasthenia gravis. Presynaptic junction disorders may be diagnosed by stimulating the nerve at very high frequencies, for example 40 Hz, and noting a dramatic increase in the size of the CMAP. Such an incremental response is seen in Eaton-Lambert syndrome.

Single-fiber electromyography (SFEMG) is an even more sensitive (but less specific) method of diagnosing disorders of the neuromuscular junction. The SFEMG method involves the use of a special needle to pick up electrical potentials from a very small area of muscle tissue, generally only one or two muscle fibers. With this method one is able to assess single or paired potentials generated from one or two muscle fibers, rather than three to five muscle fibers recorded when using a conventional EMG needle. When two single-fiber potentials are recorded at the same site, the first potential is used to activate a type of trigger, which activates the sweep on the oscilloscope screen. Measuring the time from the activation of the recording until the beginning of the second potential gives the interpotential interval. Two single-muscle fibers of the same motor unit do not necessarily fire at the same time, but rather with a small disparity. The interpotential interval between two single-fiber potentials normally is quite stable, varying only slightly on the order of 35 microseconds. The variability of the interpotential interval, known as jitter, is due to fluctuating conduction timc through terminal axons, the myoneural junction, and muscle fiber membranes. Jitter is characteristically increased in neuromuscular junction disorders as well as in some neuropathies and myopathies. The discovery of abnormally increased jitter is the most sensitive method of electrodiagnostically demonstrating a neuromuscular junction disorder, including myasthenia gravis and myasthenic syndrome (Kramer, Ruth, Johns, & Sanders, 1981; Stalberg, 1980).

SOMATOSENSORY-EVOKED POTENTIALS

Somatosensory-evoked potentials (SSEP) are occasionally useful as an adjunct to EMG and NCS in the diagnosis of neuromuscular difficulties in patients with musculoskeletal disease (Cassvan, Pease, MacLean, Ma, & Johnson, 1987b; Eisen & Aminoff, 1986). Somatosensory-evoked potentials are most commonly obtained by stimulating a peripheral mixed nerve at a frequency of approximately 2 to 5 Hz. The afferent volleys travel primarily via Ia afferents to the spinal cord and ascend the dorsal columns to synapse in the nucleus cuneatus and nucleus gracilis. The volley crosses to the contralateral side as it traverses the medial lemniscus to the thalamus, and then finally ascends to the somatosensory cortex.

With stimulation using either a surface cup or subcutaneous electroencephalographic needle electrodes, a tiny evoked response is recorded over the parietal cortex contralateral to the site of stimulation. Evoked responses can also be measured from the brachial plexus and cervicomedullary junction upon upper extremity nerve trunk stimulation as well as the lumbosacral plexus upon lower extremity stimulation. These tiny potentials can be examined only with the use of an electronic averaging system, where the time-locked evoked response emerges from background electrical noise. Somatosensory-evoked potentials are most often elicited upon stimulating the median, ulnar, tibial, and peroneal nerves.

POLYNEUROPATHY AND MONONEURITIS MULTIPLEX IN RHEUMATOID ARTHRITIS

Polyneuropathies are generalized neuropathic processes of the lower motor neuron. Electrodiagnostic studies are extremely useful in determining whether a peripheral neuropathy is present, whether the neuropathy affects predominantly motor and/or sensory fibers, and whether the pathological process is demyelinating and/or axonopathic. The development of nerve conduction studies and their application to peripheral neuropathy has been reviewed (Gilliatt, 1982).

Axonal neuropathies may display little slowing on conduction studies, but more characteristically, the CMAP may be slightly diminished in amplitude. Needle examination at rest often shows spontaneous activity in distal muscles (suggestive of denervation), and a decrease in recruited motor units is seen upon voluntary muscle contraction. These motor units may be increased in size if significant reinnervation has occurred. Demyelinating neuropathies characteristically show little denervation, but often display significant slowing of the motor and sensory nerve latency and velocity.

Mononeuritis multiplex may manifest as weakness and/or sensory loss in the distribution of various peripheral nerves rather than the symmetrical, stocking-glove distribution often accompanying peripheral neuropathy. Mononeuritis multiplex results from infarction of the nerve axon vessels that occurs when vaso nervosum are occluded due to a vasculitic process (Parry, 1985).

Peripheral nerve involvement is a common problem in the patient with rheumatological disease. (Trojaborg, 1981). Various distinct syndromes of peripheral neuropathy have been noted in patients with rheumatoid arthritis (Chamberlain & Bruckner, 1970; Edmonds, Jones, Saunders, & Sturrock, 1979; Good, Christopher, Koepke, Bender, & Tarter, 1965; Krane & Simon, 1986; Lang, Kalliomaki, Puusa, & Halonen, 1981; Massey, 1983; McCombe, Kiester, Tannenberg, Chalk, & Pender, 1991; Moritz, 1984; Pallis & Scott, 1965; Peterson, 1955; Valsrub, 1980). Chamberlain and Bruckner (1970) described two forms of peripheral nerve involvement in rheumatoid arthritis. The first group had relatively benign rheumatoid arthritis with a patchy, stocking-glove, predominantly sensory peripheral neuropathy. Electrodiagnostic studies in these patients showed marked slowing of motor conduction accompanied by a diminution or loss of sensory nerve action potentials. The second group of patients had more malignant rheumatoid arthritis and demonstrated lower greater than upper extremity motor weakness. This group displayed severe denervation on needle examination. Pallis and Scott (1965) described similar patterns of peripheral neuropathy, but did not utilize electrodiagnostic studies. McCombe et al. (1991) reported two cases of a severe motor and sensory neuropathy that developed relatively early following the onset of rheumatoid arthritis. The axonal neuropathy that was seen in association with cutaneous vasculitis responded well to immunosuppressive treatment. A case of demyelinating sensorimotor neuropathy with a course typical for chronic inflammatory polyradiculoneuropathy was also reported in association with rheumatoid arthritis (Tan, Sabre, Beyazova, Sepici, & Tan, 1993). Autonomic nervous system involvement (Edmonds et al., 1979; Valsrub, 1980) has been described. McCombe et al. (1991) found that the sympathetic skin response and heart rate variability (R to R interval) with respiration, a measure of vagal parasympathetic activity, were frequently abnormal in patients with rheumatoid arthritis. Restless leg syndrome (Reynolds, 1986; Reynolds, Blake, Spall, & Williams, 1986) has also been described in patients with rheumatoid arthritis.

Pathological studies of sural nerve biopsies have recently helped define the peripheral neuropathy of rheumatoid arthritis (Conn, McDuffie, & Dyck, 1972; Peyronnard, Charron, Beaudet, & Couture, 1982; Van Lis & Jennekens, 1977). Conn et al. (1972) studied five patients with rheumatoid arthritis and sensorimotor neuropathy documented by electrodiagnostic studies. All biopsies demonstrated axonal degeneration. This was thought to be due to immune complex deposition within vessel walls, causing an acute necrotizing arteritis, and these vasculitic vessels resulted in infarction of nerve axons. Van Lis and Jennekens (1977) described a single sural nerve biopsy from a rheumatoid arthritis patient with neuropathy in which epineural vessels were heavily infiltrated by mononuclear cells. In addition, necrotic and fibrinoid material was found in the lumen and intima, and immunoglobulins and complement were seen on immunofluorescent studies. Arterioles without necrotic and fibrinoid material showed fibrocellular proliferation and mild infiltration by inflammatory cells.

It has been suspected for many years that the peripheral neuropathy of rheumatoid arthritis is a form of mononeuropathy multiplex (Pallis & Scott, 1965). Sabin (1986) hypothesized that random infarcts of nerve axons due to vasculitic occlusion of vaso nervosum might result in a neuropathy of stocking-glove distribution. The statistical likelihood of axonal insult occurring in longer fibers is greater than that in shorter fibers (if infarcts do occur randomly). Thus, the chance that distal symptoms arise as a result of infarction of longer axons is statistically greater (Sabin, 1986).

Pharmacological treatment of rheumatoid arthritis may in itself be a cause of neuropathology of the peripheral nervous system. Fam et al. (1984) described three patients with rheumatoid arthritis who developed cranial neuropathies (cranial nerves IV, V, VI, and VII) as well as a peripheral neuropathy after treatment with gold. Pool, Feit, and Kirkpatrick (1981) reported a case of profound sensorimotor neuropathy that responded to pyridoxine in a patient treated with D-penicillamine, a known pyridoxine antagonist. A case of a pure motor demyelinating proximal neuropathy associated with penicillamine was also described. The neuropathy reversed fully with discontinuation of the drug (Pedersen & Hogenhaven, 1990). Segmental demyelination and axonal loss have been found on biopsies of patients treated with chloroquine (Estes et al., 1987).

The vasculitis of rheumatoid arthritis often manifests itself as a mononeuritis multiplex, as has been discussed above. Clinical characteristics depend on the nerve trunks involved. Onset is generally acute or subacute and may be associated with poorly localized aching pain. Proximal neuropathy predominantly affects motor nerves, whereas distal nerve trunk involvement gives a mixed involvement of the sensory and motor systems. The electrodiagnostic findings are principally those of axonal damage, namely, positive sharp waves and fibrillations on needle examination. Large-amplitude polyphasic motor units may occur later in the disorder as reinnervation occurs (Parry, 1985). Mononeuritis multiplex characteristically occurs within 1 year of the onset of systemic vasculitis. Provided that no recurrences of the systemic vasculitis occur within 18 months of the initial neurological insult, the prognosis for recovery from nerve damage is good (Chang, Bell, & Hallett, 1984).

FOCAL NEUROPATHIES

Focal neuropathies, commonly known as entrapment neuropathies, are relatively frequent in rheumatoid arthritis, particularly within the carpal tunnel. Nerve fibers may sustain focal damage through entrapment in two ways—local demyelination and axonal loss. Entrapment often results in local demyelination of nerve fibers in the vicinity of the entrapment. These changes are most notable in large myelinated sensory and motor fibers. If the myelin loss is severe enough to cause conduction block within nerve fibers, a neurapraxia has occurred. If the focal injury is more severe, axonal disruption—axonotmesis—may occur and the nerve fiber degenerates distal to the site over the ensuing days to weeks.

Within a given nerve trunk, the combination of neurapraxia and axonotmesis may occur. Neurapraxia and axonotmesis may be differentiated electrodiagnostically (Table 5–1). Nerve conduction studies demonstrate that fibers are electrically excitable distal to the lesion in neurapraxia, while degenerated fibers are not excitable in an axonotmetic lesion. On needle examination, axonotmetic lesions are implied by the findings of fibrillations and positive sharp waves when muscles innervated by the nerve in question are examined. These potentials are absent in a neurapraxic injury. Severe focal neuropathies may involve a combination of neurapraxic and axonotmetic injury in various fibers. Milder injuries may be largely neurapraxic, and the most sensitive manner of finding such an entrapment will be a loss of amplitude proximal to the entrapment site and slowing of conduction across the site of compromise (Gilliatt, 1981; Hallett, 1985).

The carpal tunnel syndrome, or entrapment of the median nerve within the carpal tunnel under the flexor retinaculum, is likely the most common nerve entrapment in rheumatoid arthritic patients. As the diagnosis of carpal tunnel syndrome is especially frequent to the electromyographer, several specialized techniques of diagnosing this disorder appear in the electrophysiological literature. Generally, (1) carpal tunnel syndrome usually involves both large sensory and motor fibers, but occasionally only one type of nerve fiber is involved; this would imply that sensory and motor studies are almost always necessary; (2) nerve conduction studies other than median should always be carried out to ensure that the median nerve slowing is due to a

Table 5–1 Electrodiagnostic Findings in Focal Neuropathy

Study	*Neurapraxia*	*Axonotmesis*
Electromyography		
Muscle at rest	Normal	Positive sharp waves Fibrillation potentials
Recruitment pattern	Decreased	Decreased
Interference pattern	Decreased	Decreased
Nerve conduction studies		
Stimulation proximal to the lesion	No CMAP elicited	No CMAP elicited
Stimulation distal to the lesion	No CMAP elicited	No CMAP elicited

focal entrapment and not a peripheral neuropathy; (3) although standard conduction latencies have been calculated for each nerve at fixed distances in normal adults, the sensitivity of the test can be increased by comparing the median study to that of an adjacent nerve (ulnar or superficial radial) or the corresponding nerve in the contralateral limb; (4) it is frequently useful to perform an electromyogram of the entire upper extremity and corresponding paraspinal muscles in addition to that of the thenar eminence; some believe that the presence of radiculopathy may predispose the patient to carpal tunnel syndrome (the "double-crush" syndrome; Hurst, Weissberg, & Carroll, 1985; Upton & McComas, 1973). Electrodiagnosis of carpal tunnel syndrome has been reviewed within the last few years (Jablecki, Andary, So, Wilkins, & Williams, 1993; Stevens, 1987).

Several studies document the occurrence of carpal tunnel syndrome in rheumatoid arthritis patients (Barnes & Currey, 1967; Brumfield, 1983; Chamberlain & Corbett, 1970; Vemireddi, Redford, & Pombejara, 1979). The entrapment may be caused by swelling (synovitis) on the volar aspect of the wrist (Brumfield, 1983; Krane & Simon, 1986). In one study, 20 patients with documented rheumatoid arthritis were examined for carpal tunnel syndrome. Eight of the forty wrists studied demonstrated findings consistent with carpal tunnel syndrome, and all improved with anti-inflammatory medication and splinting (Vemireddi et al., 1979). An older series of 45 patients with classic or definite rheumatoid arthritis demonstrated electrodiagnostic abnormalities consistent with carpal tunnel syndrome in 49% of the patients; 33% also had clinical evidence of the disorder (Barnes & Currey, 1967).

Tarsal tunnel syndrome, entrapment of the tibial nerve under the flexor retinaculum (laciniate ligament) at the ankle, has been documented in 5% to 25% of rheumatoid arthritics (Baylan et al., 1981; Grabois, Puents, & Lidsky, 1981) who did not have findings of peripheral neuropathy. The posterior interosseous nerve may be entrapped by swollen synovium at the elbow (Chang, Gowans, Granger, & Millender, 1972), the ulnar nerve at the elbow and wrist (Balagtas-Balmaseda, Grabois, Galmaseda, & Lidsky, 1983; Taylor, 1974), and the peroneal nerve and tibial nerves can be compressed in the popliteal region (Jimenea & Uddin, 1971; Krane & Simon, 1986). Digital neuropathy of the upper extremities has also been described (Massey, 1983). Winging of the scapula in rheumatoid arthritis patients may be due to disruption of the serratus anterior, and should not be confused with a palsy of the long thoracic nerve. In the former case, conduction studies and EMG examination will be normal despite classic weakness found on physical examination. Disruption of the serratus anterior has been described upon abduction and flexion at the shoulder (Meythaler, Reddy, & Mitz, 1986).

MYOPATHY

Myopathy (Buchtal, 1985) is perhaps less appreciated in rheumatoid arthritis than are peripheral or focal neuropathies, yet it has been frequently reported in the arthritis literature (Halla et al., 1984; Pitkeathly & Coomes, 1966; Steinberg & Wynn Parry, 1961; Strandberg, 1968). Electromyographic changes do not necessarily correlate with findings on muscle biopsy (Strandberg, 1968), which characteristically show diffuse inflammatory cell infiltrates and fiber necrosis (Halla et al., 1984; Pitkeathly & Coomes, 1966). Electromyographic findings are most marked in patients with elevated creatine phosphokinase (Halla et al., 1984).

A confusing picture may arise in patients treated with steroids. The treatment itself may result in a myopathy (Yates, 1963). Corticosteroids result in atrophy of skeletal muscles due to inhibition of protein synthesis, an effect most notable in fast-twitch fibers (Kelly, McGrath, Goldspink, & Cullen, 1986). The electromyogram may be extremely useful in assessing increasing weakness in a patient taking steroids. Fibrillation potentials and positive sharp waves disappear rapidly in vasculitic myopathy treated with steroids, whereas the myopathy produced by steroids produces little spontaneous activity. Recurrence of myositic weakness can be distinguished from steroid myopathy by the presence or absence of these potentials (Kimura, 1989).

Polymyositis and dermatomyositis have been described as a consequence of penicillamine therapy in two cases. One rheumatoid arthritis patient developed polymyositis 1 month after beginning the drug. Notable was the association of myocarditis, proteinuria, and hypocomplementemia, which are not typical of idiopathic polymyositis (Cucher & Goldman, 1976). A second patient developed a severe dermatomyopathy that remitted on discontinuation of the drug. Results of the muscle biopsy were compatible with a severe necrotizing myositis, and results of the skin biopsy showed atrophic epidermis and basophilic degeneration of connective tissue (Lund & Nielsen, 1983). Cloroquine or hydroxychloroquine may produce a vacuolar myopathy that may improve after discontinuation of the drug (Estes et al., 1987).

NEUROMUSCULAR JUNCTION DISORDERS

The administration of D-penicillamine as a remittive agent in rheumatoid arthritis may lead to weakness similar to myasthenia gravis (Albers, Hodach, Kimmel, & Treacy, 1980). The myasthenia picture usually resolves 3 to 6 months after discontinuation of the drug (Albers et al., 1980; Fawcett, McLachian, Nicholson, Zohar, & Mastaglis, 1982). D-Penicillamine predisposes certain paticnts to myasthenia gravis but does not directly interfere with neuromuscular transmission (Albers, Beals, & Levine, 1981; Swift, 1981). The myasthenia picture may be due to penicillamine-induced synthesis of acetylcholine receptor antibodies (Fawcett et al., 1982; Kuncl, Pestronk, Drachman, & Rechthand, 1986), whose titers fall dramatically when the drug is discontinued (Swift, 1981). One case has been reported of a myasthenia gravis picture due to administration of penicillamine that was reactivated by gold (Moore, Williams, & Hillenbrand, 1984). Both corticosteroids and azathioprine act presynaptically to disturb neuromuscular transmission; however, it is not known whether any of their effects are clinically significant (Swift, 1981).

CERVICAL SPINE IN RHEUMATOID ARTHRITIS

Rheumatoid arthritis can produce degeneration of the connective tissue structures responsible for stability of the upper cervical spine. When atlantoaxial instability is the result, anterior compression of the spinal cord may result. The patient may present with signs of a myelopathy, including pain, sensory symptoms, weakness, spastic hypertonia, and rarely fifth cranial nerve involvement. The diagnosis may be delayed if the neurological features are wrongly attributed to peripheral nerve changes (Marks, 1985; Stevens, Kendall, & Crockard, 1986).

The diagnosis of myelopathy in rheumatoid arthritis is not always clear-cut because the degree of atlantoaxial subluxation determined on plain radiographs is not closely correlated to the clinical picture (Pellicci, Ranawat, Tsairis, & Bryan, 1981). Computed myelography may add to the diagnostic impression (Stevens et al., 1986), and SSEP may be especially useful in this setting. Upon stimulation of the upper extremity, one may find that while the brachial plexus potential is of normal amplitude and latency, the evoked responses measured over the cervicomedullary junction and contralateral somatosensory cortex may show delay and loss of amplitude. Abnormalities of SSEP correlate with signs of clinical myelopathy but are more sensitive to involvement in the posterior columns than when abnormalities are located in the anterolateral spinal cord. Somatosensory-evoked potentials may detect problems in the sensory pathways that are not found on clinical testing (Chiappa & Ropper, 1982; Somatosensory, 1987). Neurological progression with corroborating laboratory studies suggests the need for rapid surgical intervention (Marks, 1985; Stevens et al., 1986).

CONCLUSION

Patients with rheumatoid arthritis may suffer from a variety of neuromuscular disorders. Electrodiagnosis may aid greatly in the diagnosis of these problems. The principal electrodiagnostic tools are electromyography, nerve conduction studies, neuromuscular junction studies, and somatosensory-evoked potentials. Electromyography is useful in detecting disease involving the motor unit and in localizing disease to a particular distribution (ie, muscle, nerve, root, or plexus). Electromyography may help to prognosticate the severity of focal nerve lesions. Nerve conduction studies identify pathology along the length of a nerve and can help localize a focal nerve lesion. Nerve conduction and electromyography may help to differentiate a demyelinating process from an axonal neuropathic process. Late responses—F waves and H reflexes—may assist in discovering nerve pathology occurring proximally in nerve trunks. Repetitive stimulation and single-fiber electromyography are used to delineate disorders of the neuromuscular junction. Somatosensory-evoked potentials can be used to verify the presence of myelopathy in the rheumatoid arthritis patient with cervical myelopathy.

Rheumatoid patients may suffer from a predominantly sensory peripheral neuropathy with a stocking-glove distribution, or a sensorimotor neuropathy with profound weakness. They may also present with asymmetrical involvement of a few nerves, mononeuritis multiplex. All these problems may be due to axonal injury resulting from the vasculitis associated with rheumatoid arthritis. Vasculitic involvement of the vaso nervosum may produce an infarction of nerve fibers supplied by the diseased vessels. Inflammatory products have been documented in nerve biopsies of afflicted patients. Peripheral nerve involvement may also occur as a result of treatment of rheumatoid arthritis by gold compounds, D-penicillamine, or chloroquine.

The most common entrapment neuropathy in rheumatoid arthritics is the familiar carpal tunnel syndrome. Diagnostic accuracy of the carpal tunnel syndrome can be improved by comparing median nerve conduction with that of adjacent upper extremity nerve trunks. Other focal neuropathies due to tenosynovitis or articular swelling may occur in arthritic patients. These include entrapment of the tibial nerve at the knee and ankle, the posterior interosseous nerve at the elbow, and the peroneal nerve at the knee, as well as digital neuropathy of the hand. Nerve conduction studies and electromyography can help determine whether a focal nerve injury is primarily axonotmetic or neurapraxic. Neurapraxic injuries carry a better prognosis.

Myopathy may be an important source of weakness in the rheumatoid patient, and can be diagnosed with the aid of electromyography. The electromyogram can also help distinguish weakness due to inflammatory myopathy from that due to steroid treatment. A myopathic picture has been associated with D-penicillamine, chloroquine, and hydroxychloroquine treatment. Neuromuscular junction abnormalities are the most common neuromuscular problem associated with D-penicillamine, however. Somatosensory-evoked potentials are a useful adjunct in assessing the patient with long-tract signs and symptoms due to rheumatoid degeneration of the upper cervical spine.

REFERENCES

Ackil, A., Shahani, B.T., Young, R.R., & Rubin, N.E. (1981). Late responses and sural conduction studies with chronic renal failure. *Archives of Neurology*, *38*, 482–485.

Albers, W., Beals, C.A., & Levine, S.P. (1981). Neuromuscular transmission in rheumatoid arthritis, with and without penicillamine treatment. *Neurology*, *31*, 1562–1564.

Albers, J.W., Hodach, R.J., Kimmel, D.W., & Treacy, W.L. (1980). Penicillamine-associated myasthenia gravis. *Neurology*, *30*, 1246–1250.

Aminoff, M.J. (Ed.). (1986a). *Electrodiagnosis in clinical neurology* (2nd ed.). New York: Churchill-Livingstone.

Aminoff, M.J. (1986b). Electromyography. In M.J. Aminoff (Ed.), *Electrodiagnosis in clinical neurology* (2nd ed.). New York: Churchill-Livingstone.

Aminoff, M.J. (1987). *Electromyography in clinical practice.* New York: Churchill-Livingstone.

Balagtas-Balmaseda, O.M., Grabois, M., Galmaseda, P.F., & Lidsky, M.D. (1983). Cubital tunnel syndrome in rheumatoid arthritis. *Archives of Physical Medicine and Rehabilitation*, *64*, 163–166.

Barnes, C.G., & Currey, H.L.F. (1967). Carpal tunnel syndrome in rheumatoid arthritis: A clinical and electrodiagnostic survey. *Annals of the Rheumatic Diseases*, *26*, 226–233.

Baylan, S.P., Paik, S.W., Barnert, A.L., Ko, K.H., Yu, J., & Persellin, R.H. (1981). Prevalence of the tarsal tunnel syndrome in rheumatoid arthritis. *Rheumatology and Rehabilitation*, *20*, 148–150.

Brown, W.F., & Bolton, C.F. (1993). *Clinical electromyography.* Stoneham, MA: Butterworth.

Brumfield, R.H. (1983). Carpal tunnel syndrome in rheumatoid arthritis. *Orthopaedic Review*, *12*, 69–71.

Buchtal, F. (1985). Electromyography in the evaluation of muscle diseases. *Neurology Clinics*, *3*, 573–598.

Cassvan, A., Pease, W.S., MacLean, I.C., Ma, D.M., & Johnson, E.W. (1987a). Electrodiagnosis: Late responses. *Archives of Physical Medicine and Rehabilitation*, *68*, S19–S22.

Cassvan, A., Pease, W.S., MacLean, I.C., Ma, D.M., & Johnson, E.W. (1987b). Electrodiagnosis: Central evoked potentials. *Archives of Physical Medicine and Rehabilitation*, *68*, S23–S27.

Chamberlain, M.A., & Bruckner, F.E. (1970). Rheumatoid neuropathy: Clinical and electrophysiological features. *Annals of the Rheumatic Diseases*, *29*, 609–616.

Chamberlain, M.A., & Corbett, M. (1970). Carpal tunnel syndrome in early rheumatoid arthritis. *Annals of the Rheumatic Diseases*, *29*, 149–152.

Chang, L.W., Gowans, J.D.C., Granger, C.V., & Millender, L.H. (1972). Entrapment neuropathy of the posterior interosseous nerve: A complication of rheumatoid arthritis. *Arthritis and Rheumatism*, *15*, 350–352.

Chang, R.W., Bell, C.L., & Hallett, M. (1984). Clinical characteristics and prognosis of vasculitic mononeuropathy multiplex. *Archives of Neurology*, *41*, 608–621.

Chiappa, K.H., & Ropper, A.H. (1982). Evoked potentials in clinical medicine. *New England Journal of Medicine*, *306*, 1205–1211.

Conn, D.L., McDuffie, F.C., & Dyck, P.J. (1972). Immunopathologic study of sural nerves in rheumatoid arthritis. *Arthritis and Rheumatism*, *15*, 135–143.

Cucher, B.G., & Goldman, A.L. (1976). D-penicillamine-induced polymyositis in rheumatoid arthritis. *Annals of Internal Medicine*, *85*, 615–616.

D'Amour, M.L., Shahani, B.T., Young, R.R., & Bird, K.T. (1979). The importance of studying sural conduction and late responses in the evaluation of alcoholic subjects. *Neurology*, *29*, 1600–1604.

Daube, J. (1986). Nerve conduction studies. In M.J. Aminoff (Ed.), *Electrodiagnosis in clinical neurology* (2nd ed.). New York: Churchill-Livingstone.

Daube, J.R. (1991). AAEM minimonograph #11: Needle examination in clinical electromyography. *Muscle and Nerve*, *14*, 685–700.

Edmonds, M.E., Jones, T.C., Saunders, W.A., & Sturrock, R.D. (1979). Autonomic neuropathy in rheumatoid arthritis. *British Medical Journal*, *2*, 173–175.

Eisen, A., & Aminoff, M.J. (1986). Somatosensory evoked potentials. In M.J. Aminoff (Ed.), *Electrodiagnosis in clinical neurology* (2nd ed.). New York: Churchill-Livingstone.

Estes, M.L., Ewing-Wilson, D., Chow, S.M., Mitsumoto, H., Hanson, M., Shirey, E., & Ratliff, N. (1987). Chloroquine neuromyotoxicity: Clinical and pathologic perspective. *American Journal of Medicine*, *82*, 447–455.

Fam, A.G., Gordon, D.A., Sarkozi, J., Blair, G.R.D., Cooper, P.W., Harth, M., & Lewis, A.J. (1984). Neurologic complications associated with gold therapy for rheumatoid arthritis. *Journal of Rheumatology*, *11*, 700–706.

Fawcett, P.R.W., McLachian, S.M., Nicholson, L.V.B., Zohar, A., & Mastaglis, F. (1982). D-Penicillamine-associated myasthenia gravis: Immunological and electrophysiological studies. *Muscle and Nerve*, *5*, 328–334.

Fischer, M.M. (1992). AAEM minimonograph #13: H reflexes and F waves: Physiology and clinical indications. *Muscle and Nerve*, *15*, 1223–1233.

Gilliatt, R.W. (1981). Physical injury to peripheral nerves—Physiologic and electrodiagnostic aspects. *Mayo Clinic Proceedings*, *56*, 361–370.

Gilliatt, R.W. (1982). Electrophysiology of peripheral neuropathies—An overview. *Muscle and Nerve*, *5*, S108–S116.

Good, A.E., Christopher, R.P., Koepke, G.H., Bender, L.F., & Tarter, M.E. (1965). Peripheral neuropathy associated with rheumatoid arthritis. *Annals of Internal Medicine*, *63*, 87–99.

Grabois, M., Puents, J., & Lidsky, M. (1981). Tarsal tunnel syndrome in rheumatoid arthritis. *Archives of Physical Medicine and Rehabilitation*, *62*, 401–403.

Halla, J.T., Koopman, W.J., Fallahi, S., Oh, S.J., Gay, R.E., & Schrobenloher, R.E. (1984). Rheumatoid myositis: Clinical and histological features and possible pathogenesis. *Arthritis and Rheumatism*, 27, 737–743.

Hallett, M. (1985). Electrophysiologic approaches to the diagnosis of entrapment neuropathies. *Neurology Clinic*, *3*, 531–541.

Hurst, L.C., Weissberg, D., & Carroll, R.E. (1985). The relationship of the double crush to carpal tunnel syndrome (an analysis of 1000 cases of carpal tunnel syndrome). *Journal of Hand Surgery [Br]*, *10*, 202–204.

Jablecki, C.K. (1985). Electrodiagnostic evaluation of patients with myasthenia gravis and related disorders. *Neurology Clinic*, *3*, 557–572.

Jablecki, C.K., Andary, M.T., So, Y.T., Wilkins, D.E., & Williams, F.H. (1993). Literature review of the usefulness of nerve conduction studies and electromyography for the evaluation of patients with Carpal Tunnel Syndrome. *Muscle and Nerve*, *16*, 392–414.

Jimenea, J., & Uddin, J. (1971). Nerve conduction studies in neuropathy associated with rheumatoid arthritis. *American Journal of Physical Medicine*, *50*, 161–168.

Kelly, F.J., McGrath, J.A., Goldspink, D.F., & Cullen, M.J. (1986). A morphological/biochemical study on the actions of corticosteroids on rat skeletal muscle. *Muscle and Nerve*, *9*, 1–10.

Kimura, J. (1989). *Electrodiagnosis in diseases of nerve and muscle* (2nd ed.). Philadelphia: F.A. Davis.

Kramer, L.D., Ruth, R.A., Johns, M.E., & Sanders, D.B. (1981). A comparison of stapedial reflex fatigue with repetitive stimulation and single-fiber EMG in myasthenia gravis. *Annals of Neurology*, *9*, 531–536.

Krane, S.M., & Simon, L.S. (1986). Rheumatoid arthritis: Clinical features and pathogenetic mechanisms. *Recent Advances in Rheumatology*, *70*, 263–284.

Kuncl, R.W., Pestronk, A., Drachman, D.B., & Rechthand, E. (1986). The pathophysiology of penicillamine-induced myasthenia gravis. *Annals of Neurology*, *20*, 740–744.

Lachman, T., Shahani, B.T., & Young, R.R. (1980). Late responses as aids to diagnosis in peripheral neuropathy. *Journal of Neurology, Neurosurgery and Psychiatry*, *43*, 156–162.

Lang, A.H., Kalliomaki, J.L., Puusa, A., & Halonen, J.P. (1981). Sensory neuropathy in rheumatoid arthritis. *Scandinavian Journal of Rheumatology*, *10*, 81–84.

Lund, H.I., & Nielsen, M. (1983). Penicillamine-induced dermatomyositis. *Scandinavian Journal of Rheumatology*, *12*, 350–352.

Ma, D.M., Pease, W.S., MacLean, I.C., Cassvan, A., & Johnson, E.W. (1987). Electrodiagnosis: Needle examination. *Archives of Physical Medicine and Rehabilitation*, *68*, S7–S12.

MacLean, I.C., Pease, W.S., Ma, D.M., Cassvan, A., & Johnson, E.W. (1987). Electrodiagnosis: Peripheral evoked potentials. *Archives of Physical Medicine and Rehabilitation*, *68*, S13–S18.

Marks, J.S. (1985). Rheumatoid neck. *British Journal of Hospital Medicine*, *33*, 96–100.

Massey, E.W. (1983). Digitalgia paresthetica with digital neuropathy in rheumatoid arthritis. *Southern Medical Journal*, *76*, 923–925.

McCombe, P.A., Kiester, A.C., Tannenberg, A.E., Chalk, J.B., & Pender, M.P. (1991). Sensorimotor peripheral neuropathy in rheumatoid arthritis. *Clinical and Experimental Neurology*, *28*, 146–153.

Meythaler, J.M., Reddy, N.M., & Mitz, M. (1986). Serratus anterior disruption: A complication of rheumatoid arthritis. *Archives of Physical Medicine and Rehabilitation*, *67*, 770–772.

Moore, A.P., Williams, A.C., & Hillenbrand, P. (1984). Penicillamine induced myasthenia gravis reactivated by gold. *British Medical Journal*, *288*, 192–193.

Moritz, U. (1984). Studies on motor nerve conduction in rheumatoid arthritis. *Acta Rheumatologica Scandinavica*, *10*, 99–108.

Oh, S.H. (1993). *Electromyography: Nerve conduction studies.* Baltimore: Williams & Wilkins.

Pallis, C.A., & Scott, J.T. (1965). Peripheral neuropathy in rheumatoid arthritis. *British Medical Journal*, *1*, 1141–1147.

Parry, G.J.G. (1985). Mononeuropathy multiplex. *Muscle and Nerve*, *8*, 493–498.

Pedersen, P.B., & Hogenhaven, H. (1990). Penicillamine-induced neuropathy in rheumatoid arthritis. *Acta Neurologica Scandinavica*, *81*, 188–190.

Pellicci, P.M., Ranawat, C.S., Tsairis, P., & Bryan, W.J. (1981). A prospective study of the progression of rheumatoid arthritis of the cervical spine. *Journal of Bone and Joint Surgery [Am]*, *63*, 342–350.

Petersen, I. (1955). An electromyographic study of the atrophied first dorsal interosseous muscle in rheumatoid arthritis. *Acta Rheumatologica Scandinavica*, *1*, 67–72.

Peyronnard, J.M., Charron, L., Beaudet, F., & Couture, F. (1982). Vasculitic neuropathy in rheumatoid disease and Sjogren syndrome. *Neurology*, *32*, 839–845.

Pitkeathly, D.A., & Coomes, E.N. (1966). Polymyositis in rheumatoid arthritis. *Annals of the Rheumatic Diseases*, *25*, 127–132.

Pool, K.D., Feit, H., & Kirkpatrick, J. (1981). Penicillamine-induced neuropathy in rheumatoid arthritis. *Annals of Internal Medicine*, *95*, 457–458.

Ravits, J.M. (1990). *Autonomic nervous system testing.* Rochester, MN: American Association of Electrodiagnostic Medicine.

Reynolds, G. (1986). Restless leg syndrome and rheumatoid arthritis. *British Journal of Medicine*, *292*, 1203.

Reynolds, G., Blake, D.R., Spall, H.S., & Williams, A. (1986). Restless leg syndrome and rheumatoid arthritis. *British Medicine Journal*, *292*, 659–660.

Sabin, T.D. (1986). Classification of peripheral neuropathy: The long and the short of it. *Muscle and Nerve*, *9*, 711–719.

Shahani, B.T., Halperin, J.J., Bouly, P., & Cohen, J. (1984). Sympathetic skin response—A method of assessing unmyelinated axon dysfunction in peripheral neuropathies. *Journal of Neurology, Neurosurgery and Psychiatry*, *47*, 536–542.

Somatosensory potentials and cervical cord disease. (1987). *Lancet*, *1*, 546–547.

Stalberg, E. (1980). Clinical electrophysiology in myasthenia gravis. *Journal of Neurology, Neurosurgery and Psychiatry*, *43*, 622–633.

Steinberg, V.L., & Wynn Parry, C.B. (1961). Electromyographic changes in rheumatoid arthritis. *British Medical Journal*, *5526*, 630–632.

Stevens, J.C. (1987). The electrodiagnosis of carpal tunnel syndrome. *Muscle and Nerve*, *10*, 99–113.

Stevens, J.M., Kendall, B.E., & Crockard, H.A. (1986). The spinal cord in rheumatoid arthritis with clinical myelopathy: A computed myelographic study. *Journal of Neurology, Neurosurgery and Psychiatry*, *49*, 140–151.

Strandberg, B. (1968). Certain muscular diseases in patients with rheumatoid arthritis. *Acta Rheumatologica Scandinavica*, *12*, 1–36.

Swift, T.R. (1981). Disorders of neuromuscular transmission other than myasthenia gravis. *Muscle and Nerve*, *4*, 334–353.

Tan, J., Sabre, A., Beyazova, M., Sepici, V., & Tan, E. (1993). Sympathetic skin response and R-R interval variation in rheumatoid arthritis. *American Journal of Physical Medicine and Rehabilitation*, *72*, 196–203.

Taylor, A.R. (1974). Ulnar nerve compression at the wrist in rheumatoid arthritis. *Journal of Bone and Joint Surgery [Br]*, *56*, 142–143.

Trojaborg, W. (1981). Electrodiagnosis in rheumatic diseases. *Clinical Rheumatic Diseases*, *7*, 349–363.

Uncini, A., Lange, D.J., Lovelace R.E., Solomon, M., & Hays, A.P. (1990). Long duration polyphasic motor unit potentials in myopathies: A quantitative study with pathological correlation. *Muscle and Nerve*, *13*, 263–267.

Upton, A.R.M., & McComas, A.J. (1973). The double crush in nerve entrapment syndromes. *Lancet*, *2*, 359–361.

Valsrub, S. (1980). Autonomic neuropathy complicating rheumatoid arthritis [Editorial]. *Journal of the American Medical Association*, *243*, 152.

Van Lis, J.M., & Jennekens, F.G. (1977). Immunofluorescence studies in a case of rheumatoid neuropathy. *Journal of Neurological Sciences*, *33*, 313–332.

Vemireddi, N.K., Redford, J.B., & Pombejara, C.N. (1979). Serial nerve conduction studies in carpal tunnel syndrome secondary to rheumatoid arthritis: Preliminary study. *Archives of Physical Medicine and Rehabilitation*, *60*, 393–396.

Yates, D.A.H. (1963). Muscular changes in rheumatoid arthritis. *Annals of the Rheumatic Diseases*, *22*, 342–347.

SUGGESTED READING

Amick, L.D. (1960). Muscle atrophy in rheumatoid arthritis: An electrodiagnostic study. *Arthritis and Rheumatism*, *3*, 54–63.

Chiappa, K.H. (1983). *Evoked potentials in clinical medicine.* New York: Raven.

DeLisa, J.A., Mackenzie, K., & Barran, M. (1987). Manual of nerve conduction velocities and somatosensory evoked potentials (2nd ed.). New York: Raven.

Endtz, L.J., Frenary, J., & Goor, C. (1983). Vasculitic neuropathy in rheumatoid arthritis. *Neurology*, *33*, 1635–1636.

Goldgood, J., & Eberstein, A. (1983). *Electrodiagnosis of neuromuscular diseases* (3rd ed.). Baltimore: Williams & Wilkins.

Johnson, E.W. (1980). *Practical electromyography.* Baltimore: Williams & Wilkins.

Ma, D.M. & Liveson, J.A. (1983). *Nerve conduction handbook.* Philadelphia: F.A. Davis.

Olney, R.K. (1992). AAEM minimonograph #39: Neuropathies in connective tissue disease. *Muscle and Nerve*, *15*, 531–542.

Warmots, J.R. (1981). Electrodiagnosis in neuromuscular disorders. *Annals of Internal Medicine*, *95*, 599–608.

CHAPTER 6

Current Medical Treatment of Rheumatoid Arthritis

Rowland W. Chang, MD, MPH, and Pamela A. Semanik, BSN, MS

This chapter discusses the general approach to and rationale for medication in rheumatoid arthritis (RA). Although commonly used antirheumatic drugs are described, this is not a comprehensive review of all accepted pharmacological preparations. The reader is referred to texts of rheumatology and other reviews for more detailed information (Cash & Klippel, 1994; Kelley, Harris, Ruddy, & Sledge, 1993; McCarty & Koopman, 1993).

Precision and specificity are terms that cannot be applied to the medical treatment of RA, unfortunately. The unknown etiology of the disease, coupled with our incomplete understanding of the pharmacological properties of all drugs with respect to the disease, limit the physician to an empirical approach to disease control. Nevertheless, much progress has been made in our understanding of the pathogenesis of RA, giving the promise of more effective drug therapy in the future.

GENERAL APPROACH TO MEDICATION USE IN RHEUMATOID ARTHRITIS

When patients first present to physicians complaining of joint pain, swelling, and stiffness, they are generally as eager for symptomatic control as for establishment of a diagnosis. Finding a medicine that will accomplish complete symptomatic relief can be quite a challenge. More realistic long-term goals of arthritis medical treatment are suppression of pain and swelling, prevention of joint deformity, and preservation of functional ability, although even these cannot be guaranteed.

In treating patients with RA, the physician is faced with a myriad of medicinal compounds from which to choose. Traditionally, a "pyramid" approach has been advocated in choosing the medication that best fits the disease activity level of the patient (Figure 6–1; Roth, 1985). Using this approach, all patients with RA receive treatment described at the base of the pyramid, which includes nonpharmacological treatments. Only those with more progressive disease are offered drugs higher on the pyramid. More recently, an "inverted pyramid" has gained acceptance, which calls for more aggressive treatment for patients with early, active inflammatory disease (Wilske & Healey, 1989).

The base of the regular pyramid includes aspirin and the nonsteroidal anti-inflammatory drugs (NSAIDs). The rationale for these agents is to suppress the pain and stiffness of RA that are a result of joint inflammation. The list of NSAIDs is already long and constantly growing. Drugs in this class are considered first-line agents and are the first to be recommended because of their relatively low toxicity rates.

In the event of severe periodic flares, a course of intra-articular, intramuscular, or oral corticosteroids may be prescribed to control the inflammation. Both NSAIDs and corticosteroids can dramatically reduce the pain and swelling of RA, but they do not alter the tissue destruction and deforming properties of the disease.

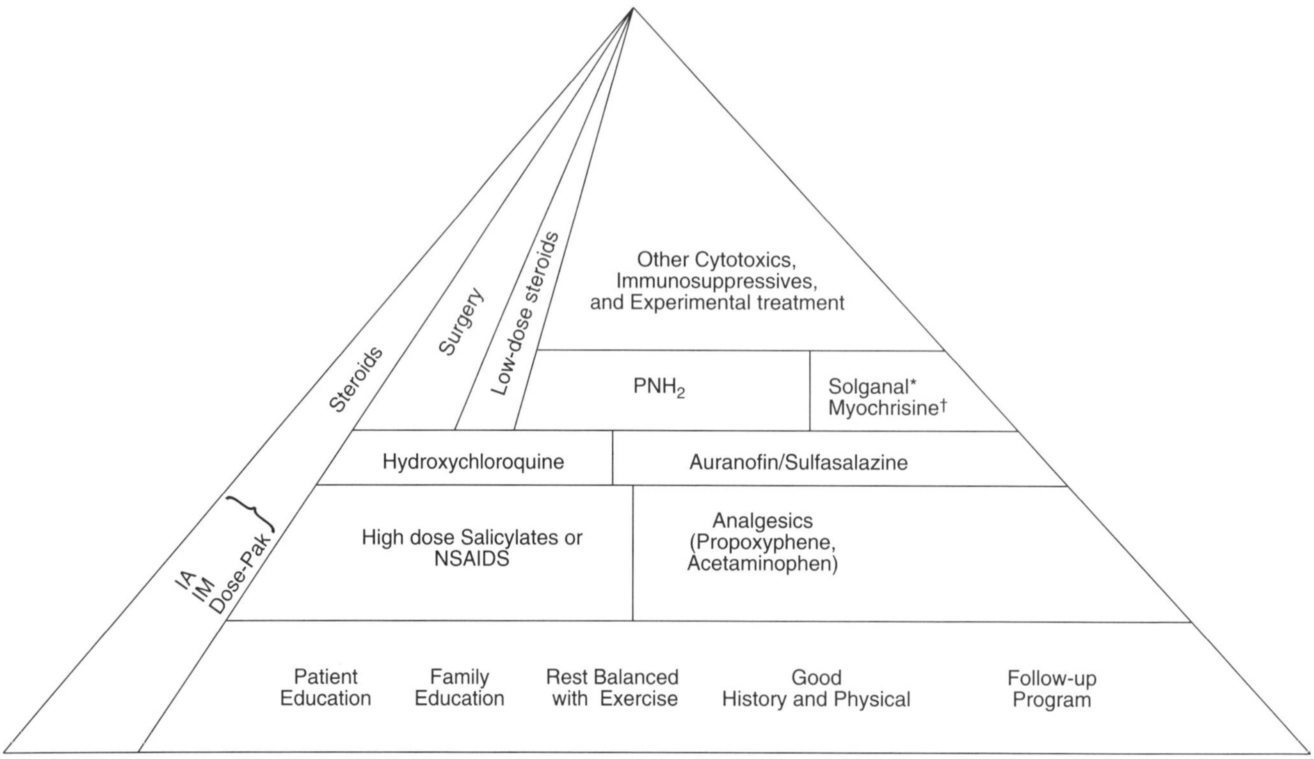

*Aurothioglucose.
†Gold sodium thiomalate.

Figure 6–1 Pyramid approach to RA therapy.

The next level of the pyramid is filled with the so-called second-line or disease-modifying antirheumatic drugs (DMARDs). The DMARDs have greater toxicity than first-line drugs, but they also have the potential to slow the tissue destruction and deformity of RA. Hydroxychloroquine, sulfasalazine, gold salts, penicillamine, and methotrexate are included in this level (Table 6–1; Pinals, Kaplan, Lawson, & Hepburn, 1986). Making the decision to add a second-line agent (generally these are given in addition to NSAIDs) involves the consideration of several factors, some of which are disease related and others patient related. A patient will be considered for a DMARD if (1) there is inadequate control of inflammatory symptoms due to persistent synovitis despite an adequate trial of NSAID therapy, (2) there is evidence of bone destruction on X-rays of the joints signaling more aggressive disease associated with a higher probability of joint deformity and dysfunction, and/or (3) recurrent flares over a period of time giving patients an aggravating "surprise element" to their disease. Patient factors that play a part in determining whether or not a DMARD is prescribed include age, responsibility, expectations, hobbies, and lifestyle. One would be more likely to suggest a DMARD to a young patient whose job required adequate suppression of hand synovitis due to RA than to an elderly patient with the same amount of synovitis but who is already severely disabled by congestive heart failure.

Unfortunately, not all patients with RA respond to or are tolerant of first-line and/or second-line agents. Immunosuppressive and cytotoxic drugs comprise the third level of the RA therapeutic pyramid. They are also thought to be disease modifiers. Azathioprine and cyclophosphamide are currently used for RA (Table 6–2). Because of the more serious side effects associated

Table 6–1 Disease-Modifying Antirheumatic Drug Therapy

Remittive Agent	*Major Side Effects*	*Initial Monitoring Schedule**	*Stable Monitoring Schedule*
Sulfasalazine (Azulfidine)	Gastrointestinal upset, nausea, leukopenia	CBC, platelet count, SMA at 3–4 wk	CBC, platelet count, SMA every 2–3 mo
Hydroxychloroquine (Plaquenil)	Gastrointestinal upset, retinal degradation, corneal deposition	Baseline eye exam before or during the first month of therapy, CBC, SMA (baseline)	CBC, SMA, eye exam every 6 mo
Gold salts (oral) (Ridaura)	Diarrhea, rash, stomatitis, proteinuria, nephrotic syndrome, cytopenia	CBC, platelet count, urinalysis every 2 wk	CBC, platelet count, urinalysis every month; SMA 20 every 6 mo
Gold salts (injectable) Aurothioglucose (Solganal)	Same as for oral gold, but with more frequent occurrence	CBC, platelet count, urinalysis every 1–2 wk	Same as for oral gold
Penicillamine (Cuprimine, Depen)	Same as for injectable gold; altered taste and smell; autoimmune reactions (myasthenia gravis, polymyositis)	Same as for injectable gold	CBC, platelet count, urinalysis every 4–6 wk; SMA 20 every 4–6 mo

*CBC = complete blood count; SMA = Sequential Multiple Analyzer.

Source: Reprinted with permission from Pinals, *Arthritis and Rheumatism*, p.1427, © 1986, J.B. Lippincott.

Table 6–2 Cytotoxic and Immunosuppressive Drugs Used for RA

	Side Effects		*Monitoring Schedule*	
Drug	*Common*	*Major*	*Initial*	*Stable*
Methotrexate	Stomatitis, abnormal liver function tests, gastrointestinal upset	Leukopenia, thrombocytopenia, anemia, interstitial pneumonitis, hepatic fibrosis, fetal toxicity	CBC, platelet count every 1–2 wk; liver function tests every 6–12 wk; creatinine every 3–12 mo; chest X-ray initially	CBC, platelet count every 1–3 mo; liver function tests every 1–3 mo; creatinine every 3–12 mo; chest X-ray every 6–12 mo
Azathoprine (Imuran)	Gastrointestinal upset, rash	Leukopenia, thrombocytopenia, anemia, hepatitis, oncogenesis	CBC, platelet count every 1–2 wk; liver function tests every 3–6 mo	CBC, platelet count every 1–2 wk; liver function tests every 3–6 mo
Cyclophosphamide (Cytoxan)	Alopecia, sterility	Leukopenia, thrombocytopenia, anemia, hemorrhagic cystitis, oncogenesis	CBC, platelet count, urinalysis every 1–2 wk; chemistry screen initially	CBC, platelet count, urinalysis; chemistry screen every 3–6 mo

with these medicines, they are generally reserved for the more refractory and aggressive cases of synovitis and systemic disease, although the apparently tolerable toxicity profile of low-dose methotrexate has many considering it a second-line agent. The immunosuppressive/cytotoxic drugs are also generally given in addition to NSAIDs.

If and when an optimal result is achieved with a particular combination of an NSAID and a DMARD or immunosuppressive drug, this regimen usually is continued indefinitely. Occasionally, doses of particular agents are reduced to lessen the probability of toxicity, but discontinuation especially of DMARDs or immunosuppressive drugs once a therapeutic response has occurred often results in the return of inflammatory symptoms and signs.

As mentioned before, the corticosteroids have possible roles at every level of the pyramid. Although high daily dosages are associated with serious side effects, low-dose daily steroids (prednisone 5 to 10 mg) are commonly used to control active synovitis while awaiting a DMARD response, or to make life tolerable for patients who cannot tolerate exposure to more toxic drugs. Steroids administered at these dosages are believed not to be associated with the more serious side effects of the same drugs at higher levels (Harris, Emkey, Nichols, & Newberg, 1983), although recent data indicate that bone may be adversely affected (Laan et al., 1993).

GENERAL PHARMACOLOGICAL CONSIDERATIONS

Individualizing drug dosages is particularly important in the medical management of RA. Occasionally, plasma levels can be helpful in establishing and maintaining therapeutic doses of medication, but only salicylate levels are routinely available. Since many patients with RA are elderly, the absorption, metabolism, and excretion processes of this age group must be kept in mind. It is also common for these patients to be taking several other medications for other conditions, making drug interactions a real possibility.

Aside from age, two other factors require attention. The first is plasma protein binding and competition of acidic drugs for protein-binding sites. Salicylates are highly protein bound when in the circulation. When administered to a patient already receiving warfarin, the salicylate may displace the warfarin, which is also a protein-bound drug. This may result in an increase in free warfarin and a potentiation of the anticoagulant effect. Aspirin may also enhance the hypoglycemic effect of the sulfonylurea antidiabetic agents by the same mechanism. In addition, when prescribing salicylates it is essential to know the serum albumin level of the patient. In patients with a depressed albumin level, the amount of unbound salicylate may be excessively high, and toxicity may ensue despite a "normal" plasma level of salicylate. The second consideration is renal function. Because NSAIDs are eliminated primarily by renal excretion, dose reduction in these drugs is necessary when treating RA in patients with renal impairment.

There are numerous other pharmacological considerations involving the drugs used in the treatment of RA, but the reader is referred to rheumatology texts and other reviews for more extensive coverage (Baker & Rabinowitz, 1986; Kelley et al., 1993; McCarty & Koopman, 1993).

REVIEW OF THERAPEUTIC AGENTS

Currently used NSAIDs, DMARDs, and cytotoxic/immunosuppressive drugs used to treat RA are listed in Exhibits 6–1 and 6–2. What follows are brief discussions of the mechanisms of action and toxicity of the more commonly utilized agents. The reader is referred to rheumatology textbooks or package inserts for more details.

Nonsteroidal Anti-Inflammatory Drugs

Generally patients with RA take a single NSAID to help reduce the pain and swelling of the inflammatory synovitis. There are many agents from which to choose (Exhibit 6–1). Although no one agent is clearly safer and more efficacious than the others, individual patient responses (both therapeutic and toxic) are unpredictable. Generally a patient develops a preference for one drug over the others, but no characteristics of the drug or the patient aid in specific NSAID choices. One approach to finding the "best" NSAID for an individual patient is to try sequentially one preparation from each chemical class (eg, salicylate, propionic acid, indole-

Exhibit 6–1 Chemical Classes of Nonsteroidal Anti-Inflammatory Drugs

1. *Salicylates*
   - Aspirin
2. *Nonacetylated salicylates*
   - Choline magnesium salicylate (Trilisate)
   - Magnesium salicylate (Magan, Mobidin)
   - Salsalate (Disalcid)
   - Sodium salicylate (Pabalate)
   - Diflunisal (Dolobid)
3. *Propionic acids*
   - Fenoprofen (Nalfon)
   - Ibuprofen (Motrin)
   - Ketoprofen (Orudis)
   - Naproxen (Naprosyn)
   - Flubiprofen (Ansaid)
   - Oxaprozin (Daypro)
4. *Indole derivatives*
   - Indomethacin (Indocin)
   - Sulindac (Clinoril)
   - Tolmetin (Tolectin)
   - Etodolac (Lodine)
5. *Phenylacetic acid*
   - Diclofenac sodium (Voltaren)
6. *Oxicams*
   - Piroxicam (Feldene)
7. *Fenamates*
   - Meclofenamate (Mellomen, Cataflam)
   - Mefenamic acid
   - Flufenamic acid
8. *Nonacidic compound*
   - Nabumetone (Relafen)
9. *Pyrrolo-pyrrole*
   - Ketorolac (Torodol)

Exhibit 6–2 Effects of Corticosteroids on Inflammation and the Immune Response

Effects on neutrophils
- Decrease in lysosomal enzyme release
- Possible increase in antibody-dependent cellular cytotoxicity

Effects on lymphocytes
- Suppression of proliferation in the mixed-leukocyte reaction
- Suppression of T lymphocyte cytoxicity
- Suppression of natural cytotoxity
- Variable effects on suppressor and helper functions
- Selective depletion of T lymphocytes

Effects on monocytes-macrophages
- Decrease in effect of lymphokines and subsequent chemotaxis, leading to blunted, delayed hypersensitivity
- Inhibition of Fc receptor binding
- Decrease in bacteriocidal activity

Other effects
- Decrease in reticuloendothelial clearance
- Inhibition of prostaglandin production
- Mild general decrease in immunoglobulin production
- Possible antagonism of histamine-induced vasodilation
- Probable inhibition of production of products of lipo-oxygenase pathway

acetic acid, oxicam) until an effective and well-tolerated drug is found. Such therapeutic trials should last 1 to 2 weeks at an appropriate anti-inflammatory dose to provide definitive information regarding efficacy and toxicity.

Salicylates

Acetylsalicylic acid (aspirin, ASA) was first synthesized more than 100 years ago and has been widely used since 1899. Its therapeutic effect is caused in part by the inhibition of the oxidation of arachidonic acid by the enzyme cyclooxygenase, which leads to reduced production of prostaglandins, known mediators of inflammation. Other mechanisms have been proposed for the anti-inflammatory, antipyretic, and analgesic properties of ASA, but it appears that much of the therapeutic and toxic effect of ASA is mediated via prostaglandin inhibition. In order to attain consistent anti-inflammatory effect, serum salicylate levels must be maintained above 15 μg/dL. This requires a minimum of eight 325-mg tablets a day divided into four doses.

The gastrointestinal (GI) tract is the major site of ASA toxicity, with frequencies of GI complaints ranging up to 40% (Baker & Rabinowitz, 1986). Heartburn, nausea, and epigastric pain are among the most common side effects. A significant number of patients (70%) will lose small amounts of blood in the stool as well. Although the prevalence of abnormal gastroscopic findings is very high, there is poor correlation between gastrointestinal symptoms and these findings.

Abnormal mucosa quickly reverts to normal on discontinuation of the drug. There is an increased incidence of gastric ulcer disease and gastritis when salicylates are consumed, but their erosive effect on duodenal mucosa is not as striking.

As mentioned previously, the mechanism for this gastric toxicity appears to be related to the very prostaglandin inhibition properties that make ASA therapeutic in RA. In animal models, prostaglandins help maintain the integrity of the mucosal barrier of the stomach and may actually inhibit acid secretion (Davenport, 1967; Gerkens et al., 1977). A reduction in these locally active prostaglandins in the stomach by ASA ingestion has been associated with the inflammatory lesions thought to be responsible for the GI toxicity. These observations have led to the development of locally active drugs that seek to mimic the action of prostaglandins in the stomach. These cytoprotective agents may decrease the risk of ulcer formation in patients on chronic ASA or NSAID therapy. The use of enteric-coated aspirin can also reduce the GI distress and microbleeding. Occasionally, however, the enteric coating leads to erratic absorption in the gut, which may result in relatively low salicylate levels (McCarty & Csuka, 1987). Other currently employed strategies to reduce the risk and extent of ASA gastric toxicity include taking the medications with meals and using a concomitant antacid (eg, sucralfate) or H_2 receptor blocker (eg, cimetidine).

The antiprostaglandin effect of ASA also explains its occasional allergic manifestations. Bronchospasm, especially in association with nasal polyps and intrinsic asthma, is a rare but well-described and potentially dangerous adverse effect of ASA. Other allergic reactions include urticaria and angioedema. Aspirin (and other prostaglandin inhibitors) are contraindicated in patients who have exhibited these allergic manifestations in the past.

Salicylates have a dose-related effect on the eighth cranial nerve, causing a high-pitched ringing with possible hearing loss. Occasionally, loss of balance, dizziness, and vertigo can occur. Hearing loss may be the only symptom, but this is more common in the elderly. Elderly patients (and some younger ones) can also experience significant central nervous system changes such as mental dullness, confusion, and disorientation. Decreasing or stopping the medication usually results in the resolution of these symptoms within a day or so.

Easy bruisability is an ASA-related phenomenon due to ASA's effect on platelet function. The ASA molecule acetylates platelet cyclooxygenase permanently, thereby rendering the platelet unable to participate normally in hemostasis for the duration of its circulating life. Once ASA is discontinued, it generally takes 7 days for bleeding times to return to normal while a new population of platelets is generated. This should be noted in patients who undergo major surgery.

Finally, ASA therapy has implications for patients with conditions associated with decreased renal blood flow (eg, intrinsic renal disease, congestive heart failure, and chronic diuretic therapy). Aspirin-induced inhibition of renal prostaglandins is related to a decrease in glomerular filtration rate and renal blood flow (Kimberly & Plotz, 1979). The clinical consequence may be a rise in levels of serum creatinine and blood urea nitrogen (BUN), which generally responds to discontinuation of the ASA.

Nonacetylated salicylates (salsalate, choline salicylate, and magnesium salicylate) are salicylate preparations with weak antiprostaglandin properties. They are anti-inflammatory, analgesic, and antipyretic but have fewer side effects caused by prostaglandin inhibition. They are particularly useful in patients with ASA or NSAID GI toxicity or allergy. The nonacetylated salicylates may also be considered for patients who require concurrent anticoagulation therapy.

Other Nonsteroidal Anti-Inflammatory Drugs

Because of the relatively high frequency of aspirin toxicity when given in anti-inflammatory doses, many nonsalicylate NSAIDs have been developed and marketed as aspirin substitutes (Exhibit 6–1). The advantages of these preparations over ASA include an improved toxicity profile (ie, less GI toxicity and tinnitus) and increased convenience, since many can be given once or twice a day instead of four times a day to maintain anti-inflammatory blood levels. The disadvantages include higher cost and the requirement of a prescription, except for low-dose ibuprofen, and naproxin, which can be purchased over the counter.

There are seven broad classes of nonsalicylate NSAIDs (Exhibit 6–1), but all are thought to inhibit prostaglandin synthesis in some way. They all differ in structure and pharmacokinetics, but rarely act synergistically with the salicylate or with each other (Greene & Winickoff, 1992).

Like ASA, these NSAIDs are absorbed from the GI tract, but in general these drugs are less toxic to the gastric mucosa. Sulindac, for example, is metabolized to its active form in the liver, so it is relatively inactive in the GI tract (Greene & Winickoff, 1992). Nonsalicylate NSAIDs have a *reversible* effect on platelets, as opposed to ASA, which irreversibly inhibits platelet cyclooxygenase; thus their effect on coagulation can be reversed more quickly.

Are nonsalicylate NSAIDs more effective than ASA in relieving the symptoms of active RA? When particular NSAIDs are compared with ASA (and the list of studies is lengthy) there are conflicting results. There is probably little difference between them. In attempting to determine a positive response to any NSAID in any given patient, a 2-week trial is suggested. If there is no response, or if toxicity occurs, it may be of benefit to switch to a different chemical class of NSAID. Patients' responses can be highly variable, so all attempts should be made to individualize therapy. Even within dosing schedules, unusual adjustments are made to make medication regimens tolerable.

Most of the toxicities and side effects associated with NSAID therapy again are related to the GI tract due to prostaglandin inhibition—microvascular blood loss and gastric ulcers. Gastrointestinal toxicity seems to be systemic in nature, and not a local phenomenon. It has been shown that indomethacin suppositories can produce just as many gastric abnormalities as their oral counterparts (Hansen, Matzen, & Madsen, 1984). Patients who experience bronchospasm when exposed to ASA may also wheeze if given the various other prostaglandin-inhibiting NSAIDs; thus these should also be avoided in such aspirin-allergic patients.

Similar to aspirin, NSAIDs can affect the central nervous system, causing mental dullness, confusion, and disorientation. Indomethacin seems to be especially capable of producing this side effect, but many of the others have been implicated as well.

Corticosteroids

Corticosteroids are potent anti-inflammatory agents that have been used to treat RA since their introduction into clinical use in the late 1940s (Hench, Kendall, Slocumb, & Polley, 1949). Although their administration can dramatically improve patients' inflammatory symptoms and signs, their prescription needs to be made with the knowledge of the potential short-term and long-term toxicity, which can be as disabling as the disease itself.

The mechanisms that account for the anti-inflammatory effects of corticosteroids are complex because of the intricacy of the inflammatory process and the numerous ways in which corticosteroids affect the process (Axelrod, 1993; Exhibit 6–2). In summary, corticosteroids decrease inflammatory cell movement and function, and in higher doses also are immunosuppressive.

Of all the glucocorticoid preparations currently available to provide variety in potency and duration of action (Table 6–3), prednisone is the most commonly used for oral administration. Prednisone is converted to a pharmacologically active compound—prednisolone—by the liver. Thus methylprednisolone occasionally is prescribed for patients with liver disease. When used intra-articularly or intramuscularly, a less soluble salt of triamcinolone or methylprednisolone is used to prolong presumably the anti-inflammatory effect.

The effect of oral or intra-articular steroids on an RA patient's joint inflammation can be immediate (within days) and dramatic. They do not appear, however, to have any impact on the disease's bone- or cartilage-destructive properties. One study has suggested that low-dose daily oral steroid therapy may hinder the development of new erosions (Byron & Kirwan, 1986), but this study has not been confirmed.

The side effects of chronic steroid use are quite staggering. They include thinning of the skin, impaired wound healing, pancreatitis, cataract formation, aggravated hypertension and/or diabetes, aseptic necrosis, acne, truncal obesity, moon faces, adrenal suppression, susceptibility to infections, and mood changes.

Two other important side effects of steroids that relate to the musculoskeletal system are myopathy and osteoporosis. One of the intrinsic problems with joint inflammation is the disuse of affected joints with ensuing muscle atrophy. Even though steroids have a calming effect on joint inflammation, they may actually contribute to existing muscle weakness (even at low doses) in both proximal and distal muscle groups (Danniskiold-Samsoe & Grimby, 1986a, 1986b). The

Table 6–3 Corticosteroid Drugs: Relative Anti-Inflammatory Strengths

Drug	*Equivalent Dose (mg)*	*Approximate Relative Strength*
Short-acting		
Cortisone	25	0.8
Hydrocortisone	20	1
Intermediate		
Prednisone	5	4
Prednisolone	5	4
Methylprednisolone	4	5
Triamcinolone	4	5
Long-acting		
Dexamethasone	0.75	30
Betamethasone	0.6	30

fluorinated steroids appear to be particularly toxic to muscle (Afifi, Bergman, & Harvey, 1968). The mechanism for this condition is unclear.

The effect of chronic corticosteroid use on bone metabolism has been recognized. It appears that pharmacological doses of steroids cause a relative calcium malabsorption in the gut, thus leading to increased resorption of bone for the body to maintain calcium homeostasis. This phenomenon is dose and duration dependent, so low-dose steroids may not have as profound an effect on bone metabolism as do higher doses. Sambrook et al. (1986) have shown that doses averaging 8 mg given for 1 to 89 months are not associated with an increased risk that the patient with RA will develop generalized osteoporosis. A recent study, however, indicates that low-dose prednisone can have adverse short-term effects on bone mineral content (Laan et al., 1993).

Patients on chronic steroid therapy should be advised to increase their dietary intake of calcium-containing products or use commercial calcium preparations. Occasionally vitamin D is prescribed to help overcome the steroid-induced calcium malabsorption. Frequent weight and blood pressure measurements are advisable, since steroids may increase hunger and aggravate a preexisting or previously borderline hypertensive condition.

The decision to initiate oral corticosteroid therapy must be made with the above-mentioned potential risks and benefits in mind. When one or two inflamed joints are causing impaired function in an RA patient, intra-articular injections commonly are performed. This is the least toxic method of steroid administration if the injections are not repeated more than three or four times a year. Commonly there is a beneficial systemic effect from the intra-articular injection due to some absorption of the steroid into the general circulation. When joints are injected with steroid preparations, response is often maximized by first aspirating the excess synovial fluid from the joint whenever possible. Patients should be advised to rest the joint for a day or two and watch for signs of infection in the joint.

Occasionally patients with RA will experience severe, but transient, disabling flares of increased joint inflammation. These can be managed by the use of episodic oral or intramuscular steroids. During severe flares, it may be necessary to prescribe doses as high as 30 or 40 mg, then taper the dose by 5 to 10 mg/d when the desired symptom control is attained. An alternative to this is the administration of a single intramuscular injection of a long-acting corticosteroid (eg, 40–80 mg of triamcinolone acetonide).

Finally, there are RA patients whose chronic inflammatory joint disease is at such a high level of activity that carrying on the activities of daily living is difficult if not impossible. Such patients are often candidates for DMARD therapy, but as is mentioned below, DMARDs often take months before an initial effect is noted. Low-dose corticosteroids are used in such a situation, when the patient needs to be "tided over" until other more long-acting agents take effect. When steroids are used for this reason, the dosage usually ranges between 5 and 10 mg/d, although higher doses are occasionally needed. This more chronic use of oral corticosteroids is associated with a higher probability of steroid toxicity than intra-articular use or occasional oral or intramuscular use. Thus it requires thoughtful risk-benefit consideration.

Disease-Modifying Antirheumatic Drugs

Between 50% and 75% of all RA patients do not achieve acceptable symptom relief with NSAIDs alone. Most of these patients with more persistent and aggressive synovitis are appropriate candidates for DMARD therapy. The choice of the specific DMARD for any individual patient again depends on risk-benefit considerations. If the symptoms and functional deficits associated with the rheumatoid synovitis are not overwhelming, then the traditional DMARDs are typically considered first. However, when treating a patient with severe, aggressive, and disabling synovitis, there is a growing tendency to consider methotrexate, a faster-acting remittive agent, early in the course to achieve a more timely therapeutic response.

The other immunosuppressives, while not generally considered as first-choice remittive agents, are used in patients who have failed therapeutic trials of the more traditional DMARDs.

Antimalarials

Rheumatoid arthritis has been treated with the antimalarials since 1951. The dosage used for RA was up to 20 times greater than that needed for malaria, however, and subsequent reports of retinal damage associated with antimalarial therapy led to its decreased use. Modern daily dose limitations and frequent ophthalmological surveillance has brought these drugs back into favor for RA. The most commonly used of these drugs is hydroxychloroquine (Plaquenil). Its exact mechanism of action in RA therapy is not known, but it has been demonstrated that the antimalarials inhibit lysosomal enzymes, inhibit leukocyte chemotaxis, and are mildly immunosuppressive (Rynes, 1993).

A rare, but serious side effect associated with hydroxychloroquine use is retinopathy. The lesion is thought to be caused by the deposition of chloroquine in the melanin-containing tissues of the eye. Occasionally visual acuity loss can result. The early changes of this phenomenon can be detected by retinoscopy; thus baseline and follow-up eye examinations before and during hydroxychloroquine therapy are required. The recommended frequency of periodic eye exams ranges from every 3 months to annually. There is no single retinal function test that stands out as a predictor of visual trouble development with the use of hydroxychloroquine, and so the drug is usually discontinued on the basis of macular pigmentary changes alone.

Hydroxychloroquine may also deposit its unchanged salts into the cornea in up to 46% of treated patients (Maksymowych & Russell, 1987). Although 50% are asymptomatic, patients experiencing this side effect may complain of seeing halos around lights. The effect is entirely reversible.

The most common side effects are GI disturbances, such as abdominal cramping, bloating, and diarrhea. Some of these can be minimized by administering the drugs with milk or meals. Rashes are also an occasional problem. Patients with psoriasis should be warned that their skin disease may flare while under antimalarial treatment.

The usual dosage of hydroxychloroquine is 200 mg to 400 mg/d, depending on the patient's weight and level of disease activity, for up to 6 months. If no clinical improvement is noted at this time, the drug is usually discontinued or supplemented with another drug.

How effective is hydroxychloroquine in producing remission of disease activity in RA patients? The long-term studies give favorable ratings to hydroxychloroquine, with response rates as high as 80% in some studies that examined clinical improvement (Freedman & Steinberg, 1960). However, associated slowing of radiological progression of disease activity associated with antimalarial use has been only tenuously demonstrated (Maksymowych & Russell, 1987). Conclusions derived from such studies are limited by small patient populations and methodological shortcomings. Nevertheless, the relative ease in patient administration and patient tolerance make the antimalarials attractive in the treatment of less aggressive forms of RA.

Gold Compounds

In the early 1900s it was believed that RA and tuberculosis had a common infectious etiology. Since gold salts were thought to be useful in the treatment of tuberculosis, they began to gain attention as a possible treatment for RA (Forestier, 1935). Subsequently, they have become very popular in the treatment of this disease.

Originally, gold was available by injection only. With the release of auranofin in 1985, oral gold has become an alternative for patients that eliminates the need for weekly injections. The therapeutic and toxicity profiles of injectable and oral gold are sufficiently different, making both methods of administration useful in the overall management of RA.

Two injectable gold compounds differ from each other mostly in terms of toxicity. Gold sodium thiomalate (Myochrysine), a water-soluble formulation, is generally associated with an increased incidence of vasomotor reactions when compared with aurothioglucose (Solganol). However, Solganol is based in sesame oil, making it a more viscous preparation that may result in more painful injections, inexact dosing, and lumps at the site of injection (Baker & Rabinowitz, 1986).

The mechanism by which gold exerts its effects against RA is not well understood. Gold has been found to have multiple effects on the immune system, to have antimicrobial actions, and to inhibit the actions of several lysosomal enzymes. It appears that gold's inhibition of macrophage function in terms of antigen presentation capability and angiogenesis factor production are the major reasons for its clinical efficacy in RA (Koch, Cho, Burrows, Leibovich, & Polverini, 1988; Lipsky & Ziff, 1977; Vernon-Roberts, Dore, Jessop, & Henderson, 1976).

Clinically, the best result of successful gold therapy is the gradual appearance of disease remission, which is reflected in both the disappearance of joint inflammation and improvement in functional status. Complete remission occurs in less than 20% of cases. However, gold improves disease activity in between 60% and 70% of patients who tolerate treatment (Empire Rheumatism Council, 1961) and is thought to be capable of retarding the destructive properties of RA (Sigler et al., 1974). The proportion of people who derive benefit increases as the length of treatment increases (Lockie & Smith, 1985).

Between 25% and 50% of patients treated with injectable gold must discontinue treatment because of toxicity (Srinivasan, Miller, & Paulus, 1979). The most common side effect of gold is rash, which is usually mild, pruritic, and limited to the extremities. Most providers attribute any new rash to gold therapy until proven otherwise. Therapy can be interrupted until the rash resolves, then reinstituted.

Mouth ulcers (stomatitis) also occur in a significant number of patients taking all forms of gold. If only one or two ulcers are present patients fare well. A whole mouthful of ulcerations can be quite incapacitating, however, so therapy should be suspended while multiple lesions heal.

The most common serious complication of gold treatment is proteinuria, which occurs in about 25% of patients and is usually reversible (Gottlieb & Gray, 1978). True nephrotic syndrome is rare. Gold treatment can also cause reversible leukopenia and thrombocytopenia. Rarely, aplastic anemia is encountered. Thus, gold is contraindicated in patients with significant renal or hematopoietic dysfunction.

Vasomotor reactions to Myochrysine can range from lightheadedness to syncope. Anaphylaxis has also been reported, but is less common. Vasomotor reactions usually occur in the first 10 to 15 minutes after injection, so it is advisable to have the patient stay in the office for at least this long after the first two injections.

Oral gold is capable of producing the side effects mentioned earlier, but they occur less frequently (Davis, Menard, Thompson, Harth, & Beaudet, 1985). It does have the added ability to irritate the gut, with diarrhea being the most common complaint. Usually, patients notice only a general softening of stools. One or two diarrheal stools per day are tolerable, but sometimes patients experience as many as six stools per day. Antidiarrheal agents are sometimes used to counteract this side effect. Bulk formers such as bran or fiber can absorb extra fluid from the colon, thereby slowing diarrhea in these patients.

The usual protocol for initiating intramuscular gold therapy is to give one test dose of 10 mg followed by weekly injections of between 25 mg and 50 mg, until a cumulative dose of 1 g is reached. If clinical benefit is noted, subsequent injections are given every 2 to 3 weeks for 2 to 3 months, then monthly. Before each injection, the patient must be questioned about side effects and monitored with a CBC, platelet count, and urinalysis to check for toxicity. Patients usually prefer to have the injection site rotated from side to side, since gold is usually administered as a deep injection into the gluteal muscles.

Oral gold therapy is usually initiated with one 3-mg capsule daily for 1 to 2 weeks, then increased to two capsules daily. Taking oral gold in split doses may help decrease GI irritation. Toxicity is monitored monthly by checking a CBC, platelet count, and urinalysis, as with injectable gold. After 3 to 6 months of therapy, the dosage may be increased to 9 mg/d in nonresponding patients, provided there is no evidence of toxicity.

Penicillamine

Penicillamine (Cuprimine, Depen) is an oral agent that is also used in the treatment of Wilson's disease. Its mechanism of action in RA is unclear. Penicillamine has some immunological capabilities, such as down-regulating the function of lymphocytes, but its effect may be related to its chelating properties, to its effects on collagen cross-linking, sulfhydryl and disulfide interchange, and/or nucleophilic addition (Jaffe, 1993).

Clinically, patients who are able to tolerate therapy do obtain benefit as evidenced by a reduction in the number of swollen joints and subjective complaints, although onset of action is usually 3 to 4 months (Hill, 1977; Multicenter Trial Group, 1973). There is equivocal evidence that penicillamine slows the progression of bone erosions (Shiokawa et al., 1977).

Many of penicillamine's toxicities are similar to those of gold. Most of the problems occur within the first 18 months of treatment (Balme & Huskisson, 1975). Bone marrow depression, proteinuria, and nephrotic syndrome are the most serious side effects. Penicillamine can also cause rash and/or mouth ulcers in up to 44% of patients (Jaffe, Scheinberg, & Sternlieb, 1981). Many patients also complain of loss of taste, which usually improves with continued therapy after about 3 months. There is also a small possibility that an autoimmune syndrome such as myasthenia gravis or systemic lupus erythematosus may occur. While many of the toxicities tend to be dose related, they can occur at any time and at any dose (Cooperative Systematic Studies of the Rheumatic Disease Group, 1987).

To limit toxic side effects associated with penicillamine, it may be critical to adjust the dose appropriately, beginning with either 125 mg/d or 250 mg/d. It is thought that this low-dose introduction of the drug, along with cautious escalation of the dose by no more than 125 mg every month, may significantly reduce toxic side effects (Jaffe, 1975). After 4 to 6 months at a daily dosage of 750 mg to 1000 mg, the clinical benefit or lack thereof should be evident. If benefit is perceived, the maintenance dose may be adjusted downward to improve tolerance further.

During surveillance visits, patients should be asked about skin rash and mouth ulcers and monitored for hematological and renal toxicities. When glomerulonephritis develops as a consequence of penicillamine therapy, it usually subsides when the drug is withdrawn, although signs of it may persist for months. Patients should be instructed to take the drug on an empty stomach if possible, and to avoid taking it with iron, since penicillaminc (a chelating agent) will interfere with its absorption. Finally, many patients allergic to penicillin question whether they will have a similar reaction to penicillamine. The use of penicillamine in patients with a history of hypersensitivity to penicillin is not contraindicated (Bell & Graziano, 1983).

Sulfasalazine

Recently, sulfasalazine has regained attention as a second-line agent in RA. A Swedish physician inspired the development of sulfasalazine (Azulfidine) over 50 years ago when he proposed that RA had a bacterial etiology. Even though clinical results seemed promising, the drug fell into disuse when a single uncontrolled trial showed it to be less effective than gold in the control of RA. The drug was thereafter able to establish a good safety record as a first-line agent in the treatment of inflammatory bowel disease, for which it continues to be used today. Fairly recent controlled trials involving sulfasalazine have been encouraging in the long-term treatment of RA, thus leading to the resurgence of interest in this drug as a DMARD (Amos et al., 1986; Bax & Amos, 1985; Pinals et al., 1986). It is not well understood how sulfasalazine exerts its effect against RA. Its disease-modifying abilities seem similar to those of gold; however, sulfasalazine is both less toxic and less expensive than gold, as well as more convenient to administer.

There is some debate over whether sulfasalazine has the potential to slow the development of bony erosions in RA. Data on this subject are rather sparse, but the results of one small study (Pullar, Hunter, & Capell, 1987) suggest that over a 2-year period, sulfasalazine may slow the progression of radiologically evident disease of the hands. No significant difference was seen in large joint radiographs between the treatment and placebo groups. During the first year of this study, radiological progression took place at about the same rate in both treatment and control groups, improving in the treatment group only during the second year.

Most patients who experience major toxicity with sulfasalazine therapy do so within the first 3 months of treatment (Amos et al., 1986), and these are usually self-limiting after the discontinuation of the drug. The most common side effect is GI upset, which is usually expressed as nausea, vomiting, abdominal pain, or any combination of the above. Gastrointestinal disturbances accounted for the greatest number of therapy withdrawals in a long-term drug safety study (Amos et al., 1986). In the same study, mucocutaneous reactions resulting in pruritic maculopapular eruptions constituted the second most common reason for drug withdrawal. Neutropenia and leucopenia have also been documented in conjunction with sulfasalazine therapy (Amos et al., 1986; Farr, Symmons, Blake, & Bacon, 1986) in both severe and mild forms, but the effects seem to resolve readily after discontinuation of the drug. Sulfasalazine is contraindicated in patients who are allergic to sulfa-based medications.

Sulfasalazine is usually initiated at 1 g/d in divided doses, progressing to a maximum dose of 3 g/d over a period of 3 to 4 months. Many patients are maintained at 2 g/d in divided doses. The use of enteric-coated tablets helps reduce treatment withdrawal due to GI upset. Blood counts and serum chemistries are recommended at baseline and at 6- to 8-week intervals initially. Eventually, an every-3-month monitoring schedule may be reached, making this therapy more attractive to patients who find the monthly monitoring associated with most other DMARD inconvenient or unacceptable.

Immunosuppressives

Increased understanding of the role of immune dysfunction in the pathophysiology of RA has led to the use of immunosuppressive drugs, especially in refractory cases. Clinical benefits have been observed in controlled trials, although alteration of immune function has not always been clearly correlated with improvement in clinical status (Clements & Davis, 1986; Wilkins, 1985). Owing to the relatively small doses of these drugs used in RA, it is possible that they exert their action by an anti-inflammatory mechanism as well.

Even in small doses, there is reasonable concern that all of the drugs (methotrexate, azathioprine, and cyclophosphamide) have the potential to suppress bone marrow function and induce opportunistic infections. In addition, their long-term use in cancer chemotherapy has been associated with malignancy. Whether this malignancy risk applies in the treatment of RA is unclear presently. Each of these drugs is discussed separately, although many of the side effects and monitoring practices are very similar among them.

Methotrexate

Methotrexate is probably the most widely used immunosuppressive drug at this time because of its safety record and ease of administration. It is a folate antagonist, commonly used in severe psoriasis as well as in the treatment of cancer (but in much larger doses for cancer). Methotrexate can be administered orally or parenterally. It exerts its effect by damaging proliferating cells, but has little effect on resting cells. Clinically, studies have shown that methotrexate can produce significant improvement in the symptoms associated with RA, and its ability to retard radiological progression of disease has been demonstrated (Kremer & Lee, 1988; Weinblatt et al., 1988). One of the most popular aspects of methotrexate therapy is its rapid onset of action compared with most other drugs used in the treatment of RA. Patients can usually expect to notice a decrease in disease symptoms within 1 to 2 months after initiating therapy. Unfortunately, long-lasting remissions have not been attained with methotrexate. Patients often suffer a severe flare of arthritis symptoms after discontinuation of methotrexate, even if they have taken it faithfully for several months or years. One small-scale study that randomized patients doing well on methotrexate to a continuing methotrexate group or a placebo group had to be discontinued when all of the patients in the placebo group experienced significant deterioration in multiple clinical parameters after only 1 month off methotrexate (Kremer, Rynes, & Bartholomew, 1987).

Approximately 63% of patients taking methotrexate in another study experienced minor side effects, while 9.7% of patients experienced major side effects (severe infection, cytopenia, respiratory failure, seizures, and GI bleeding; Gispen et al., 1987). The most common minor side effects associated with methotrexate use are mainly gastrointestinal: anorexia, nausea, vomiting, and diarrhea, but rarely do they lead to the discontinuation of the drug. Stomatitis is also fairly common, presenting as a burning, erythematous, painful erosion within a few days of drug ingestion. Usually, stomatitis can be controlled with the administration of folinic acid (1 mg/d for 3 days) on the days when methotrexate is not given. Rarely, alopecia is reported as a side effect of methotrexate use, but this is usually a general thinning of the hair, as opposed to frank baldness (Weinblatt, 1985). Routine monitoring of renal function is recommended with methotrexate therapy, since the primary route of excretion is renal, and renal insufficiency can lead to toxic levels of the drug (Weinblatt, 1985).

Major methotrexate toxicity is relatively rare but can manifest in several ways. Hematological complications resulting from methotrexate use include leukopenia, thrombocytopenia, and very occasionally anemia. Administration of methotrexate to women during the first 4 to 12 weeks of pregnancy may cause any one of several birth defects, and may even result in fetal wastage (Weinblatt, 1985). Women capable of conceiving should always be counseled regarding this potential side effect, and should be encouraged to use a reliable form of contraception while receiving methotrexate. It has not been shown that methotrexate therapy in RA increases these patients' risk of developing a malignancy (Weinblatt, 1985).

Pulmonary toxicity can occur with methotrexate therapy. This phenomenon has been noted more often in cancer patients, but can occur in patients on the lower doses of methotrexate used in the treatment of psoriasis, polymyositis, and RA (Weinblatt, 1985). The most common symptoms of methotrexate lung disease are nonproductive cough, fever, and dyspnea, all of which may precede radiographic abnormalities by several weeks. A chest X-ray may eventually exhibit diffuse bilateral interstitial infiltrates. There does not seem to be any relationship between cumulative dose, route of administration, duration of therapy, age or sex, and the development of pulmonary toxicity (Weinblatt, 1985). Nor is there any clinical or laboratory feature that can predict this usually reversible but potentially fatal complication of therapy (Carson, Cannon, Egger, Ward, & Clegg, 1987). In the management of methotrexate lung disease, it is recommended that the drug be withheld, respiratory support be initiated, the possibility of infection ruled out, and corticosteroids be administered (Weinblatt, 1985).

Finally, methotrexate has been associated with hepatic fibrosis, which cannot always be screened for adequately by the routine liver function tests, and occasionally is detectable only by liver biopsy. This phenomenon appears to be not only less prevalent but also less severe in RA patients than in patients being treated for psoriasis (Pinals, 1988). Recent studies have suggested that liver biopsies are necessary only if liver function tests have been persistently elevated during monthly surveillance (Kremer et al, 1994).

Dosage of methotrexate ranges generally between 5 mg/wk and 20 mg/wk usually given orally in "pulse" doses, that is, on 1 or 2 days per week. Dividing the prescribed dose over 2 days seems to decrease the incidence of GI intolerance in some patients, as does intramuscular administration, which is an alternative route of administration. Monthly monitoring should include a CBC, platelet count, and liver function tests. Relative contraindications for methotrexate use include preexisting liver disease, obesity, alcoholism, diabetes, and renal disease.

Azathioprine

Azathioprine (Imuran) is another immunosuppressive drug used in the treatment of RA. It is also used in renal transplant patients to decrease the incidence of rejection, as well as other connective tissue diseases. Azathioprine suppresses B cell proliferation and antibody production. Its onset of action is rather slow, with maximum responses achieved in about 4 to 6 months. Clinical studies have shown azathioprine to be as efficacious as the other DMARD (Paulus et al., 1984); however, it does not seem to halt the progression of bony erosions seen on X-ray (Urowitz, Gordon, Smythe, Pryzanski, & Ogryzlo, 1973).

Side effects associated with azathioprine are nausea, vomiting, and leukopenia, and possibly an increased risk of infection in patients on higher doses. Azathioprine has been associated with an increased risk of malignancy in the renal transplant population (Hoover & Fraumeni, 1973). It is still controversial, however, as to whether the same risk exists in the RA population treated with this agent.

Daily doses of azathioprine range between 50 mg and 200 mg orally. Renal disease and concomitant allopurinol therapy may require dosage adjustment (drug levels can be increased drastically if given with allopurinol; Baker & Rabinowitz, 1986). Standard monitoring includes monthly CBC and platelet counts and quarterly liver function tests.

Cyclophosphamide

Because of the potential for serious toxicity, cyclophosphamide (Cytoxan) is usually reserved for patients with more refractory or systemic illness. Radiographic studies have convincingly shown that cyclophosphamide decreases bony erosion formation in RA, but this effect unfortunately seems to require toxic dosage levels (O'Brien, 1986). This drug exerts its effect by acting on the S phase of cell division, thus reducing the numbers of lymphocytes and the production of immunoglobulins (Cupps, Edgar, & Fauci, 1982).

Cyclophosphamide has several serious side effects associated with its use in RA treatment. Alopecia and bone marrow toxicity can occur, along with pulmonary and myocardial toxicity at higher dosages. This drug also damages the germinal epithelium of both sexes, which can lead to azoospermia in men and amenorrhea in most women. The most common serious side effect of cyclophosphamide therapy is the ability of its metabolites to damage the transitional epithelium of the bladder, which can lead to fibrosis, hemorrhagic cystitis, and even malignancy. Avoiding prolonged exposure to the metabolites is particularly crucial. This can be accomplished by having the patient drink large volumes of fluid, which should result in frequent voiding.

Cyclophosphamide is usually taken orally in doses ranging from 50 mg to 150 mg daily. Dosage adjustments in renally impaired patients may be necessary. As with the other immunosuppressives, monthly CBC and platelet counts are essential.

Combination Therapy

Csuka, Carrera, and McCarty (1986) first suggested the idea that lower than standard doses of two or more compounds given simultaneously in the treatment of RA might possibly result in improvement of disease while reducing toxicity risks. These investigators hoped to reduce toxicity while providing a remission of sufficient duration to promote damaged tissue healing. They studied cyclophosphamide, azathioprine, and hydroxychloroquine sulfate in 31 patients with RA refractory to conventional therapy. After 43 months, 16 patients achieved complete remission, 7 achieved near remission, and 7 patients were left with partial disease activity. Only one patient experienced no response whatsoever. The clinical improvements included the disappearance of rheumatoid nodules in seven patients, the discontinuation of prednisone in 50% of the patients who started the protocol on prednisone, and some recortication of erosions on serial X-rays in 20 patients (although progression of existing erosions was noted in 11 instances, sometimes coinciding with evidence of healing in others).

Adverse effects experienced by this group included cancer development in three patients (the absolute risk of malignancy from combined therapy is unclear) and erythroleukemia in one. Other side effects that necessitated withdrawal of the drug included thrombocytopenia, stomatitis, diarrhea, pneumonia, and the development of leg ulcers. Hydroxychloroquine was discontinued in five patients because of possible early macular changes. Unfortunately, disease recurrence always followed even prolonged remission after withdrawal of drug therapy. Most patients, however, were responsive to traditional RA therapy after the recurrence of postprotocol disease activity.

The authors concluded that the combined use of remittive agents may be useful in the treatment of severe RA, that cyclophosphamide should be replaced with a nonalkylating agent to reduce the risk of malignancy, and that further controlled trials are necessary to determine the appropriate use of the combined remittive approach in the treatment of severe RA. Trials of other combinations of therapeutic agents have also been completed, but as yet no favored one has emerged (Seminars in Arthritis and Rheumatism Supplement, 1993).

THE FUTURE: IMMUNOMODULATING AGENTS

Recent knowledge about the role of cytokines and adhesion molecules in the pathophysiology of RA has led to a new generation of potential therapeutic agents aimed at modulating the synthesis and biological activities of these molecules. Although early data have been encouraging with some of these agents, larger clinical trials need to be done before they become available for use in patients with RA.

CONCLUSION

Rheumatoid arthritis is a chronic, progressive, potentially crippling disease with no known etiology or complete cure. Advancing medical technology and a greater understanding of the immune response in disease has enabled the medical profession to offer RA patients a growing number of pharmacological preparations that have the potential to control the arthritic process. Effecting a maximal response sometimes requires the addition of drugs from two or three different levels of drug classes. At each level, potential benefits must be weighed against the potential risks to the patient. Since therapy is usually long term, requiring vigilant follow-up and laboratory monitoring, it is crucial to involve patients in decision making whenever possible, and to provide them with complete information regarding their medication. A well-informed patient is a critical team member who can make an important contribution to the optimal management of this chronic and potentially disabling disease.

REFERENCES

Afifi, A.K., Bergman, R.A., & Harvey, J.C. (1968). Steroid myopathy: Clinical, histologic, and cytologic observation. *John Hopkins Medical Journal, 123*, 158–174.

Amos, R.S., Pallor, T., Bax, D.E., Situnayaki, D., Capell, H.A., & McConkey, B. (1986). Sulphasalazine for rheumatoid arthritis: Toxicity in 774 patients monitored for one to eleven years. *British Medical Journal, 293*, 420–424.

Axelrod, L. (1993). Glucocortoids. In W.N. Kelley, E.D. Harris, S. Ruddy, & C.B. Sledge (Eds.), *Textbook of rheumatology* (4th ed. pp. 779–796). Philadelphia: Saunders.

Baker, D.G., & Rabinowitz, J.L. (1986). Current concepts in the treatment of rheumatoid arthritis. *Journal of Clinical Pharmacology, 26*, 2–21.

Balme, H.E., & Huskisson, E. C. (1975). Chronopharmacology of penicillamine and gold. *Scandinavian Journal of Rheumatology, 4* (Suppl. 8), 21.

Bax, D.E., & Amos, R.S. (1985). Sulphasalazine: A safe effective agent for prolonged control of rheumatoid arthritis: A comparison with sodium aurothiomalate. *Annals of the Rheumatic Diseases, 44*, 194–198.

Bell, C.L., & Graziano, F.M. (1983). The safety of administration of penicillamine to penicillin-sensitive individuals. *Arthritis and Rheumatism, 26*, 801–803.

Byron, M.A., & Kirwan, J.R. (1986). Corticosteroids in rheumatoid arthritis: Is a trial of their "disease modifying" potential feasible? *Annals of the Rheumatic Diseases, 46*, 171–173.

Carson, C.W., Cannon, G.W., Egger, M.J., Ward, J.R., & Clegg, D.O. (1987). Pulmonary disease during the treatment of rheumatoid arthritis with low dose pulse methotrexate. *Seminars in Arthritis and Rheumatism, 16*, 186–195.

Cash, J.M., & Klippel, J.H. (1994). Second-line drug therapy for rheumatoid arthritis. *New England Journal of Medicine, 330*, 1368–1375.

Clements, P.J., & Davis, J. (1986). Cytotoxic drugs: Their clinical application to the rheumatic diseases. *Seminars in Arthritis and Rheumatism, 15*, 231.

Cooperative Systematic Studies of the Rheumatic Disease Group. (1987). Toxicity of long-term low dose D-penicillamine therapy in rheumatoid arthritis. *Journal of Rheumatology, 14*, 67–73.

Csuka, M., Carrera, G.F., & McCarty, D. J. (1986). Treatment of intractable rheumatoid arthritis with combined cyclophosphamide, azathioprine, and hydroxycloroquine. *Journal of the American Medical Association, 255*, 2315–2319.

Cupps, T.R., Edgar, L.C., & Fauci, A.S. (1982). Suppression of human B lymphocyte function of cyclophosphamide. *Journal of Immunology, 128*, 2453–2457.

Danneskiold-Samsoe, B., & Grimby, G. (1986a). Muscle morphology and enzymes in proximal and distal muscle groups of lower limb from patients with cortico-steroid treated rheumatoid arthritis: The relationship to maximal isokinetic muscle strength. *Clinical Science, 71*, 685–691.

Danneskiold-Samsoe, B., & Grimby, G. (1986b). The influence of prednisone on the muscle morphology and muscle enzymes in patients with rheumatoid arthritis. *Clinical Science, 71*, 693–701.

Davenport, H.W. (1967). Salicylate damage to the gastric mucosal barrier. *New England Journal of Medicine, 276*, 1307–1310.

Davis, P., Menard, H., Thompson, J., Harth, M., & Beaudet, F. (1985). One year comparative study of gold sodium thiomalate and auranofin in the treatment of rheumatoid arthritis. *Journal of Rheumatology, 12*, 60–67.

Empire Rheumatism Council. (1961). Gold therapy in rheumatoid arthritis: Final report of a multicenter controlled trial. *Annals of the Rheumatic Diseases, 20*, 315–341.

Farr, M., Symmons, P.M., Blake, D.R., & Bacon, P.A. (1986). Neutropenia in patients with inflammatory arthritis treated with sulphasalazine. *Annals of the Rheumatic Diseases, 45*, 761–764.

Forestier, J. (1935). Rheumatoid arthritis and its treatment by gold salts. *Journal of Laboratory and Clinical Medicine, 20*, 827–831.

Freedman, A., & Steinberg, V.L. (1960). Chloroquine in rheumatoid arthritis: A double blindfold trial of treatment for one year. *Annals of the Rheumatic Diseases, 19*, 243–250.

Gerkens, J.F., Shand, D.G., Flexner, C., Nies, A.S., Oates, J.A., & Data, J.L. (1977). The effect of indomethacin and aspirin on gastric blood flow and secretion. *Journal of Pharmacological and Experimental Therapeutics, 203*, 646–651.

Gispen, J.G., Alarcon, G.S., Johnson, J.J., Acton, R.T., Barger, B.O., & Koopman, W.J. (1987). Toxicity to methotrexate in rheumatoid arthritis. *Journal of Rheumatology, 14*, 74.

Gottlieb, N.L., & Gray, R.G. (1978). Diagnosis and management of adverse reactions from gold compounds. *Journal of Analytical Toxicology, 2*, 173–177.

Greene, J.M., & Winickoff, R.N. (1992). Cost-conscious prescribing of nonsteroidal anti-inflammatory drugs for adults with arthritis: A review and suggestions. *Archives of Internal Medicine, 152*, 1995–2002.

Hansen, T.M., Matzen, D., & Madsen, P. (1984). Endoscopic evaluation of the effect of indomethacin capsules and suppositories on the gastric mucosa in rheumatic patients. *Journal of Rheumatology, 11*, 484–487.

Harris, E.D., Emkey, R.D., Nichols, J.E., & Newberg, A. (1983). Low dose prednisone therapy on rheumatoid arthritis: A double blind study. *Journal of Rheumatology, 10*, 713–721.

Hench, P.S., Kendall, E.C., Slocumb, C.H., & Polley, H.F. (1949). The effect of a hormone of the adrenal cortex (17-hydroxy-11-dehydrocorticosterone: compound E) and of pituitary adrenocorticotropic hormone on rheumatoid arthritis. *Proceedings of the Staff Meetings of the Mayo Clinic, 24* (8), 181–197.

Hill, H.F.H. (1977). Treatment of rheumatoid arthritis with penicillamine. *Seminars in Arthritis and Rheumatology, 6*, 361–366.

Hoover, R., & Fraumeni, J.F., Jr. (1973). Risk of cancer in renal transplant recipients. *Lancet, 2*, 55–57.

Jaffe, I.A. (1975). The technique of penicillamine administration in rheumatoid arthritis. *Arthritis and Rheumatism, 18*, 513–520.

Jaffe, I.A. (1993). D-Penicillamine. In W.N. Kelley, E.D. Harris, S. Ruddy, & C.B. Sledge (Eds.), *Textbook of rheumatology* (4th ed., pp. 760–766). Philadelphia: Saunders.

Jaffe, I.A., Scheinberg, H., & Sternlieb, I. (1981). Proceedings of the International Symposium of Penicillamine. *Journal of Rheumatology, 8* (Suppl. 7), 1–181.

Kelley, W.N., Harris, E.D., Ruddy, S., & Sledge, C.B. (Eds.). (1993). *Textbook of rheumatology* (4th ed.). Philadelphia: Saunders.

Kimberly, R.P., & Plotz, P.H. (1979). Aspirin induced depression of renal function. *New England Journal of Medicine, 296*, 1418–1421.

Koch, A.E., Cho, M., Burrows, J., Leibovich, S.J., & Polverini, P.J. (1988). Inhibition of production of macrophage derived angiogenic activity by the anti-rheumatic agents gold sodium thiomalate and auranofin. *Biochemistry and Biophysics Research Communications, 154*, 205–211.

Kremer, J.M., Alarcon, G.S., Lightfoot, R.W., Willkens, R.F., Furst, D.E., Williams, H.J., Dent, P.B., & Weinblatt, M.E. (1994). Methotrexate for rheumatoid arthritis: Suggested guidelines for monitoring liver toxicity. *Arthritis and Rheumatism, 37*, 316–328.

Kremer, J.M., & Lee, J.K. (1988). A long-term prospective study of the use of methotrexate in rheumatoid arthritis: Update after a mean of fifty-three months. *Arthritis and Rheumatism, 31*, 577–589.

Kremer, J.M., Rynes, R.I., & Bartholomew, I. E. (1987). Severe flare of rheumatoid arthritis after discontinuation of long-term methotrexate therapy. *American Journal of Medicine, 82*, 781–786.

Laan, R.F.J.M., Van Riel, P.L.C.M., Van de Platte, L.B.A., Van Erning, L.J.T.O., Van't Hof, M.A., & Lemmens, J.A.M. (1993). Low-dose prednisone induces rapid reversible axial bone loss in patients with rheumatoid arthritis: A randomized controlled study. *Annals of Internal Medicine, 119*, 963–968.

Lipsky, P.E., & Ziff, M. (1977). Inhibition of antigen- and mitogen-induced human lyphocyte proliferation by gold compounds. *Journal of Clinical Investigation, 59*, 455–466.

Lockie, L.M., & Smith, D.M. (1985). Forty-seven years experience with gold therapy in 1,019 rheumatoid arthritis patients. *Seminars in Arthritis and Rheumatism, 14*, 238–246.

Maksymowych, W., & Russell, A.S. (1987). Antimalarials in rheumatology: Efficacy and safety. *Seminars in Arthritis and Rheumatism, 16*, 206–221.

McCarty, D.J., & Csuka, M.E. (1987). Aspirin in the treatment of chronic inflammatory arthritis [Letter to the editor]. *Journal of the American Medical Association, 257*, 1331.

McCarty, D.J., & Koopman, W.J. (Eds.). (1993). *Arthritis and allied conditions* (12th ed.). Philadelphia: Lea & Febiger.

Multicenter Trial Group. (1973). Controlled trial of D-penicillamine in severe rheumatoid arthritis. *Lancet, 1*, 275–276.

O'Brien, W.M. (1986). Radiological evaluation of erosions: A quantitative method for assessing long-term remittive therapy in rheumatoid arthritis. *British Journal of Clinical Pharmacology, 22*, 1735–1825.

Paulus, H.E., Williams, H.J., Ward, J.R., Reading, J.C., Egger, M.J., Coleman, M.L., Samuelson, C.O., Jr., Wilkens, R.F., Guttadauria, M., & Alarcon, G.S. (1984). Azathioprine versus D-penicillamine in rheumatoid arthritis patients who have been treated unsuccessfully with gold. *Arthritis and Rheumatism, 27*, 721–727.

Pinals, R.S. (1988). Rheumatoid arthritis: A pharmacologic overview. *American Family Physician, 37*, 145–152.

Pinals, R.S., Kaplan, S.B., Lawson, J. G., & Hepburn, B. (1986). Sulphasalazine in rheumatoid arthritis: A double-blind placebo-controlled trial. *Arthritis and Rheumatism, 29*, 1427–1434.

Pullar, T., Hunter, J.A., & Capell, H.A. (1987). Effect of sulphasalazine on the radiological progression of rheumatoid arthritis. *Annals of the Rheumatic Diseases, 46*, 398–402.

Roth, S.H. (Ed.). (1985). *Rheumatic therapeutics*. New York: McGraw-Hill.

Rynes, R.I. (1993). Antimalarial drugs. In W.N. Kelley, E.D. Harris, S. Ruddy, & C.B. Sledge (Eds.), *Textbook of rheumatology* (4th ed., pp. 731–742). Philadelphia: Saunders.

Sambrook, P.N., Eismon, J.A., Yeates, M.G., Pocock, N.A., Eberl, S., & Champion, G.D. (1986). Osteoporosis in rheumatoid arthritis: Safety of low dose corticosteroids. *Annals of the Rheumatic Diseases, 45*, 950–953.

Seminars in Arthritis & Rheumatism. (1993). Limitations of randomized clinical trials to recognize possible advantages of combination therapies in rheumatic diseases. *Seminars in Arthritis & Rheumatism, 23* (2, Suppl. 1), 2–10.

Shiokawa, Y., Horiuchi, Y., Honma, M., Kageyama, T., Okada, T., & Azuma, T. (1977). Clinical evaluation of D-penicillamine by multicenter double-blind comparative study in chronic rheumatoid arthritis. *Arthritis and Rheumatism, 20*, 1464–1472.

Sigler, J.W., Bluhm, G.B., Duncan, H., Sharp, J.T., Ensign, D.C., McCrum, W.R. (1974). Gold salts in the treatment of rheumatoid arthritis: A double blind study. *Annals of Internal Medicine, 80*, 21–25.

Srinivasan, R., Miller, B.L., & Paulus, H.E. (1979). Long-term chrysotherapy in rheumatoid arthritis. *Arthritis and Rheumatism, 22*, 105–110.

Urowitz, M.B., Gordon, D.A., Smythe, H.A., Pryzanski, W., & Ogryzlo, M.A. (1973). Azathioprine in rheumatoid arthritis: A double-blind, cross-over study. *Arthritis and Rheumatism*, *16*, 411–418.

Vernon-Roberts, B., Dore, J.L., Jessop, J.D., & Henderson, W.J. (1976). Selective concentration and localization of gold in macrophages of synovial and other tissues during and after chrysotherapy in rheumatoid patients. *Annals of Rheumatic Diseases*, *35*, 477–486.

Weinblatt, M.E. (1985). Toxicity of low dose methotrexate in rheumatoid arthritis. *Journal of Rheumatology*, *12* (Suppl. 12), 35–39.

Weinblatt, M.E., Trentham, D.E., Fraser, P.A., Holdsworth, D.E., Falchuk, K.R., Weissman, B.N., & Coblyn, J.S. (1988). Long-term prospective trial of low dose methotrexate in rheumatoid arthritis. *Arthritis and Rheumatism*, *31*, 167–175.

Wilkins, R.F. (1985). Immunomodulating agents. In S.H. Roth (Ed.), *Rheumatic therapeutics* (pp. 331–332). New York: McGraw-Hill.

Wilske, K.R., & Healey, L.A. (1989). Remodeling the pyramid—A concept whose time has come. *Journal of Rheumatology*, *16*, 565–567.

SUGGESTED READING

Wilske, K.R., & Campbell, P.M. (1987). Network Physician Organization and guidelines for reviewers of rheumatic disease care. *Bulletin on the Rheumatic Diseases*, *37*, 1–10.

CHAPTER 7

Heat and Cold in the Management of Rheumatoid Arthritis

Karen W. Hayes, PhD, PT

HEAT

Effects of Heat

The primary reason for using heat in patients with rheumatoid arthritis (RA) is to decrease pain and stiffness in the joints. Heat decreases pain by washing out pain-producing metabolites with improved blood flow (Lehmann & DaLateur, 1982a) and by temporarily increasing the threshold of the pain-carrying fibers (Lehmann, Brunner, & Stow, 1958). An additional mechanism of pain relief may be the decrease of muscle guarding via effects on the muscle spindle and the golgi tendon organs (Lehmann & DeLateur, 1982a; Mense, 1978). In addition to pain relief, heat can decrease the stiffness associated with joint diseases (Gersten, 1955; Lehmann, Masock, Warren, & Koblanski, 1970). Wright and Johns (1961) found that when the skin temperature over the joints of asymptomatic hands was elevated to 45°C by exposure to infrared radiation, stiffness decreased 20%. Stiffness was also found to decrease with hot water immersion in patients with RA (Backlund & Tiselius, 1967). On the negative side, there is concern that heat may exacerbate the acute inflammatory processes associated with RA (Feibel & Fast, 1976; E.D. Harris & McCroskery, 1974).

Therapeutic Heat Application

Superficial heat can be delivered by infrared lamps, hot packs, heating pads, liquid paraffin, agitated baths, steam cabinets, or warm air circulated through soft, solid particles. All of the superficial heat sources produce electromagnetic waves in the infrared spectrum. These waves penetrate only a few millimeters and produce most of their effects through elevation of skin temperature and subsequent reflex mechanisms. Many superficial heat methods are convenient for home use, and the practitioner should be certain that they are used only with thorough patient education programs.

Deep heat is delivered by conversion of electrical or sound energy via shortwave diathermy (SWD), microwave diathermy (MWD), or ultrasound (US). Deep heat is effective at elevating temperature in muscle and subcutaneous connective tissue and thus produces its effect in different target tissues than superficial heat. In animals, US has been shown to produce increased extensibility in deeply seated connective tissue if combined with a prolonged, low-load, mechanical stretch (Gersten, 1955; Lehmann et al., 1970). The deep-heating agents have more inherent hazards associated with

The author thanks Mary Keen, MD, for her contributions to an earlier version of this chapter.

Source: Reprinted with permission from *Arthritis Care and Research*.

their use and should not be recommended to patients for home use.

Traditionally, most heat treatments are delivered for 20 to 30 minutes to allow the body time to develop maximal heat loss responses such as increased blood flow. After 30 minutes, equilibrium is reached, and the responses are not as strong (Stillwell, 1965). Little research has been performed examining optimal treatment times for specific problems. Intensity of treatment depends on the strength of the desired effects; mild heat produces small change, and stronger heat produces more marked effects. Therapeutic temperatures are considered to be 40°C to 45°C. Ultrasound differs from the other agents in that it is usually delivered for 5 to 10 minutes at intensities between 0.5 W/cm^2 and 3.0 W/cm^2.

Contraindications often are not studied formally. Traditionally, heat has been used with caution or not used in conditions that prevent adequate thermoregulatory responses or impair judgment of heat intensity, or in conditions that would be aggravated or spread by heating. Generalized heat is not used or is used with caution in cases of cardiac insufficiency, impaired cognition, fever, or infection. Localized heat may also be hazardous in conditions involving impaired arterial circulation, impaired sensation, local hemorrhage, malignancy, or inflammation (Lehmann & DeLateur, 1982a).

COLD

Effects of Cold

Cold can also decrease pain and muscle guarding by decreasing nerve conduction velocity or blockading nerve impulses, especially in the smaller nerve fibers; that is, A-delta, A-gamma, and C fibers (Lehmann & DeLateur, 1982b). Recent evidence suggests that part of the effectiveness of cold in decreasing pain may be through the release of endorphins (Utsinger, Bonner, & Hogan, 1982). Cooling decreases blood flow and capillary pressure by causing vasoconstriction and may thereby decrease inflammatory responses and swelling. In contrast to heat, cold has been found to increase connective tissue stiffness. Both Wright and Johns (1961) and Backlund and Tiselius (1967) found increased stiffness in subjects with and without RA when their hands were immersed in ice water. Joint motion can be increased using cold, however, through its pain-relieving action. If motion is limited by pain, either heat or cold may be useful; if it is limited by stiffness, heat may be preferable.

Therapeutic Cold Application

Cold treatments are delivered by means of packs, baths, vapocoolant sprays, or ice massage (a block of ice rubbed over the affected site). Any of the methods may be combined with mobility exercises if desired. The selection of method depends on the depth of the target, the size and accessibility of the part, the strength of the stimulus necessary, and the requirements for positioning. Ice packs and ice massage are very cold stimuli, capable of producing anesthesia. Many commercial packs, on the other hand, are not cold enough to produce true numbness.

Treatment times vary with the goal of treatment. Deeply seated targets, especially if the patient has more than 2 cm of superficial fat, are not cooled in less than 20 to 30 minutes (Lehmann & DeLateur, 1982b). Skin anesthesia, on the other hand, is produced within about 7 minutes (Waylonis, 1967). Treatments of more than 10 minutes will allow tissue temperature to decrease for up to 1 hour post-treatment; with less than 10 minutes of treatment, tissue temperature will return to pretreatment levels in about 10 minutes (Hollander, 1974).

The traditional precautions and contraindications for the use of cold are similar to those listed for heat, such as inadequate thermoregulatory responses and cardiac or vascular insufficiency. In addition, cold is used with extreme caution or not at all with regenerating peripheral nerves, open wounds after 48 hours, hypersensitivity to cold as demonstrated by Raynaud's phenomenon, or cold urticaria (Lehmann & DeLateur, 1982b).

HEAT AND COLD AND RHEUMATOID ARTHRITIS

To determine whether the use of heat and cold is appropriate for patients with RA, several issues must be examined. For example, E.D. Harris and McCroskery (1974) raised the concern that the disease process might be aggravated and that the joint might be further damaged by heating. Do the heating or cooling agents penetrate to the joint and alter intra-articular temperature (IAT)? Is there evidence that the use of heat or cold affects the disease process? If heat and cold do not have deleterious effects on the course of the disease, do they produce significant clinical relief? If there is an impact on the course or clinical symptoms, do heat and cold affect patients differentially depending on the stage of disease? Do patients with RA respond to heat and cold in the same manner as people without RA? Last, if heat and cold are safe and effective to use in patients with RA, do patients with RA express a preference for heat or for cold?

Intra-Articular Temperature of Joints

Role of Intra-Articular Temperature and Blood Flow

Both skin and IAT of patients with RA have been demonstrated to be elevated over that of nondiseased joints by as much as 3.3°C (Horvath & Hollander, 1949). Patients with active synovial reactions demonstrate warmer skin and joint temperature than those with more quiescent conditions. Therefore, there appears to be a positive relationship between both surface and joint temperatures and amount of synovial reaction.

Blood flow is closely correlated with temperature, increasing in response to increased temperature. Using radioactive tracers, R. Harris, Millard, and Banerjee (1958) found a close relationship between blood flow in the knees and clinical evidence of joint involvement in RA. Radioactive clearance was slower for asymptomatic subjects and patients with RA whose knees were unaffected than for patients with major or severe involvement of the knees. The accelerated clearance indicates increased blood flow in the more involved knees.

Because synovitis in RA is associated with both increased joint temperature and blood flow, the effect of increased joint temperature on synovial tissues has been examined in vitro. Studies of the effect of temperature on degradation of cartilage collagen by rheumatoid synovial collagenase demonstrated that collagenolysis was much greater at higher temperatures. At temperatures found in joints with active RA (36°C), collagenolysis was four times greater than at temperatures found in nondiseased knee joints (30°C to 33°C). Collagenolysis was negligible at 30°C (E.D. Harris & McCroskery, 1974). Temperatures greater than 39°C were not studied, so no conclusion can be drawn regarding whether temperatures in the therapeutic range would produce further lysis. When temperatures in the periarticular structures are in therapeutic range, however, IAT may well be in the range at which increased collagenolysis occurs.

Castor and Yaron (1976) addressed the issue of further increase in temperature. They studied nondiseased and rheumatoid synovial cell cultures and the effect of exposure to different temperatures on hyaluronic acid, lactic acid, and glucose production. These products are indicators of synovial metabolic activity, a function of blood flow and inflammation. They found that hyaluronate synthesis, glucose uptake, and lactate production increased dramatically at increased temperatures (32°C to 38°C) in both nondiseased and rheumatoid cell cultures but decreased sharply at 41°C, which is in the therapeutic temperature range. Thus, relatively small changes in joint temperatures caused significant changes in synovial metabolic activity. Both low and high temperatures were associated with lower metabolic activity.

Findings that heat might accelerate joint collagen degradation associated with RA have led to suggestions that perhaps externally applied heat, if it reached the intra-articular space, might actually be deleterious and should not be used (Feibel & Fast, 1976). Although evidence exists that relates elevated joint temperature to collagen destruction (E.D. Harris & McCroskery, 1974), these data were gathered in vitro and may not be relevant clinically. The pattern of lysis and metabolic activity needs further clarification. Although lysis and metabolism increase with increasing temperature, metabolic activity decreases at higher temperatures (Castor & Yaron, 1976) well below the maximum therapeutic temperature of 45°C.

Because elevated IAT and blood flow have been found to correlate closely with the synovial reaction of RA, an agent that decreases IAT or blood flow might decrease the inflammatory process associated with RA. Increased IAT might increase inflammatory activity initially but slow it with further increase in temperature. These suppositions support clinical trials of heat and cold. However, whether clinical heating and cooling agents actually alter the IAT and whether or not alteration of IAT is deleterious must be examined.

Intra-Articular Temperature and Blood Flow

Effects of Superficial Heating

Hot packs, radiant heat, melted paraffin, and Fluidotherapy, a dry heat composed of small particles through which warm air is blown, have been studied for their effects on tissue temperatures and joint blood flow. Hot packs applied to the skin directly over the knee joint for 4 minutes depress IAT by as much as 1.2°C in both asymptomatic subjects and patients with RA. However, 5 to 10 minutes after removal of the hot packs, IAT rises reflexively about 0.8°C, and returns to pretreatment levels within 20 minutes (Horvath & Hollander, 1949). The initial decrease in temperature may be due to reciprocal blood flow between the skin and the deeper structures, shunting blood from deeper structures to the surface as surface vessels dilate. This pattern of reflexive cooling of deeper tissues during short bouts of superficial heating may not occur when standard clinical treatment times of 20 to 30 minutes are used. Knee IAT in patients with RA has been shown to increase about 1°C after 15 minutes of heating with hot packs and remain elevated for 1 hour after treatment was terminated (Weinberger, Fadilah, Lev, & Pinkhas, 1989).

Radiant heat has been shown to cause a 40% increase in blood flow in the knees of asymptomatic subjects, 22% in subjects with mild RA, and a decrease in blood flow of 24% in subjects with more severe RA (R. Harris, 1963). However, the elevation of IAT following radiant heating to the knee joint and surrounding tissue in patients with RA is minimal (Hollander & Horvath, 1949). Radiant heat is absorbed in the superficial layers of the skin and is not transmitted to deeper layers, so it is not surprising that IAT does not change. Changes in blood flow could represent the shunting of blood between the deeper tissues and the skin.

Paraffin is another source of superficial heat that has been shown to produce increases of IAT under certain conditions. In the knees of subjects with RA, IAT increased 1.7°C when paraffin was applied over the knee joint as a pack at 54.5°C, but increased very little (0.4°C) when paraffin was applied at 64.5°C (Hollander & Horvath, 1949). This difference in temperature increase may be due to the difference in the thickness of the paraffin layers. The thermal energy transfer produced by paraffin applications depends on the thickness of the paraffin layer coating the joint, which in turn is controlled by the temperature of the paraffin. Hotter applications melt the layers applied earlier, resulting in a thin layer of wax. Heat is lost to the environment easily, and only superficial temperature change may be produced. Thicker layers, which build up when cooler temperatures of wax are used, may produce greater temperature increases because the paraffin provides greater insulation.

Fluidotherapy has been used to study the capsular and muscular temperatures in the hands and feet (Borell, Parker, Henley, Masley, & Repinecz, 1980). Intra-articular temperature has not been reported. Operating at 47.8°C for an unreported period of time, this agent has produced capsular temperature increases as high as 9°C and muscular temperature increases of 5°C.

Hot packs, radiant heat, paraffin treatments, and Fluidotherapy are all forms of infrared energy that penetrate only a few millimeters. If tissue is slightly compressed (as with hot pack treatments) or if the heating agent prevents convective or radiant heat loss (as with paraffin, hot pack, or Fluidotherapy treatments), heat may penetrate slightly more deeply. If joints are superficial, such as those of the hands and feet, the intra-articular spaces can be heated with superficial heat. The interior of the knee joint is insulated by thicker structures except at the joint line. Superficial heat would be expected to elevate IAT more in the joints of the hands and feet than in the knee. In patients with severe RA, the hypertrophy of the synovial lining may also serve to prevent heat from reaching the joint. Thus, in response to superficial heat, IAT appears to increase only slightly and might decrease as a result of shunting warm blood to the surface (Hollander & Horvath, 1949).

Effects of Deep Heating

Microwave diathermy applied for 15 minutes over the knee joint has caused an increase of IAT of 0.6°C to 4.7°C in patients with RA (Hollander & Horvath, 1949). Intra-articular temperature also increased substantially in one asymptomatic subject and two patients with rheumatoid knee joints after 20 minutes of heating with inductive SWD wrapped around the knee joint, but the increase depended on disease activity. Intra-articular temperature increased 5.7°C in the asymptomatic subject, 5.4°C in the subject with quiescent RA (initial IAT 30°C), but only 2.6°C in the subject with more active RA (initial IAT 35.9°C; Hollander & Horvath, 1949). Shortwave diathermy produces the greatest increase of joint temperature of all heating procedures discussed but produces less increase in patients with active RA than in less involved patients.

The effect of SWD on blood flow in knee joints follows a similar pattern. Shortwave diathermy was applied using condenser electrodes to either side of the knee joint. Asymptomatic subjects showed a 100% increase in blood flow following heating; subjects in early stages of RA showed a 60% increase, but subjects with more severe disease showed a mean decrease in blood flow of 25% (R. Harris, 1961). Subjects who showed decreases in blood flow had initially high circulation, and SWD decreased circulation to levels comparable to postheating values of the asymptomatic and less involved groups, a reduction similar to that produced by intra-articular injection of cortisone. Although change in blood flow has not been correlated with symptomatic change, a reduction of synovial hyperemia might lead to clinical improvement (R. Harris, 1961).

Although not heavily studied, a pattern is suggested. Patients with active knee disease demonstrate increased IAT and blood flow as a result of their disease. With deep heating they have only a small increase or sometimes a decrease in IAT and blood flow, suggesting that deep heating may actually serve to normalize these variables in subjects with RA. The slight increase in IAT, however, is still greater than the increase in IAT produced by superficial heating.

Effects of Cooling

Intra-articular temperature of the knee in asymptomatic subjects and in patients with RA increases in response to treatment with cold packs applied directly over the knee joint for 4 minutes and continues to increase subsequent to removal for another 6 minutes (Horvath & Hollander, 1949). Cold applied for a short period increases joint temperature, but prolonged cooling (more than 10 minutes) with packs or compresses over the knee joint reduces IAT 2°C to 3°C for as long as several hours (Hollander, 1974).

Blood flow in knees of control subjects following application of vapocoolant spray has been shown to decrease sharply (about 40%; R. Harris, 1963). Subjects with mild RA showed a 45% reduction with a rapid return to pretreatment values, and patients with severe, active RA showed a reduction of at least 50% with a more prolonged return to pretreatment values. Local cooling might, therefore, be of some value in RA.

The work just reviewed (R. Harris, 1961; R. Harris et al., 1958; Hollander, 1974; Hollander & Horvath, 1949; Horvath & Hollander, 1949) provides some insight about the responses of joint structures to heat and cold applications directly over the joint. The generalizability of these studies is questionable, however, because the studies had small sample sizes and did not control or discuss somatotype or stage of disease. Baseline IATs and the magnitude of response to hot packs and cold packs differed markedly in summer and winter (Horvath & Hollander, 1949).

The ability of the various heating and cooling agents to elevate IAT in humans has been studied only on joints of the hands, feet, and the knees. Hip joint temperature in pigs has been measured following exposure to US and shown to increase (Lehmann, McMillan, Brunner, & Blumberg, 1959), but inflamed hip joints or human hip joints and their responses have not been studied.

To summarize, in superficial joints of humans, even the superficial heating agents are capable of elevating IAT. Superficial heat raises IAT only slightly when applied for prolonged periods and appears to cool the joint reflexively if applied for less than 10 minutes (Horvath & Hollander, 1949). Deeper heat is capable of substantially increasing IAT in knees and joints of the hands and feet, especially in asymptomatic subjects and patients with quiescent RA. For patients with active RA, local heat via SWD appears to lower blood flow to normal values, albeit temporarily (R. Harris, 1961). Intra-articular temperature is elevated to a lesser extent in patients with active RA than in asymptomatic subjects but is still higher than that produced by superficial heat. Hollander (1974) stated that treatment of inflamed joints with the various forms of SWD and US nearly always exacerbated the inflammation. He suggested that superficial heating of a joint for less than 10 minutes or cooling a joint for more than 10 minutes reduces the inflammatory process and spares the joint further destruction, at least temporarily. However, none of the previous studies report histological evidence suggesting impact on disease progression, nor do they document clinical effects of heating or cooling.

Does the Use of Heat or Cold Alter the Disease Process?

In light of the concern regarding the effect of IAT on the course of RA, the effects of heating and cooling on the disease process should be studied. However, there have been few attempts to study the effect of heat or cold on thc disease process in humans. In one prospective study, R. Harris and Millard (1955) found no change in erythrocyte sedimentation rate (ESR) following treatment of the hands with paraffin bath. In another prospective study, Mainardi, Walter, Spiegel, Goldkamp, and Harris (1979) investigated whether heat accelerated the destructive process of RA as measured by radiography. After determining that an electric mitten was capable of elevating joint temperature in the second metacarpophalangeal joint in a single individual without disease, one hand of patients with RA was heated for 30 minutes twice a day for 2 years. The other hand served as control. Patients were evaluated radiographically for joint destruction initially, at 1 year, and at the end of the study. Relying on the data from the single asymptomatic subject, IAT was not measured in patients. At the end of the 2-year study, 12 of the 17 patients showed evidence of disease progression on radiographs, but there was no significant difference between control and experimental hands. The authors concluded that the application of heat, capable of elevating IAT in an asymptomatic subject, did not affect the progression of the disease as determined radiographically.

This conclusion is somewhat suspect for several reasons. First, the control was not independent. Contralateral responses to heat are known to occur (Lehmann & DeLateur, 1982b; Woodmansey, Collins, & Ernst, 1938) and may have masked differences between the hands. Second, the small sample size may have prevented differences from being detected. Third, radiographic indicators may not be sensitive enough to demonstrate difference in progression.

Other investigators have examined the effect of cold on synovial fluid. Twenty-four subjects with knee synovitis received an ice bag above and below the knee joint for 20 minutes three times a day for 4 weeks (Kangilaski, 1981). Synovial fluid was examined both before and after the course of treatment and demonstrated no changes in pH, white blood cell (WBC) count, T and B lymphocytes, total protein levels, or immune complexes. The investigators concluded that ice did not alter the synovial fluid. If joint fluid constituents are good indicators of disease activity, this study indicates that ice has no effect on the progression of the disease.

Still other investigators have attempted to demonstrate effects of heat and cold on disease progression in animals. Dogs with experimentally produced inflammation in their knee joints have been treated with 4 hours of cold or superficial heat to the joint (Dorwart, Hansell, & Schumacher, 1974). Fluid temperature, WBC counts, joint volume, enzymatic activity (synovial fluid lactate dehydrogenase, lysozyme), and vascularity were measured among other variables. Cold decreased WBC count, fluid volume, and temperature (by 3°C), but did not alter phagocytosis or enzymatic activity. Changes were temporary, lasting less than 24 hours. Conversely, heat increased temperature (by 1°C), WBC count, phagocytosis, and vasodilatation. There were no differences in enzymatic activity or the number of damaged synovial cells. Therefore, the inflammation of acute synovitis may be relieved by cold and slightly aggravated by heat but without apparent damage. However, the dosage used for both heat and cold differed substantially from that used clinically, and dogs have less soft tissue coverage than humans, making them more susceptible to thermal stimuli.

In summary, in spite of evidence that superficial IAT can be changed with most agents and that heating synovial tissues can increase collagen lysis (E.D. Harris & McCroskery, 1974), there is very little evidence to clarify the impact of alteration of joint temperature on disease progression. Synovial fluid appears to be unaltered by cold (Kangilaski, 1981); ESR is unchanged with superficial heat (R. Harris & Millard, 1955); radiographic changes may not be accelerated by heating (Mainardi et al., 1979); and blood flow in the joint appears to be normalized by deep heat (R. Harris, 1961). Enzymatic activity may not be changed with either heat or cold (Dowart et al., 1974). None of these findings suggests deleterious effects of heat on disease progression. The use of cold appears to produce no deleterious effects and perhaps some positive ones on the disease activity. However, in these few studies, sample sizes were small, did not have independent control groups, or both. Subjects may not have been followed for an adequate period of time for changes to appear. Measures used may not have been true indices of disease activity or may not have been sensitive enough to detect change. No histological samples from diseased joints exposed to heat or cold were studied to detect any changes in the collagen. Until this kind of work is done, there is inadequate evidence to support the presence or absence of damage as a result of heating joints. Assuming that there is no harm to the joint from either heat or cold treatment, the effects of either type of treatment on clinical outcomes such as pain and joint motion should be examined.

Symptomatic Relief

Symptomatic responses to heat and cold treatments have been more extensively studied than effects on disease progression. In general, both heat and cold are used for a variety of treatment goals, but cold has been studied little in this population. Cold usually is expected to decrease pain but may increase stiffness. However, significant improvements in range of motion (ROM), as well as strength, function, pain, sleep duration, and oral analgesic intake have resulted from 20-minute cold treatments to the knee joint structures (Kangilaski, 1981).

Studying 10 patients with RA, Halliday-Pegg, Littler, and Littler (1969) also found improvements in pain and stiffness following cold treatment. They studied the effect of exercises following 5-minute ice packs to one surface of the knee and elbow joints or 10-minute intermittent ice immersion to the proximal interphalangeal and metacarpophalangeal joints. Outcome measures were pain, tenderness, stiffness, ROM, and skin temperature. Descriptive data indicated that perceived stiffness improved both immediately after treatment and over the course of treatment in all patients. Pain improved in a similar fashion for 93% of the patients. Ice was not beneficial for complaints of tenderness. For some subjects, ROM improved immediately after treatment and improvement was retained; however, this effect was countered by a number of subjects whose mobility deteriorated following ice treatment. Hands accounted for most of the unfavorable results. Effects appeared to be most beneficial when skin temperature fell 7°C or less. Those patients whose ROM increased may have experienced decreased pain, whereas those whose ROM worsened may have experienced increased connective tissue stiffness with colder skin temperatures. Reported data are difficult to interpret because the investigators did not include a control group or relate symptomatic changes to specific joints and skin temperatures. Outcome measures were not clearly defined.

In contrast, the use of cold on the hands of patients with RA following surgery produced no change in hand volume or pain (Rembe, 1970). Thirty subjects were randomly assigned to a control group or to a group that received ice baths. Pain reports did not differ between the two groups. Hands decreased in volume in the cold-treated group, but the difference was not statistically significant. The small sample size may have prevented the differences from reaching significance. The results of this study, taken with those just discussed, suggest that cold may be effective in decreasing pain for patients with RA. It may also be useful to increase ROM, especially if the limitation results from pain. Cold apparently has no effect on tenderness or swelling.

Heat treatments also have been studied for effectiveness in providing symptomatic relief. Heat is generally expected to decrease both pain and stiffness. In a randomized study, paraffin baths were shown to improve ROM and pain (Hawkes, Care, Dixon, Bird, & Wright, 1985). Daily treatments of the hands with paraffin and exercise were compared with daily treatment using US, faradic bath, and exercise or US and exercise alone. There was no untreated control group. Subjects were assessed on grip strength, interphalangeal joint circumference, visual analogue pain scale, articular index, ROM, dexterity, and functional measures. Compared with pretreatment measures, all groups improved significantly by 3 weeks. There were no differences among groups except for functional scores that were significantly lower for the group receiving US, faradic bath, and exercise. Although the small sample size may have prevented detection of differences among groups, the authors suggested that with no major differences in efficacy being apparent, paraffin and exercises that can be done at home are the most cost effective and convenient treatment.

In contrast, R. Harris and Millard (1955) did not find positive effects of paraffin bath in their controlled, randomized study of RA patients with hand involvement. Ninety subjects were divided into a control group and two experimental groups that received a six-layer paraffin glove at 43.3°C for 20 minutes per day for 3 or 6 weeks. Patients were evaluated weekly for 6 weeks for tenderness, pain, swelling, grip strength, and dexterity. Data were consolidated to assign an overall grade of progress. Patients also ranked their improvement on a 5-point scale. Although only descriptive statistics were reported, all three groups changed very little and in a similar fashion. At the end of 6 weeks the group receiving 3 weeks of paraffin treatment had improved the least and the group receiving 6 weeks of paraffin improved slightly more than the other two groups. The authors concluded that paraffin treatments were of little value in the treatment of RA. The usual treatment temperature for paraffin bath is 52.2°C (Hayes, 1992), however, and wax gloves cool quickly (Stimson, Rose, & Nelson, 1958). Perhaps continuous immersion in warmer paraffin would produce changes because the tissue temperature can be maintained at a higher level for a longer time.

More recently, Dellhag, Wollersjö, and Bjelle (1992) conducted a controlled, randomized trial of paraffin bath treatments alone compared with exercise alone and in combination with paraffin bath treatments. They also included an untreated control group. Fifty-two patients with RA of the hands and wrists were treated three times a week for 4 weeks. At the end of the treatment period, flexion and extension ROM and grip function in the nondominant hand had improved significantly in the group receiving paraffin bath and exercise. Flexion ROM in the dominant hand, pain on unresisted movement, and stiffness had improved significantly in the group receiving exercise only. The groups receiving paraffin alone and the control groups did not exhibit any changes. A between-group analysis demonstrated that exercise with and without paraffin contributed to increased ROM and decreased pain compared with the controls. Grip function was better in the group receiving the combined treatment compared with all other groups. Except for grip function, paraffin added little benefit to treatment compared with exercise alone.

It is unclear whether the evaluators were blinded to group assignment in this study; it also has a small sample size. The study does suggest, however, that exercise may be the intervention that is most beneficial for patients.

Mainardi and associates (1979) also found no change in clinical signs of inflammation, joint tenderness, swelling, and grip strength following treatment to the hand with superficial heat. In addition, most of their patients did not feel it provided long-term benefit or effect on morning stiffness.

Ultrasound was used by Newman and Murphy (1952) to treat patients with a variety of rheumatological diseases, including RA. These patients had not responded to other forms of management. Joint areas of 14 patients with RA involving the knees, wrist, and elbows were treated with 20 minutes of US at 2.5 W/cm^2 to 3 W/cm^2, three times a week for 1 month. Of the 14 patients, 8 had decreased swelling and stiffness, 4 had decreased tenderness, and 10 had increased mobility and decreased pain. Symptoms of four of the subjects were unchanged. No patient developed increased symptoms. No statistical analysis was done in this uncontrolled study. The dosage of US used by Newman and Murphy (1952) is strong and long. It is possible that, if the dose were closer to that commonly used clinically, results would have been less favorable. Clinicians may want to consider more aggressive dosage for the periarticular structures of this patient population but should try to avoid focusing the treatment directly over inflamed joints.

These studies using heat for symptomatic management of patients with RA suggest that heat may be effective in decreasing pain and stiffness, perhaps increasing mobility and function. Dosage should be adequately strong to produce the effects desired, especially to decrease stiffness. Heat appears to have little effect on tenderness, swelling, or strength.

Given that both heat and cold can improve pain and joint motion, the effectiveness of heat and cold in managing symptoms should be compared. Kirk and Kersley (1968) compared hot packs and ice in treating the knee joints of patients with RA. Twenty knees of 14 subjects were treated in a crossover study with five daily treatments of ice and five daily treatments of hot packs separated by a week without treatment. Evaluations of pain, stiffness, ROM, knee circumference, and skin temperature were made before intervention, at crossover, and at the end of the trial. Pain, stiffness, and ROM improved with both heat and cold, with no significant difference between the two methods. Knee circumference and knee skin temperature decreased slightly with both heat and cold.

Utsinger and colleagues (1982) treated the knee joints of 100 patients with RA for a week with 20-minute ice packs followed by a week of evaluation, a week of 20-minute hot pack treatment, and another week of cold treatments. Outcome measures were ROM, strength, circumference, pain, function, and sleep duration. All subjects improved on at least one outcome measure, and the authors concluded that both heat and cold were effective in decreasing pain and improving function.

A pilot study that compared ice to hot packs in treating patients with RA affecting the shoulder also found no differences between heat and cold (Williams, Harvey, & Tannenbaum, 1986). Eighteen subjects were randomly assigned to receive a 20-minute hot pack or a 20-minute ice pack to the shoulder joint area. Both groups received exercise for the cervical spine and both upper extremities. Subjects were evaluated blindly for pain and ROM using the McGill Pain Questionnaire and an electrogoniometer before intervention and after 3 weeks of treatment three times per week. The majority of patients in both groups experienced decreases in pain levels. There were no significant differences between groups for either pain or ROM; the group that received ice showed a slightly greater pain reduction whereas the group receiving heat had slightly better joint motion, a result not surprising in light of previous work on joint stiffness (Wright & Johns, 1961).

In summary, both heat and cold appear to be effective in managing pain, stiffness, and limitation of motion (Kirk & Kersley, 1968; Utsinger et al., 1982; Williams et al., 1986). Heat may be more effective for joint motion, and cold may be better for pain reduction (Williams et al., 1986). Neither seems to be particularly effective in decreasing tenderness or swelling.

Few of these studies were well controlled or had adequate sample sizes. None of the studies appeared to consider the effect of the amount of adipose tissue on the outcomes of their studies. The amount of soft tissue, especially adipose tissue, affects the depth of penetration of heating or cooling agents. Treatments were applied to the skin overlying the involved joint. Because these studies were clinical, they did not include measurements of actual temperature change in tissues deep to the skin, so it is unclear whether periarticular or articular structures actually experienced altered temperatures. Controlled, randomized, blinded studies with large samples and controls for soft tissue thickness will shed more light on the efficacy of these agents in controlling clinical symptoms.

Disease Stage

Heat and cold appear to be effective for many patients with RA, but the results have been inconsistent. Perhaps the inconsistency is due to patients being in different stages of disease or having different levels of disease activity at the time of study. Several investigators have recorded disease stage and activity and related them to clinical response, inflammatory response, and blood flow. A major problem in summarizing these studies is that terms have not been defined consistently. Acute, active, severe, advanced, and chronic have all been used. Each of these terms could have a different meaning to different investigators. In general, disease stage is a severity measure relating to the extent of anatomical damage. Disease activity relates to the amount of inflammation.

In patients with acute disease, cold has been equally or more effective than heat in increasing motion and decreasing pain (Kirk & Kersley, 1968; Utsinger et al., 1982). Hollander and Horvath (1949) argue that heat aggravates patients with active inflammation. Patients with advanced disease appear to achieve more improvement in ROM with heat than cold (Williams et al., 1986). These conclusions are extended in animal studies of acute and chronic inflammatory response in dogs (Dowart et al., 1974). Cold decreases the tissue response in acute inflammation but has no effect on chronic inflammation.

Joint blood flow has been studied in relation to disease stage and activity and found to decrease in response to SWD in patients with severe, active disease (R. Harris, 1961). Asymptomatic subjects and subjects with inactive disease demonstrated marked increase in joint blood flow. Subjects with active disease already had high blood flow, and SWD decreased these values to within normal limits.

Because no clinical studies have specifically addressed disease stage and activity, data are not sufficient to resolve whether patients respond differently depending on these factors. Until further information is available, it is probably wise to use cold with acute patients and heat only when patients are not actively inflamed. Research must be conducted comparing responses to heat and cold of subjects with active and inactive disease. Patients may also differ in their responses to treatment depending on other characteristics of the disease. Determining differential response to treatment is fundamental to selecting proper management methods.

Physiological Responses

If heat and cold have symptomatic benefit for patients with RA, it is important to be certain that there are no physiological responses demonstrated by patients with RA that might prove harmful. Several authors have suggested that patients with RA have a higher frequency of vasomotor instability than subjects without the disease (Naide, Sayen, & Comroe, 1945; Short, Bauer, & Reynolds, 1957; Steinbrocker & Samuels, 1941). The instability has been attributed to an overactive sympathetic nervous system (Short et al., 1957).

Disturbed vasomotor responses of patients with RA affect their tolerance and ability to respond appropriately to heat and cold. Patients with RA have slower vasodilatation in the feet when exposed to warm environments (Martin, Roth, Elkins, & Krusen, 1946). Subjects with RA are unable to tolerate extended periods of cold exposure. Although there is not a constant deficit in vasomotor response, patients with RA have more sluggish vasoconstriction in response to cold and complain of increased stiffness (Martin et al., 1946). Sluggish vasoconstriction is worse in women than in men (Woodmansey et al., 1938).

Patients with RA experience lower skin temperatures during local cold exposure and return to baseline temperature significantly more slowly. The vasoconstriction following local cold treatment is more marked and prolonged in patients with RA than in subjects without disease (Fricke & Gersten, 1952). Vasospasm in response to cold exposure is not uncommon in patients with RA (Naide et al., 1945; Short et al., 1957; Steinbrocker & Samuels, 1941). Smokers with RA who receive local cold treatments experience more pain during treatment than nonsmoking patients with RA, presumably because smoking aggravates the vasospasms already present (Helliwell, Wallace, & Evard, 1989). Because of the concern for the vasomotor responses of these patients, when using cold, clinicians should monitor these patients closely to ensure that the vascular supply to the skin remains adequate to maintain tissue integrity.

Changes in vasomotor responses to generalized cold and warm exposures are also characteristic of aging (Wagner & Horvath, 1985). Age could confound studies investigating thermoregulation. In any of the studies cited, the oldest subject with disease was 54, and the majority of the subjects in all studies were in their 20s and 30s, making age an unlikely cause for change in vascular response. None of these studies specifically examined the relationship between change in vascular response and age.

In addition to vasomotor instability, patients with RA may have other systemic manifestations of connective tissue disease. Vasculitis can occur in patients at any stage of the disease process and in patients with minimal impairment or deformity. By affecting the small arterioles, vasculitis may affect response to heat and cold agents by preventing the vasomotor responses necessary to lose or conserve heat. Vasculitis in patients with RA is frequently associated with peripheral neuropathy, presumably ischemic in origin (Dyck, Conn, & Okazaki, 1972). Peripheral neuropathy may further impair vasomotor responses to heat or cold as well as cause sensory impairment, predisposing a patient to thermal injury.

To summarize, patients with RA are not as tolerant of high or low temperatures as those who do not have the disease (Fricke & Gersten, 1952; Martin et al., 1946; Woodmansey et al., 1938). This difference in response appears to be unrelated to the aging process. These patients should be monitored closely to ensure an adequate vascular response to maintain tissue viability locally and core temperature generally when heat and cold treatments are used. Serious problems have not been reported, but further research to determine the extent of the risk for these patients is indicated.

Preference for Heat or Cold

Both heat and cold have been shown to be effective in symptomatic management of RA, many times for the same therapeutic goal. Assuming that patients exhibit no vascular or neurological conditions prohibiting the use of either heat or cold, the preference of the patient may be the best determinant for treatment selection. In Kirk and Kersley's study (1968) subjects improved in mobility and pain measures with both treatments. There were no significant differences in effectiveness between treatments, although the tendency was in favor of cold. Similarly, patients preferred ice to heat by a margin that was not statistically significant.

In the study by Williams et al. (1986), both heat and cold produced positive changes in pain reduction and mobility. However, in spite of effective pain reduction and mobility improvement with ice, at the end of the study most of the subjects in the ice group asked to be treated with heat.

Of the subjects studied by Utsinger et al. (1982), 50 preferred heat, 32 preferred cold, and 18 had no preference. Subjects who preferred cold were, in general, more inflamed and earlier in the course of their disease. Both heat and cold appeared to be effective in the symptomatic management of patients with RA. Preference may be related to perceived benefit.

There appear to be no major differences between heat and cold in clinical outcome or patient preference. Historically, heat has been preferred, and patients still may select heat if given the choice. However, in the few studies that have examined this issue, once cold has been tried and results have been positive for a particular patient, cold is often preferred. Symptomatic relief appears to be more of a concern to some patients than the comfort of the treatment.

CONCLUSION

Several issues regarding the use of heat and cold treatments with patients with RA have been explored in this review. Heat can increase IAT if applied for more than 10 minutes, and prolonged cold application can cool the joint. It remains unclear, however, whether heat applied to involved joints is deleterious; consequently, heat applied to inflamed joints would best be avoided until this issue is resolved. Both heat and cold appear to contribute to improved pain, muscle guarding, stiffness, and limitation of motion, but not to tenderness or swelling. The research suggests the use of cold during the acute phase to decrease inflammation and pain. During the chronic phase, both heat and cold have been effective depending on the therapeutic goal in question. The vasomotor responses of patients with RA often are different from those of patients without disease and should be monitored carefully to ensure tissue integrity and core temperature stability. Patients with RA often prefer the agent that provides them with the most benefit.

Many questions remain regarding the use of heating and cooling agents for patients with RA. For example, the question of effectiveness of heat or cold depending on disease stage or activity is as yet unclear. Cold has been shown to have positive effects during the acute phase, but evidence does not consistently show negative effects of heat in the acute phase. The issue of whether joints of patients with RA are damaged by heating also requires further study. Future research in this area should control for body size and type and provide control groups, adequate sample sizes, blinded evaluators, and clear definitions of outcome measures, disease stage, and disease activity.

Heat and cold treatments have a role in the management of patients with RA, but the selection of treatment must be carefully made, considering the disease stage, disease activity, the safety of the agent, the effectiveness of the treatment, the need to continue the treatment at home, and the patient's preferences. The studies reviewed in this paper can help health professionals make informed decisions regarding the safest and most cost-effective treatment.

REFERENCES

Backlund, L., & Tiselius, P. (1967). Objective measurement of joint stiffness in rheumatoid arthritis. *Acta Rheumatologica Scandinavica*, *13*, 275–288.

Borrell, R.M., Parker, R., Henley, E.J., Masley, D., & Repinecz, M. (1980). Comparison of in vivo temperatures produced by hydrotherapy, paraffin wax treatment, and Fluidotherapy. *Physical Therapy*, *60*, 1273–1276.

Castor, C.W., & Yaron, M. (1976). Connective tissue activation: VIII, The effects of temperature studied in vitro. *Archives of Physical Medicine and Rehabilitation*, *57*, 5–9.

Dellhag, B., Wollersjö, I., & Bjelle, S. (1992). Effect of active hand exercise and wax bath treatment in rheumatoid arthritis patients. *Arthritis Care Research*, *5*, 87–92.

Dorwart, B.B., Hansell, J.R., & Schumacher, H.R., Jr. (1974). Effects of cold and heat on urate crystal-induced synovitis in the dog. *Arthritis and Rheumatism*, *17*, 563–571.

Dyck, P.J., Conn, D.L., & Okazaki, H. (1972). Necrotizing angiopathic neuropathy: Three-dimensional morphology of fiber degeneration related to sites of occluded vessels. *Mayo Clinic Proceedings*, *47*, 461–475.

Feibel, A., & Fast, A. (1976). Deep heating of joints: A reconsideration. *Archives of Physical Medicine and Rehabilitation*, *57*, 513–514.

Fricke, F.J., & Gersten, J.W. (1952). Effect of contrast baths on the vasomotor response of rheumatoid arthritis patients. *Archives of Physical Medicine*, *33*, 210–216.

Gersten, J.W. (1955). Effect of ultrasound on tendon extensibility. *American Journal of Physical Medicine*, *34*, 362–369.

Halliday-Pegg, S.M., Littler, T.R., & Littler, E.N. (1969). A trial of ice therapy and exercise in chronic arthritis. *Physiotherapy Canada*, *55*, 51–56.

Harris, E.D., Jr., & McCroskery, P.A. (1974). The influence of temperature and fibril stability on degradation of cartilage collagen by rheumatoid synovial collagenase. *New England Journal of Medicine*, *290*, 1–6.

Harris, R. (1961). Effect of short wave diathermy on radio-sodium clearance from the knee joint in the normal and in rheumatoid arthritis. *Archives of Physical Medicine*, *42*, 241–249.

Harris, R. (1963). The effect of various forms of physical therapy on radiosodium clearance from the normal and arthritic knee joint. *Annals of Physical Medicine*, *7*, 7–10.

Harris, R., & Millard, J.B. (1955). Paraffin-wax baths in the treatment of rheumatoid arthritis. *Annals of the Rheumatic Diseases*, *14*, 278–282.

Harris, R., Millard, J.B., & Banerjee, S.K. (1958). Radio-sodium clearance from the knee joint in rheumatoid arthritis. *Annals of the Rheumatic Diseases*, *17*, 189–195.

Hawkes, J., Care, G., Dixon, J.S., Bird, H.A., & Wright, V. (1985). Comparison of three physiotherapy regimens for hands with rheumatoid arthritis. *British Medical Journal*, *291*, 1016.

Hayes, K.W. (1992). *Manual for physical agents* (4th ed.). Norwalk, CT: Appleton & Lange.

Helliwell, P., Wallace, F., & Evard, F. (1989). Smoking and ice therapy in rheumatoid arthritis. *Physiotherapy*, *75*, 551–552.

Hollander, J.L. (1974). Collagenase, cartilage and cortisol [Editorial]. *New England Journal of Medicine*, *290*, 50–51.

Hollander, J.L., & Horvath, S.M. (1949). The influence of physical therapy procedures on the intraarticular temperature of normal and arthritic subjects. *American Journal of the Medical Sciences*, *218*, 543–548.

Horvath, S.M., & Hollander, J.L. (1949). Intraarticular temperature as a measure of joint reaction. *Journal of Clinical Investigation*, *28*, 469–473.

Kangilaski, J. (1981). "Baggietherapy": Simple pain relief for arthritis knees [News]. *Journal of the American Medical Association*, *246*, 317–318.

Kirk, J.A., & Kersley, G.D. (1968). Heat and cold in the physical treatment of rheumatoid arthritis of the knee: A controlled clinical trial. *Annals of Physical Medicine*, *9*, 270–274.

Lehmann, J.F., Brunner, G.D., & Stow, R.W. (1958). Pain threshold measurements after therapeutic application of ultrasound, microwaves and infrared. *Archives of Physical Medicine*, *39*, 560–565.

Lehmann, J.F., & DeLateur, B.J. (1982a). Therapeutic heat. In J.F. Leymann (Ed.), *Therapeutic heat and cold* (3rd ed.). Baltimore: Williams & Wilkins.

Lehmann, J.F., & DeLateur, B.J. (1982b). Cryotherapy. In J.F. Leymann (Ed.), *Therapeutic heat and cold* (3rd ed.). Baltimore: Williams & Wilkins.

Lehmann, J.F., Masock, A.J., Warren, C.G., & Koblanski, J.N. (1970). Effect of therapeutic temperatures on tendon extensibility. *Archives of Physical medicine*, *51*, 481–487.

Lehmann, J.F., McMillan, J.A., Brunner, G.D., & Blumberg, J.B. (1959). Comparative study of the efficiency of shortwave, microwave and ultrasonic diathermy in heating the hip joint. *Archives of Physical Medicine*, *40*, 510–512.

Mainardi, C.L., Walter, J.M., Spiegel, P.K., Goldkamp, O.G., & Harris, E.D., Jr. (1979). Rheumatoid arthritis: Failure of daily heat therapy to affect its progression. *Archives of Physical Medicine and Rehabilitation*, *60*, 390–393.

Martin, G.M., Roth, G.M., Elkins, E.C., & Krusen, F.H. (1946). Cutaneous temperature of the extremities of normal subjects and of patients with rheumatoid arthritis. *Archives of Physical Medicine*, *27*, 665–682.

Mense, S. (1978). Effects of temperature on the discharges of muscle spindles and tendon organs. *Pfluegers Archiv European Journal of Physiology*, *374*, 159–166.

Naide, M., Sayen, A., & Comroe, B.I. (1945). Characteristic vascular pattern in patients with rheumatoid arthritis. *Archives of Internal Medicine*, *76*, 139–142.

Newman, M.K., & Murphy, A.J. (1952). Application of ultrasonics in chronic rheumatic diseases. *Journal of the Michigan State Medical Society*, *51*, 1213–1215.

Rembe, E.C. (1970). Use of cryotherapy on the postsurgical rheumatic hand. *Physical Therapy*, *50*, 19–23.

Short, C.L., Bauer, W., & Reynolds, W.E. (1957). *Rheumatoid arthritis: A definition of the disease and a clinical description based on a numerical study of 293 patients and controls.* Cambridge, MA: Harvard University Press.

Steinbrocker, O., & Samuels, S.S. (1941). The arterial circulation of the lower extremities in chronic arthritis. *Journal of Laboratory and Clinical Medicine*, *26*, 974–980.

Stillwell, G.K. (1965). General principles of thermotherapy. In S. Licht (Ed.), *Therapeutic heat and cold* (2nd ed.). Baltimore: Williams & Wilkins.

Stimson, C.W., Rose, G.B., & Nelson, P.A. (1958). Paraffin bath as thermotherapy: An evaluation. *Archives of Physical Medicine*, *39*, 219–227.

Utsinger, P.D., Bonner, F., & Hogan, N. (1982). The efficacy of cryotherapy (CR) and thermotherapy in the management of rheumatoid arthritis (RA) pain: Evidence for an endorphin effect [Abstract]. *Arthritis and Rheumatism*, *25*, S113.

Wagner, J.A., & Horvath, S.M. (1985). Influences of age and gender on human thermoregulatory responses to cold exposures. *Journal of Applied Physiology*, *58*, 180–186.

Waylonis, G.W. (1967). The physiologic effects of ice massage. *Archives of Physical Medicine*, *48*, 37–42.

Weinberger, A., Fadilah, R., Lev, A., & Pinkhas, J. (1989). Intra-articular temperature measurements after superficial heating. *Scandinavian Journal of Rehabilitation Medicine*, *21*, 55–57.

Williams, J., Harvey, J., & Tannenbaum, H. (1986). Use of superficial heat versus ice for rheumatoid arthritic shoulder: A pilot study. *Physiotherapy Canada*, *38,* 8–13.

Woodmansey, A., Collins, D.H., & Ernst, M.M. (1938). Vascular reactions to the contrast bath in health and in rheumatoid arthritis. *Lancet*, *2*, 1350–1353.

Wright, V., & Johns, R.J. (1961). Quantitative and qualitative analysis of joint stiffness in normal subjects and in patients connective tissue diseases. *Annals of the Rheumatic Diseases*, *20*, 36–46.

CHAPTER 8

Exercise for the Person with Rheumatoid Arthritis

Sharon V. Feldmann, MS, PT

Until recently, exercise has been perceived as detrimental to the patient with rheumatoid arthritis (RA). Health care professionals feared that movement of joints with RA could cause further joint destruction and exacerbation of the disease process because of the increased stresses that exercise places on joint and periarticular structures. More recent evidence, however, suggests that carefully prescribed and monitored exercise is not detrimental, but might actually inhibit some of the articular and systemic effects of the disease (Nordemar, Ekblom, Zachrisson, & Lundqvist, 1981).

MUSCULOSKELETAL EFFECTS OF RHEUMATOID ARTHRITIS

As mentioned in earlier chapters, RA can have multiple effects on the musculoskeletal system. Pain is a common symptom in RA and may be local or diffuse. Pain is known to have an inhibitory effect on neuromuscular function, and can lead to self-imposed immobilization as well. Immobilization can lead to further pain because of impaired circulation and lack of disposal of metabolic waste products in various tissues.

Joint swelling is another common symptom of RA. The inflammatory nature of the disease often leads to joint effusion, which can have secondary effects on joint function. Swelling can cause altered joint positions in static postures and during movement, and as such can cause abnormal stresses on joint structures during activity. Increased joint pressure from swelling might also inhibit neuromuscular function, further altering joint mechanics and stresses.

Stiffness and loss of motion can affect both joint and periarticular structures. Again, changes in joint mechanics due to loss of motion can lead to abnormal stresses on involved tissues, causing damage not directly related to the disease process. Decreased motion can also lead to disuse atrophy of involved muscles, contributing to weakness, another common complaint in patients with RA.

Weakness is believed to be due to a combination of disuse and primary disease process (Ekdahl & Broman, 1992). Muscular control is an essential element in joint stability, and in the rheumatoid joint this muscular stabilization is especially important. Without adequate strength in the muscles surrounding involved joints, the resultant instability can lead to further joint damage.

Fatigue is a more systemic effect that is a cardinal symptom of RA. It can be caused by a decrease in aerobic capacity, that is, a decrease in the efficiency of the cardiovascular system. This symptom, too, is believed to be a combination of primary disease process and general deconditioning due to immobility (Ekdahl & Broman, 1992).

Many of the symptoms associated with RA, including stiffness, loss of motion, weakness, fatigue, and sometimes pain, are also sequelae of immobilization in the general population. One must question whether these symptoms in the patient with RA are a direct result of the disease process alone or whether the self-imposed or medically prescribed immobility intended to slow disease activity also contributes.

The ultimate concern of any patient is loss of function. The pain, swelling, stiffness, weakness, and fatigue associated with RA can all contribute to loss of function in patients with the disease. Obviously, the more symptoms present, the more function tends to be impaired. The main goal of any treatment regimen should be to maintain or restore the highest level of function possible. This means addressing each potential cause of limitation.

BENEFITS OF EXERCISE FOR RHEUMATOID ARTHRITIS

The benefits of exercise in the general population are well documented (Astrand, 1987), and the application to RA is becoming more widely studied (Semble, Loeser, & Wise, 1990). It is possible that each of the major signs and symptoms of RA may be affected by exercise as a treatment modality.

Pain

Exercise causes a release of β-endorphins; endogenous opiates that have analgesic effects. Plasma endorphin levels have been shown to increase in response to increased intensity and frequency of exercise (Astrand, 1987). Ekdahl, Ekman, Andersson, Melander, and Svensson (1990) suggest that exercise can have a direct effect on pain due to RA via this β-endorphin mechanism.

Pain may be modulated directly by another mechanism as well. Joint receptors that are stimulated by joint movement are believed to have inhibitory effects on pain signals arising from the same joint. Stenstrom, Lindell, Swanberg, Harms-Ringdahl, and Nordemar (1990) suggest the use of functional training (ie, physical exercise) as a primary modality in the treatment of pain caused by RA.

Swelling

Joint swelling can be affected by movement, especially by weight-bearing activity, which causes alternating compression and decompression of joint surfaces. Several studies have shown that vigorous exercise can lead to a decrease in the number of swollen joints in subjects with RA (Lyngberg, Danneskiold-Samsoe, & Halskov, 1988; Perlman et al., 1990).

Loss of Motion

Exercise can have beneficial effects on mobility of periarticular structures, including joint capsule, ligament, tendon, and muscle. Movement of joint and periarticular tissues produces stresses necessary to cause changes at the cellular level that lead to improved mobility, as well as increased tensile strength to better withstand day-to-day stresses (Astrand, 1987).

Osteoporosis

Bone is another periarticular tissue that can be affected beneficially by exercise. Both immobility and the primary disease processes associated with RA can cause decreased bone density. Some medications used in the treatment of RA, especially corticosteroids, can also contribute to demineralization. Weight-bearing exercise is known to place adequate stresses on bone to stimulate calcium absorption into bone and increase density and compressive strength.

Weakness

Weakness caused by disuse or immobilization of muscles can be reversed with strengthening exercise. Muscle proteins increase, and the strength of connective tissue within and around muscles can also be increased with this type of training (Astrand, 1987).

Fatigue

Fatigue is a symptom that can be affected positively by exercise as well. Aerobic exercise, which stresses the cardiovascular and respiratory systems, can cause changes in cardiac and vascular tissue, as well as in muscle at the cellular level. All of these changes lead to more efficient transport of oxygen and nutrients to working tissues and transport of waste products away from them. Increased functional capacity and less fatigue for the system results. This effect has been shown to occur in subjects with RA (Minor, Hewett, Webel, Anderson, & Kay, 1989; Perlman et al., 1990).

A well-rounded exercise program, then, will include elements to affect pain, swelling, stiffness, weakness, and fatigue. A program that includes flexibility training, strength training, and cardiovascular conditioning should address all of these symptoms. The inclusion of specific functional training as part of the exercise program can optimize the patient's function further. For example, for the patient who wishes to improve stair-climbing ability, climbing stairs should be included in the program. This principle of specificity of training is discussed later.

EXERCISE ASSESSMENT

Before prescribing an exercise program for the patient with RA, the patient's disease activity, functional status, resources, and expectations must be evaluated. Start with a medical work-up to determine the current level of disease activity as well as the patient's functional status. Because inflammation waxes and wanes in RA, reassess the patient's status at each visit. The amount of joint inflammation will determine the appropriate level of exercise activity at a given time.

Functional ability can also be formally measured by using patient self-report questionnaires. The Arthritis Impact Measurement Scale (AIMS; Meenan, Gertman, & Mason, 1980) and the Health Assessment Questionnaire (HAQ; Fries, Spitz, Kraines, & Holman, 1980) are examples of patient surveys that have been documented as valid and reliable measures of patient status and can also be used to document changes in status over time.

Cardiovascular function can be assessed using maximal treadmill stress tests. Patients with RA, however, might have difficulty performing such tests, especially if lower extremity joints are involved. Submaximal bicycle or upper extremity ergometer tests can give reliable information on which to base an exercise prescription, while minimizing musculoskeletal stresses and possible patient apprehension (Figure 8–1). Both the YMCA and the American College of Sports Medicine (ACSM) have published submaximal bicycle protocols (Heyward, 1991) that are relatively easy to administer in the clinic, yet accurately predict maximal functional capacities.

In the patient with known cardiovascular disease or in one who is at risk for disease, even submaximal stress testing should be carried out under the supervision of a physician (ACSM, 1991). In the absence of these factors, however, an experienced therapist or exercise physiologist can safely perform submaximal exercise testing. The practitioner experienced in treating RA will be able to modify equipment and patient positioning as necessary to limit effects of joint and muscle limitations. Patients with assistive devices or orthotics should use these devices during testing to get an accurate picture of overall function.

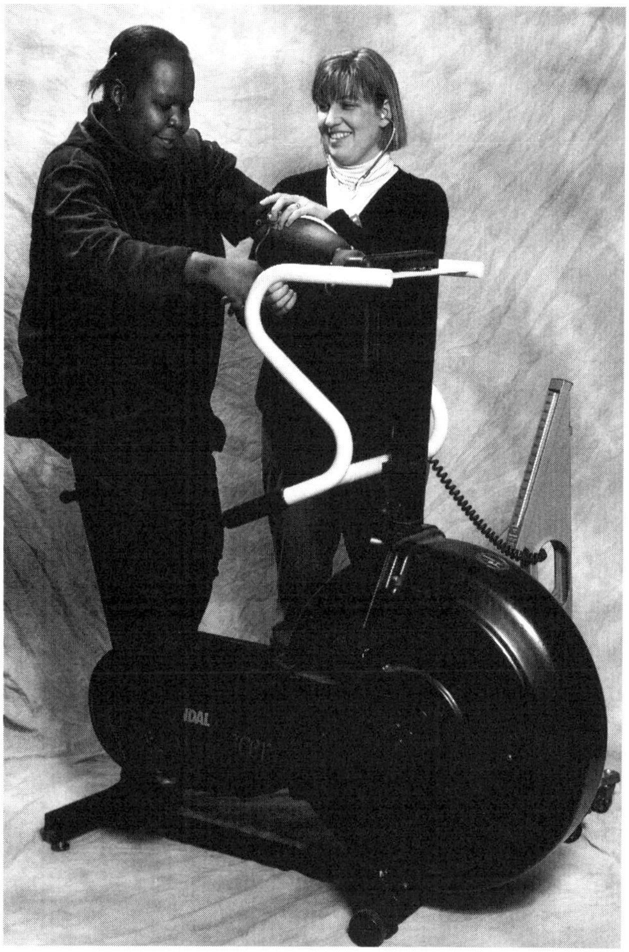

Figure 8–1 Exercise testing can provide a basis for exercise prescription. The patient with RA can be positioned to account for deformities.

Joint mobility and muscle flexibility should be assessed to determine a starting level and the need for stretching versus maintenance range of motion (ROM) exercises. Areas of hypermobility or instability also should be identified, because exercises will need to be modified to prevent further damage. Goniometric measurements can be used to document joint mobility and muscle flexibility (Figure 8–2). Joint instability measurement is usually somewhat more subjective based on the tester's interpretation of joint stress tests such as drawer tests at the knee.

Muscle strength can be assessed using isokinetic equipment or the more traditional manual techniques (Figure 8–3). The one-time or 10-repetition maximal tests are frequently used to determine baseline strength in the general population, but should be used with caution in the patient with RA. Joint mobility, both limited and excessive, must be considered in this type of test, as it requires movement of a resistance through a ROM. The traditional manual muscle test is an isometric test, and is a safer alternative. This method is not as exact in determining a baseline level for starting a strength-training program using weights, but in a clinical setting where patient outcomes are the primary focus a ballpark starting point is adequate.

The patient's goals and resources should also be determined before prescribing an exercise program. The patient who is very apprehensive about exercising may need more supervision and guidance than one who is used to and more comfortable with exercising. The patient who has limited resources should not be set up on a program involving complicated or expensive equipment.

SPECIAL CONSIDERATIONS FOR EXERCISE FOR THE PATIENT WITH RHEUMATOID ARTHRITIS

Several considerations must be weighed before an exercise program can be prescribed for the patient with RA. Rheumatoid arthritis is not a homogeneous disease, and as such, does not affect two patients alike. Exercise prescription must be individualized, taking into account each patient's specific problems and goals.

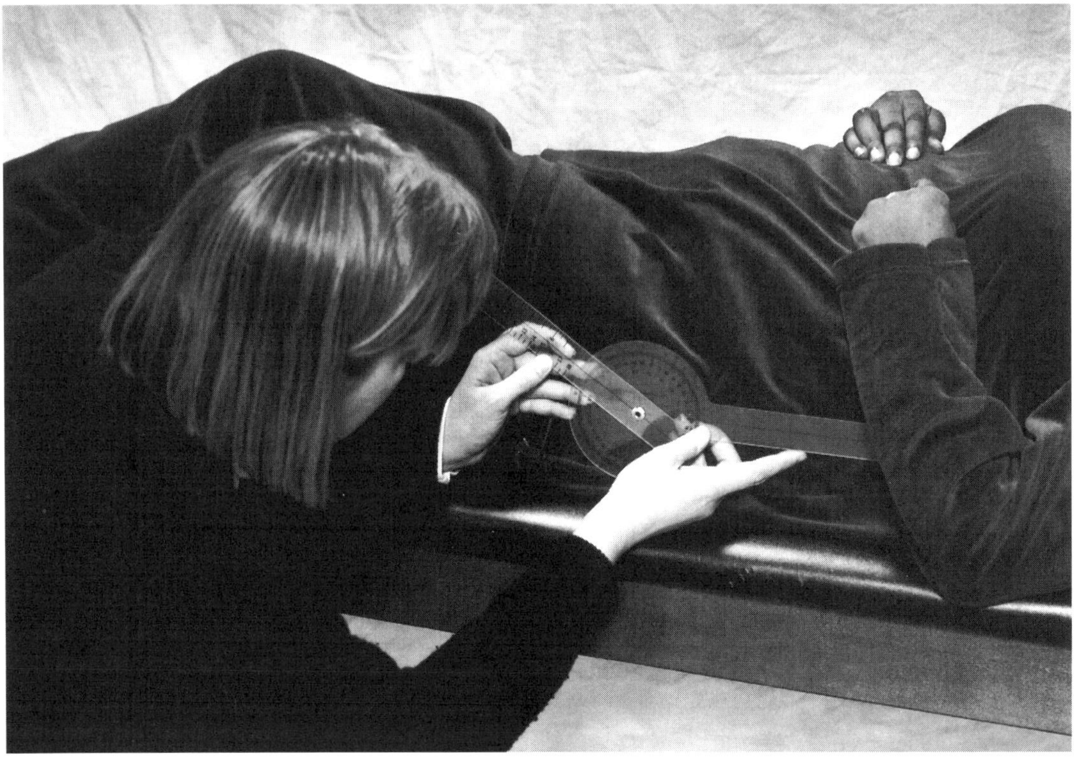

Figure 8–2 Goniatric measurements, such as that for hip flexion shown here, provide indicators for setting exercise goals.

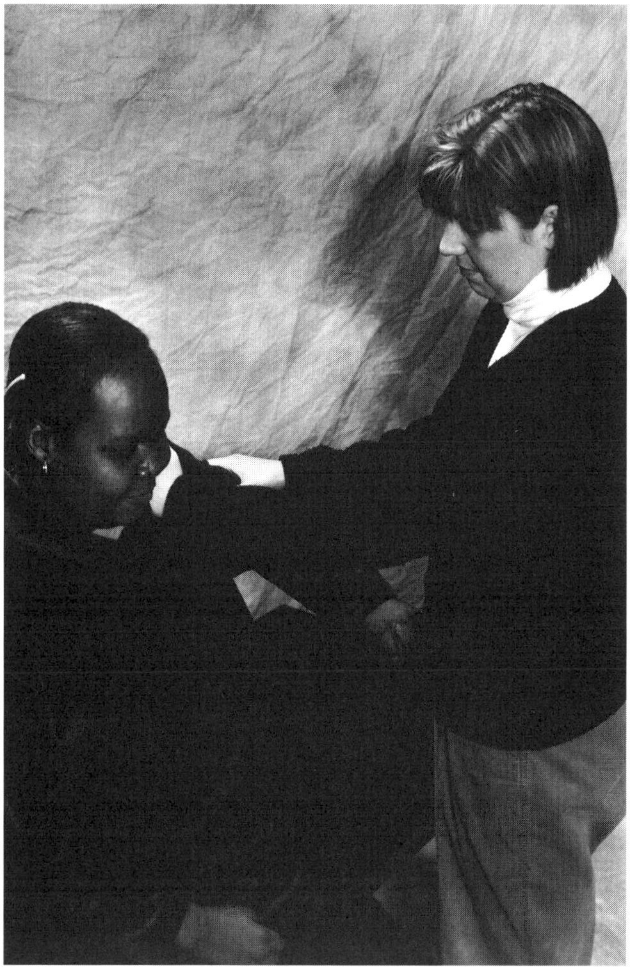

Figure 8–3 Manual muscle testing provides baseline strength measures that guide exercise prescription.

Based on the evaluation of cardiovascular function, strength, and flexibility, and the patient's functional status, goals, and resources, an exercise prescription can be made. The prescription should include intensity, duration, and frequency for each component of the program. In addition, patients must be taught some basic principles. They must understand their own limitations and realize that their performance will probably vary from day to day. Joints that are acutely inflamed should not be exercised vigorously, but should be moved through gentle ROM to prevent the effects of immobility until the flare has subsided. Patients must learn to recognize the signs of an acute flare so that they can modify their routines appropriately.

Likewise, patients must learn awareness of their bodies' responses during and after exercise. Acute joint pain brought on during exercise is usually a sign of excessive stress to tissues and should be avoided. More vague exercise-induced pain is generally acceptable, provided it does not last more than 2 hours after the exercise session. Other signs of excessive exercise include undue fatigue, increased weakness, increased swelling, or decreased ROM (Hicks, 1990). Exercise intensity should be modified according to the body's response to each activity.

Each patient should also be aware of the importance of proper posture and alignment while exercising (Figure 8–4). Maintenance of good alignment is essential to minimize stress on joints as well as to maximize effi-

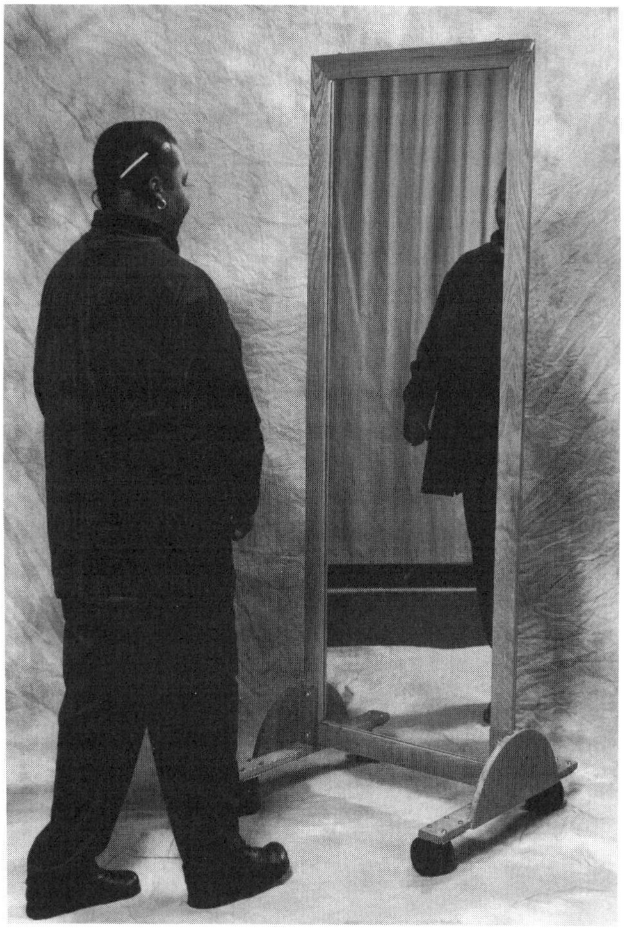

Figure 8–4 Viewing posture in a mirror enhances patient awareness of correct alignment.

ciency of movements. The use of slow, controlled movements will ensure maintenance of correct alignment and body mechanics during exercise. This will enhance patient safety while exercising, and patients will be less likely to experience postexercise soreness as well. Using mirrors and videotaping during exercise sessions are good ways to help patients become aware of their body positions.

To encourage patients' ongoing participation the exercise practitioner must make the program realistic and enjoyable. While it might be unrealistic to expect every patient to join an expensive health club, the local community center is probably an accessible and affordable option. Exercising in groups or pairs may make exercise sessions more enjoyable (Figure 8–5). Exercising together facilitates socialization and peer support, and patients tend to motivate each other.

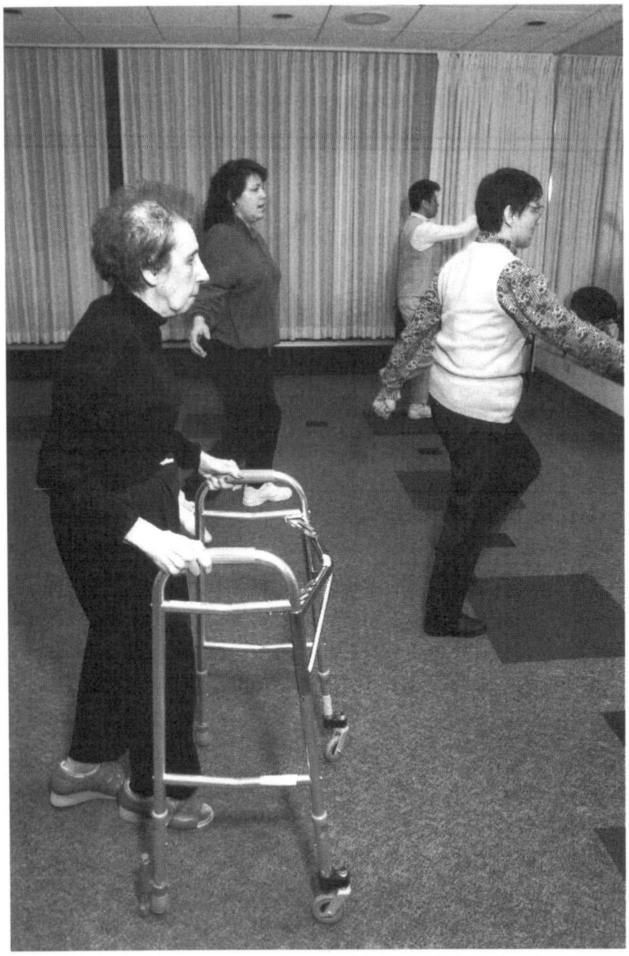

Figure 8–5 Specialized exercise classes are offered for patients with chronic diseases, including those with RA.

STRENGTHENING EXERCISE FOR THE PATIENT WITH RHEUMATOID ARTHRITIS

Strengthening exercises involve contraction of muscle against a resistance. Muscle contractions are classified as isometric, concentric, or eccentric. In an isometric contraction no joint movement occurs as the muscle contracts. Pushing the arm against an immovable object would involve isometric contraction. Concentric contraction involves shortening of a muscle while moving a resistance. Stepping up a step involves concentric contraction of the quadriceps muscle as the knee joint is extended. Eccentric contraction involves lengthening of the muscle while moving a resistance. Eccentric contractions are generally thought of as control mechanisms during dynamic activity. Stepping down a step involves eccentric contraction of the quadriceps muscle as it controls the speed of knee flexion.

The principle of specificity states that improvement in muscular strength will be specific to the muscle being trained and to the type of contraction used (Astrand, 1987). This means that if specific functional goals have been determined, the exercise program should include these specific activities. To use the example of improving stair-climbing ability, exercises to include might be abdominal sets (isometric contraction), stepping up a step (concentric contraction), and stepping down a step (eccentric contraction).

Because isometric strengthening does not involve moving a joint through its full ROM, this method previously was thought to be ideal for strengthening in the patient with RA and was taught exclusively. Although strength gains can be made with isometric training, these gains occur only at the joint angle at which the exercise is performed, with little carryover to other points in the range of joint motion (Astrand, 1987). Isometric strengthening of the limbs, then, has very limited functional use, as most functional activities involve movement of joints through various degrees of motion. Ekdahl, Andersson, Moritz, and Svensson (1990) have shown that dynamic training results in greater increases in functional capacity than does static training.

Isometric contractions in the trunk and proximal muscles, however, can be very useful because this is the way these muscles typically function. The concept of "postural set" involves the contraction of muscles to maintain spinal and pelvic stability during dynamic activity of the extremities. Isometric strengthening of abdominal, pelvic, spinal, and shoulder girdle musculature is important to maintain the stable bases on which dynamic activity of the limbs can take place.

In determining the strength-training program, then, all three types of muscle contraction should be included. Isometric or stabilization exercises for pelvic and spinal muscles and concentric and eccentric exercises for the quadriceps and hamstrings would constitute a complete lower extremity program. The exception to including all three types of contraction occurs when the patient is experiencing increased joint activity (ie, an acute flare). Under this circumstance it is unadvisable to move the inflamed joint through its full ROM because additional joint damage may occur. It is advisable, however, to maintain isometric contractions of the surrounding musculature to prevent the effects of immobility from occurring while the joint is being rested. Once the flare has subsided dynamic activity can be resumed.

As mentioned earlier, the exercise prescription should include not only the type of activity, but also the intensity, duration, and frequency of activity as well. Intensity is a measure of the amount of resistance the working muscle is moving. Intensity is determined by the initial assessment and by the patient's subsequent response to the exercise.

Resistance is anything that resists movement of the limb or body part that causes the involved muscle to perform work. Resistance can be simply the weight of a limb being moved against gravity, or resistance can be applied by an external force such as a weight. Resistance can be increased or decreased in a number of different ways.

The weight of a limb against gravity can be a resistance in weaker muscles. If a muscle is so weak that it cannot move a body part against gravity, a change in the position of the body so that the part can be moved in a plane in which gravity is eliminated will decrease the resistance and improve the patient's ability to move the part actively. The use of equipment such as slings or powder boards can assist in holding an extremity in gravity-eliminated positions so that this type of exercise can be performed (Figure 8–6). Manual assistance can also be applied to allow some active movement when this cannot be performed completely independently.

For increases in strength to occur, the principle of overload must be applied. This principle states that a muscle must work against a resistance greater than that to which it is accustomed. As strength gains occur, resistance must be increased accordingly so that overload of the muscle will continue.

Since most functional activity occurs in gravity-resisted postures, muscles should be progressed to working against gravity as soon as they are able. Once these

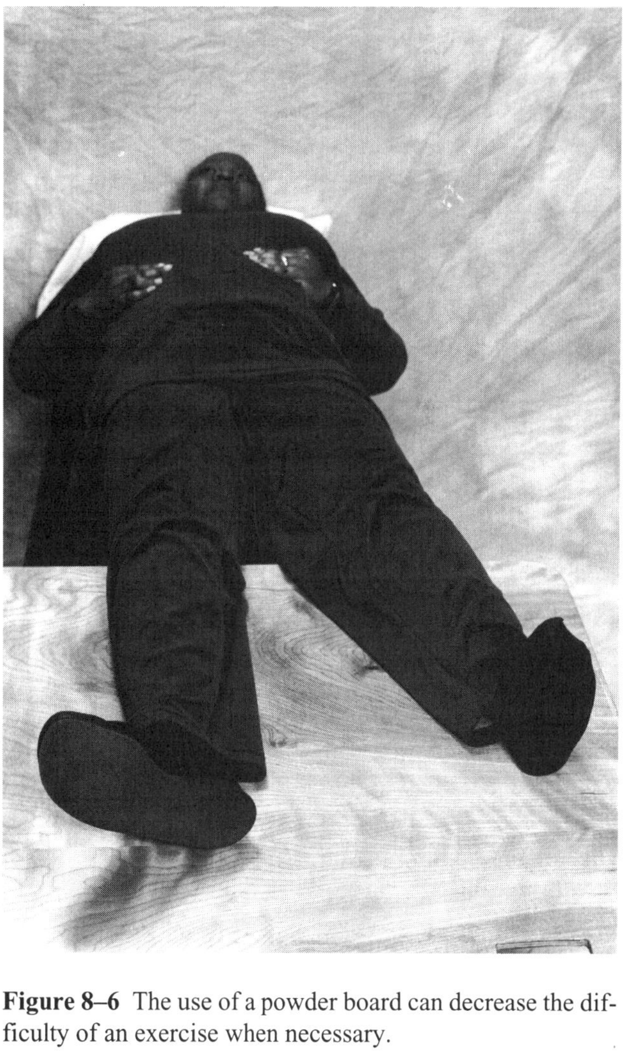

Figure 8–6 The use of a powder board can decrease the difficulty of an exercise when necessary.

positions are achieved the resistance can be increased further with the use of external resistance devices such as elastic bands, hand-held weights, resistance-training machines, water in a therapeutic pool, or the patient's own body weight (Figure 8–7). No method of providing resistance is better than another per se. Each patient's abilities and resources must be considered. The goal is to continue to overload the muscle as long as strength gains are desired.

Determining appropriate intensity is often a trial-and-error procedure. As a general rule, exercise-induced pain that lasts longer than 2 hours after exercise indicates that the intensity was too great. Additionally, difficulty performing the exercise with the body in good alignment or in a smooth, controlled manner is also an indication that the intensity is too great (ie, the resistance is too much for safe, effective performance of the activity). It is extremely important for patients to understand these concepts so that they will use them and exercise safely.

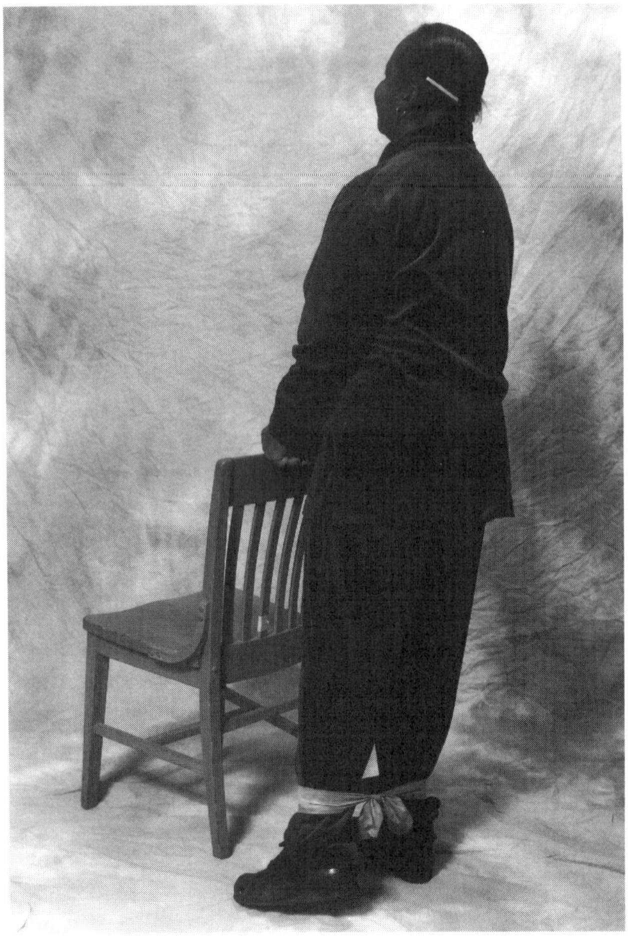

Figure 8–7 The use of resistance, such as the elastic band shown here, can enhance a patient's strengthening program.

Duration of exercise is the measure of how long the exercise is performed, and should also be included in the exercise prescription. With strengthening exercise, duration can refer to the number of repetitions performed (concentric or eccentric activities) or to the length of time a contraction is held (isometric activities). Duration is inversely related to intensity; that is, a more intense exercise will be performed for fewer repetitions and vice versa. In the patient with RA for whom joint safety is of major concern, lower intensities with longer durations are advised. Activities of longer duration facilitate muscular endurance as well as strength. Endurance is an important component in the ability to perform most functional activities. As a basic guideline, 10 to 12 repetitions of an exercise are advised.

In the very debilitated patient this many repetitions might be too ambitious a guideline at first. In this situation duration may be decreased, but frequency could be increased. Frequency is the third component of the exercise prescription and refers to the number of times an exercise session is performed, usually stated as times per day or times per week. If a patient is unable to tolerate the recommended intensity or duration initially, frequency can be increased. For example, if a muscle is fatigued after four repetitions the muscle can be rested and the exercise repeated at a later time that day. Thus a very weak muscle can be exercised several times per day in shorter sessions until endurance improves.

If a patient is able to exercise for 10 to 12 repetitions with resistance, a frequency of three or four times per week is recommended for strength training. A day of rest between sessions is recommended to allow for muscle recovery and to prevent exercise-induced injury.

Because the RA patient's performance can vary from day to day, the exercise prescription should be considered a guideline, not an absolute. Patients and exercise practitioners must understand the importance of symptom-guided activity and be able to modify the program appropriately.

FLEXIBILITY EXERCISE FOR THE PATIENT WITH RHEUMATOID ARTHRITIS

Flexibility, the second component of the exercise program, is defined as the ability of a joint to move through its full ROM. It is determined by the length of the soft tissue structures surrounding a joint: muscle, joint capsule, tendon, and ligaments. The exercise practitioner will determine from the initial assessment whether stretching is needed to increase tissue length or joint ROM or whether the current range is adequate and just needs to be maintained.

For stretching to increase soft tissue length, the overload principle is applied again. The tissue must be lengthened to a point beyond which it is accustomed for gains to occur. Intensity of the stretch is determined by the sensation of resistance or stretch felt. The patient should stretch the tissue to this point. This should not be a painful sensation, rather a sense that the tissue has reached its length limit. At this point the stretch should be held for a duration of 10 to 30 seconds. Static stretching in this way is considered the safest way to increase ROM. Ballistic stretching, or bouncing at the end of the range, is contraindicated because it is likely to cause damage to muscle and other soft tissue. A frequency of three to five repetitions of each stretching exercise is recommended.

The principle of specificity also applies to flexibility training. The effects of stretching are very specific to the tissue and direction of the stretch. If increases in ankle dorsiflexion are desired, for example, stretching of the plantar flexors and posterior soft tissue will be required. A complete flexibility program includes all of the major muscle groups as well as any problem areas specific to the individual. The anterior chest, lumbar spine, hip flexors, hamstrings, and plantar flexors tend to be less flexible in the patient with RA.

Once again, alignment and posture are of utmost importance in RA patients performing stretching exercises (Figure 8–8). Patients must also know when to stop stretching for increased length, that is, when full ROM has been achieved. Stretching in improper alignment or overstretching could lead to hypermobility of joints, potentially causing further joint damage. Once full ROM has been achieved patients should continue to stretch at this end range, but should push no further.

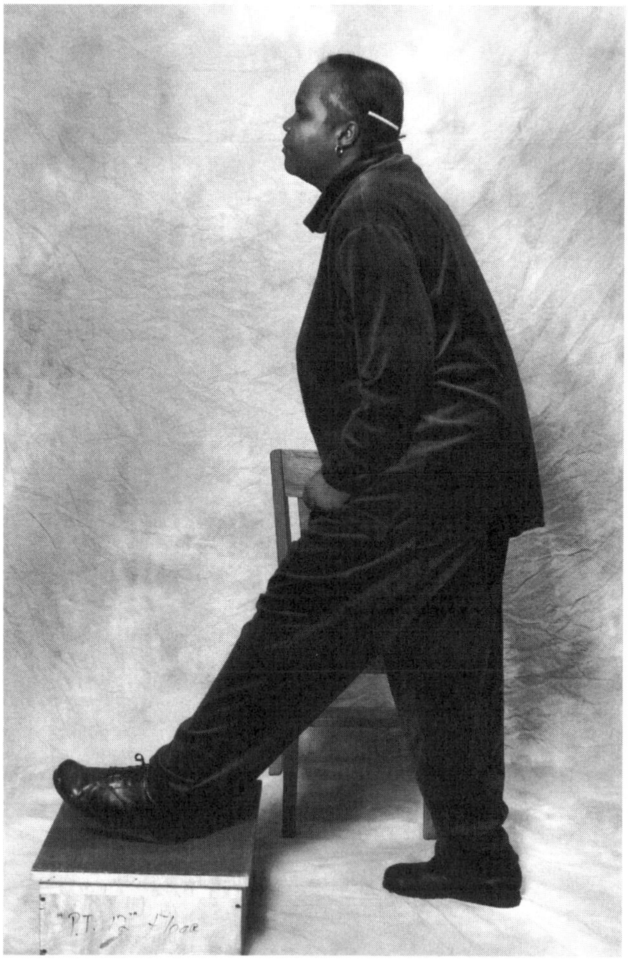

Figure 8–8 Correct alignment is necessary when performing flexibility exercises such as this hamstring stretch.

A frequency of three to five times per week is recommended for flexibility exercise.

It is also recommended that soft tissue be warmed up prior to stretching, as tissue with greater temperature has been shown to be more flexible than cooler tissue. Soft tissue can be warmed up by performing low-intensity aerobic activity for a few minutes prior to the stretching routine. Because of the relaxing nature of flexibility activities, stretching is often included as part of the cool-down period following more intense aerobic exercise.

CARDIOVASCULAR EXERCISE FOR THE PATIENT WITH RHEUMATOID ARTHRITIS

Aerobic exercise or cardiovascular training is the third component of the comprehensive exercise program. Aerobic exercise can be beneficial for all patients, but especially for those who demonstrate significant fatigue or loss of functional capacity.

Cardiovascular activities stress the heart and vascular system to increase efficiency in delivering oxygen to working body parts. Aerobic activities are those that involve large muscle groups in rhythmical, sustained movements (Figure 8–9). Examples include walking, jogging, biking, rowing, swimming, or dancing, among others. Note that both weight-bearing and non–weight-bearing activities can be considered aerobic, and that both types can be used safely for training in the patient with RA (Perlman et al., 1990; Minor et al., 1989).

Activity selection for the RA patient will depend on a number of factors, including the extent of involvement of the lower extremities and the degree of disease activity. Other factors to be considered are patient resources and interests. Patients should have a few exercise options, so that the same joints are not stressed repeatedly. This can also fend off exercise dropout due to boredom. For example, a patient might walk 2 days per week and participate in an aquatic aerobic exercise class 1 day per week.

Intensity of cardiovascular exercise can be measured in several ways. The most common approach is to measure heart rate. Based on the evaluation of the patient's initial cardiovascular function, a target heart rate range can be determined. Using the YMCA or ACSM protocols for exercise testing, the individual's maximal heart rate is estimated. The target exercise range is expressed as a percentage of this maximal heart rate. The ACSM recommends that individuals in the general population exercise at a level between 55% and 90% of the maximal heart rate, while studies on RA patients have recommended target ranges of 50% to 70% of the maximal rate (Semble et al., 1990). More fit people will have to exercise at higher intensities in order to see increases in

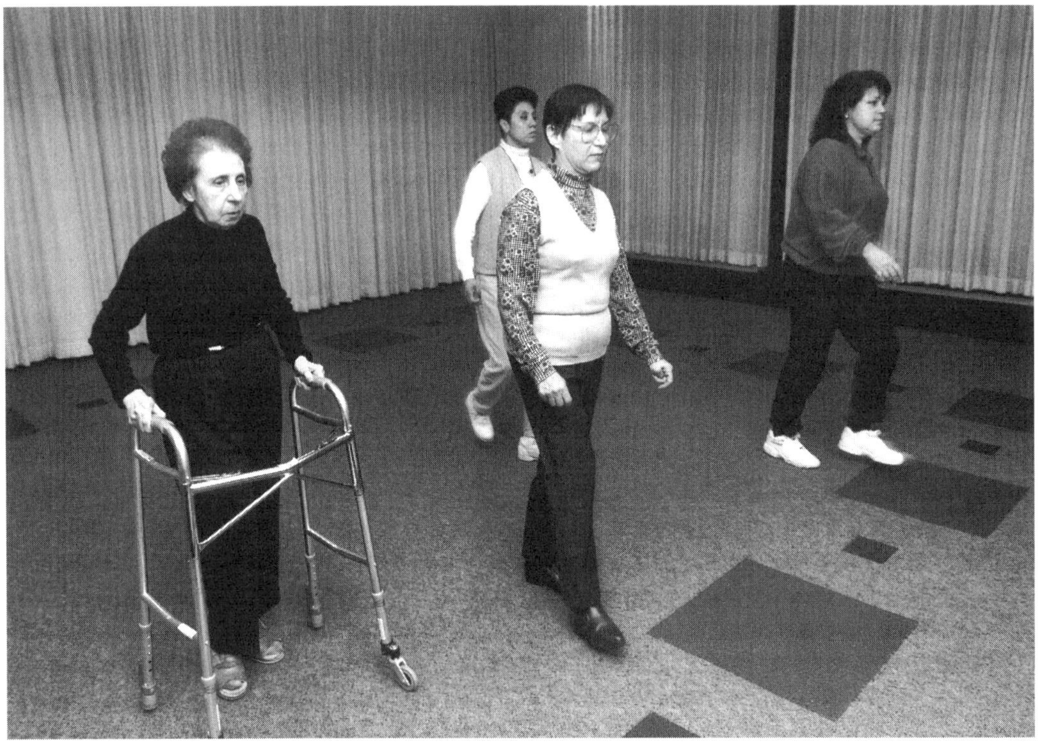

Figure 8–9 Aerobic exercise is an important component of a well-rounded exercise program.

fitness level. Conversely, patients who are less fit to begin with can exercise at lower intensities and still show increases in functional capacity.

If the maximal heart rate has not been determined by a graded exercise test, a target heart rate range can be determined based on a formula using the patient's age. The formula estimates a person's maximal heart rate to be 220 minus his or her age, and the target range is determined from that figure. For example, the maximal heart rate of a 60-year-old patient would be estimated at 220 – 60, or 160 beats per minute. If the exercise prescription called for a range of 60% to 70% maximal, the target heart rate will be between 96 and 112 beats per minute. The patient is instructed to exercise at an intensity great enough to increase the heart rate to this level, then maintain it for the duration of the exercise. Patients are taught to find and count their pulse, usually at the radial or carotid artery, to monitor their exercise intensity.

Sometimes using heart rate as a measure of intensity is not possible or practical. Patients whose disease involves their hands might not be able to feel their pulse. Other patients could be on cardiac medication, such as β-blockers, which maintain their heart rate at a very low level. In these instances, exercise intensity can be measured using the Rating of Perceived Exertion (RPE; Heyward, 1991). This is a visual scale that allows patients to determine subjectively their exercise intensity. The scale has been found to be a valid and reliable estimate of exercise intensity once users are familiar with it. The RPE scale can be used during the cardiovascular assessment, and a target exercise range can be determined based on the maximum achieved during the test. Patients must be instructed to use the scale, and should practice with supervision to ensure accurate use independently.

A third very simple way to monitor exercise intensity is the "talk test." This test states that patients should be able to maintain a conversation while carrying on the exercise program. Intensity is too high if patients are winded to the point that they cannot continue talking during the activity. This method is a simple way of keeping intensity from going too high in patients who might have difficulty grasping the concepts of monitoring pulse or RPE. It does not, however, help to determine whether exercise is intense enough to have cardiovascular benefits.

Regardless of the means of monitoring immediate exercise intensity, patients should always monitor postexercise response to the activity in terms of its effect on the joints. As mentioned earlier, exercise-induced pain lasting greater than 2 hours after the activity is an indication that the activity was too intense.

Duration of the aerobic activity will depend somewhat on the intensity. A duration of 15 to 60 minutes is recommended for the general population to see cardiovascular changes. In the population with RA, shorter durations performed more frequently have been found to be equally effective. For example, patients who do not tolerate 15 minutes of continuous exercise could get the same benefit from three bouts of 5 minutes each, with brief rest periods between bouts (Ekblom & Nordemar, 1993). This could allow adequate training for cardiovascular improvement while minimizing risk to joints. As always, the patient's response to the program will help determine these parameters.

Frequency of the aerobic sessions should be limited to three times per week, preferably with a day of rest between sessions. Again, this minimizes overuse trauma to joints and soft tissue structures, but allows for maximum improvement in cardiovascular function (Heyward, 1991).

CONCLUSION

This chapter emphasizes specific training parameters for the components of strength, flexibility, and cardiovascular function. The benefits of recreational exercise in the overall fitness picture should also be considered (Hicks, 1990). Activities such as golf, tennis, or dancing combine the different fitness components, and are often more interesting and enjoyable than isolated exercise sessions. Recreational exercise allows for socialization, as well as a sense of accomplishment that can have psychological benefits in addition to the physical ones. These types of activities can help reinforce the gains made in specific areas of strength, flexibility, or endurance by incorporating them into functional activities. After all, the primary goal with any treatment program is to improve our patients' overall function.

It is clear that well-planned and monitored exercise can have many benefits for the patient with rheumatoid arthritis. In addition to the specific musculoskeletal benefits, participants in a comprehensive program can experience improved functional ability in their everyday lives as well. When this population's special needs are taken into consideration, the exercise practitioner can prescribe safe and effective programs for almost any individual.

REFERENCES

American College of Sports Medicine. Preventive and Rehabilitative Exercise Committee. (1991). *Guidelines for exercise testing and prescription* (4th ed.). Malvern, PA: Lea & Febiger.

Astrand, P. (1987). Exercise physiology and its role in disease prevention and rehabilitation. *Archives of Physical Medicine and Rehabilitation, 68*, 305–309.

Ekblom, B., & Nordemar, R. (1993). Rheumatoid arthritis. In J. S. Skinner (Ed.), *Exercise testing and exercise prescription for special cases* (2nd ed., pp. 113–126). Malvern, PA: Lea & Febiger.

Ekdahl, C., & Broman, G. (1992). Rheumatoid arthritis: A comparative study with healthy subjects. *Annals of the Rheumatic Diseases, 51*, 35–40.

Ekdahl, C., Andersson, S.I., Moritz, U., & Svensson, B. (1990). Dynamic versus static training in patients with rheumatoid arthritis. *Scandinavian Journal of Rheumatology, 19*, 17–26.

Ekdahl, C., Ekman, R., Andersson, S.I., Melander, A., & Svensson, B. (1990). Dynamic training and circulating levels of corticotropin-releasing factor, beta-lipotropin and beta-endorphin in rheumatoid arthritis. *Pain, 40*, 35–42.

Fries, J.F., Spitz, P., Kraines, R.G., & Holman, H.R. (1980). Measurement of patient outcome in arthritis. *Arthritis and Rheumatism, 23,* 137–145.

Heyward, V.H. (1991). *Advanced fitness assessment & exercise prescription* (2nd ed.). Champaign, IL: Human Kinetics Books.

Hicks, J.E. (1990, October). Exercise for patients with inflammatory arthritis. *Journal of Musculoskeletal Medicine,* 40–56.

Lyngberg, K., Danneskiold-Samsoe, B., & Halskov, O. (1988). The effect of physical training on patients with rheumatoid arthritis: Changes in disease activity, muscle strength and aerobic capacity: A clinically controlled minimized cross-over study. *Clinical and Experimental Rheumatology, 6*, 253–260.

Meenan, R.F., Gertman, P.M., & Mason, J.H. (1980). Measuring health status in arthritis: The arthritis impact measurement scales. *Arthritis and Rheumatism, 23,* 146–152.

Minor, M. A., Hewett, J.E., Webel, R.R., Anderson, S.K., & Kay, D.R. (1989). Efficacy of physical conditioning exercise in patients with rheumatoid arthritis and osteoarthritis. *Arthritis and Rheumatism, 32*, 1396–1405.

Nordemar, R., Ekblom B., Zachrisson, L., & Lundqvist K. (1981). Physical training in rheumatoid arthritis: A controlled long-term study. *Scandinavian Journal of Rheumatology, 10,* 17–23.

Perlman, S.G., Connell, K.J., Clark, A., Robinson, M.S., Conlon, P., Gecht, M., Caldron, P., & Sinacore, J.M. (1990). *Dance-based aerobic exercise for rheumatoid arthritis.* Atlanta: Arthritis Health Professions Association.

Semble, E.L., Loeser, R.F., & Wise, C.M. (1990). Therapeutic exercise for rheumatoid arthritis and osteoarthritis. *Seminars in Arthritis and Rheumatism, 20,* 32–40.

Stenstrom, C.H., Lindell, B., Swanberg, E., Harms-Ringdahl, K., & Nordemar, R. (1990). Functional and psychosocial consequences of disease and experience of pain and exertion in a group of rheumatic patients considered for active training. *Scandinavian Journal of Rheumatology, 19*, 374–382.

SUGGESTED READING

Eichner, E.R. (1990). The hematology of inactivity. *Rheumatic Disease Clinics of North America, 16*, 815–825.

Ekdahl, C. (1992). Postural control, muscle function and psychological factors in rheumatoid arthritis. *Scandinavian Journal of Rheumatology, 21*, 297–301.

Gerber, L.H., & Huritz, S.R. (1986). Biomechanical principles pertinent to rehabilitation of patients with rheumatic disease. In G.E. Ehrlich (Ed.), *Rehabilitation management of rheumatic conditions* (2nd ed., pp. 65–76). Baltimore: Williams & Wilkins.

McCubbin, J.A. (1990). Resistence exercise training for persons with arthritis. *Rheumatic Disease Clinics of North America, 16*, 931–943.

Namey, T.C. (1990). Adaptive bicycling. *Rheumatic Disease Clinics of North America, 16*, 871–886.

Pincus, T., Summey, J.A., Soraci, S.A., Jr., Wallston, K.A., & Hummon, N.P. (1983). Assessment of patient satisfaction in activities of daily living using a modified Stanford health assessment questionnaire. *Arthritis and Rheumatism*, *26*, 1346–1353.

Stenstrom, C.H., Lindell, B., Swanberg, P., Harms-Ringdahl, K., & Nordemas, R. (1991). Intensive dynamic training in water for rheumatoid arthritis functional class two: A long-term study of effects. *Scandinavian Journal of Rheumatology*, *2D*, 358–365.

Swezey, R.L. (1978). *Arthritis: Rational therapy and rehabilitation.* Philadelphia: Saunders.

CHAPTER 9

Hand Splinting in Rheumatoid Arthritis: A Perspective on Current Knowledge and Directions for Research

Judith A. Falconer, PhD, MPH, OTR/L

Splints, external supports applied to body parts, are commonly prescribed for patients with rheumatoid arthritis to decrease inflammation, relieve pain, protect a joint, prevent or correct deformity, or improve function. Most major textbooks in rheumatology and rehabilitation recommend splinting in one form or another, and the majority of physicians, nurses, occupational therapists, physical therapists, and patients will often consider a splint for relief from symptoms and prevention or correction of pain, deformity, and disability or dysfunction associated with rheumatoid arthritis of the hand. Despite the widespread use of splints, splinting practices and beliefs in its efficacy vary widely among clinicians.

The majority of an extensive body of literature on splinting describes specific splinting principles, designs, materials, and training programs. Observations and experiences of experts and other forms of case-report or case-series studies are the primary sources of clinical evidence for the efficacy of splints. A few splints such as the resting wrist-and-hand splint (Gault & Spyker, 1969), compression gloves (Askari, Moskowitz, & Ryan, 1974; Culic, Battaglis, Wichman, & Schmid, 1979; Swezey, Spiegel, Cretin, & Clements, 1979), or splints (McKnight & Schomburg, 1982), and the static wrist working splint (Backman & Dietz, 1988) have been studied under controlled clinical conditions. Although the results have been generally positive, few splints or splint protocols have been empirically studied.

The theoretical support and indirect evidence for splinting are perhaps stronger than either the clinical or the empirical evidence of the efficacy, but are less well represented in the literature. In this chapter, the theoretical rationale for the use of splints, based on a model that hypothesizes synovial inflammation and proliferation as primary causal factors in hand pain and deformity, is briefly reviewed. The purposes of the review are to provide a broad perspective on nonsurgical hand splinting and to suggest some directions for future research based on this perspective.

HAND DYSFUNCTION

A modern view of rheumatoid arthritis regards the pathology of the synovium in two somewhat separate but related components: inflammation and proliferation (E.D. Harris, 1990). Inflammation, the initial process, is manifested by inflammatory joint effusion, which increases articular pressure, stretches and weak-

The author thanks Rowland W. Chang, MD, MPH, and Russell Foley, MS, PT, for their thoughtful comments and recommendations on an earlier draft of this chapter.

ens joint-supporting structures, and causes pain. To reduce pain, the inflamed joint assumes a position whereby it is anatomically positioned to accommodate the greatest volume of fluid, intra-articular pressure is lowest, and the joint capsule and other soft tissues are slack (Eyring & Murray, 1964; Favreau & Laurin, 1963). In progressive cases of rheumatoid arthritis, the synovium remains inflamed, proliferates, and becomes destructive to articular cartilage, subchondral bone, and surrounding soft tissues. At this stage, the pathological synovium, called pannus, further increases intra-articular pressure, stretches and weakens the already lax joint-supporting structures, and leads to further joint instability. The joint in this state loses the ability to withstand internal and external forces acting on it, thereby causing secondary biomechanical as well as primary pathophysiological derangement of the joint. Muscle weakness caused by neurological inhibition due to pain, or by the misuse, disuse, or adaptive shortening of soft tissues further exacerbates the joint's inability to withstand forces. Normal anatomical and biomechanical characteristics of the joint, activity patterns, and an unknown affinity for synovitis at some joints more so than others partially explain the fact that this process tends to produce patterns of deformity commonly called the zigzag, boutonniere, swan-neck, and thumb type I, II, and III deformities (Nalebuff, 1963; Swezey, 1971). Although initially impaired by pain, hand function is compromised further by mechanical derangement of the joint.

Although a chronic disease by definition, rheumatoid arthritis is characterized by periods of acute inflammation interspersed throughout the disease course. The relative importance of each factor in this model of hand dysfunction (for example, inflammation, intra-articular pressure, muscle weakness, joint derangement, or activity patterns) shifts, depending on the inflammatory state and the destructiveness of the pannus. For example, during acute periods of inflammation, the inflammation may dictate muscle weakness, joint derangement, and hand dysfunction; whereas in chronic periods (relatively little inflammation), joint derangement and activity patterns may assume more important mediating roles in muscle weakness and hand dysfunction.

In theory, if a splint (or any modality) disrupts this process, then it may help to relieve symptoms and to maintain structural and functional integrity of the rheumatoid joint and, consequently, function of the hand and upper extremity. The purpose, design, and efficacy of the splint, however, may vary depending on the inflammatory severity, duration, and destructiveness of the rheumatoid process.

ACUTELY INFLAMED RHEUMATOID JOINT

The rationale for splinting an acutely inflamed joint is both biomechanical and physiological. By externally supporting, positioning, and restricting motion of the inflamed joint, the splint reduces the pain, stress, and deformity caused by abnormal muscle action, positional factors, and external loads. For example, the resting hand-and-wrist splint, a rigid, volar support, immobilizes the hand and wrist, and positions the wrist in slight extension, the second through fifth metacarpophalangeal (MCP) joints in midflexion, the proximal (PIP) and distal interphalangeal (DIP) joints in extension, the thumb carpometacarpal (CMC) joint in flexion and abduction, and MCP and interphalangeal (IP) joints in extension in order to counter the deforming forces. The biomechanical rationale for splinting an acutely inflamed joint, however, does not separate the relative importance of pathophysiological processes from the secondary effects of mechanical stressors in the etiology of pain and deformity. If the primary inflammatory and proliferative processes are the major determinants of tissue damage, then splinting the inflamed rheumatoid joint may reduce pain by relieving stress, but may not substantially prevent deformity.

Splints, however, may also help quiet the primary inflammation and limit the destructiveness of the process. Joint motion increases intra-articular temperature, which may exacerbate inflammatory disease (Hollander & Horvath, 1949); conversely, joint immobilization may help to remit inflammatory disease. Some empirical support exists for the hypothesis that local (splinting) and general (bed rest) immobilization or rest reduces disease activity.

Controlled clinical studies of local immobilization of the upper limb (Gault & Spyker, 1969) and knee (R. Harris & Copp, 1962) have revealed that immobilization by splinting reduces disease activity and causes only transient loss of range of motion or strength. Gault and Spyker (1969) reported significant reduction in disease activity of the upper limbs of seven subjects who were continuously splinted for 3 weeks, as compared with each subject's nonsplinted limb. R. Harris and Copp (1962) found reduction in disease activity and knee symptoms in 18 patients who wore knee plaster casts for 4 weeks, but they were unable to find a differential benefit between complete immobilization of one knee randomly selected and partial immobilization of the other knee of each subject. Differential effects of splinting on weight-bearing and non–weight-bearing joints, marginal differences between complete and partial immobilization as compared to no immobilization, and general effects of disease that were uncontrolled in these studies may have confounded the results. R. Harris and Copp (1962) described marked symmetry of changes in each pair of joints and emphasized the importance of general over local factors such as splinting in control of disease activity.

Studies of general rest enforced by bed rest (Lee, Kennedy, Anderson, & Buchanan, 1974), bed rest and splinting (Partridge & Duthie, 1963), and hospitalization (Mills, Pinals, Ropes, Short, & Sutcliffe, 1971) produced conflicting evidence about the relationship between rest and disease activity. Partridge and Duthie (1963), Lee et al. (1974), and Mills et al. (1971) reported the reduction of disease and no long-term negative consequences in patients following general rest. Partridge and Duthie (1963), however, found only slight differences between 34 hospitalized patients who were completely immobilized by bed rest and plaster splints for 4 weeks and 34 control hospitalized patients who were allowed daily periods of activity over 4 weeks of bed rest. Lee et al. (1974) found that 16 patients hospitalized for 4 weeks with 13 hours of bed rest per day had significantly less disease activity than 14 patients who were managed as outpatients and allowed unrestricted activity; however, the improvement was not dramatic. Mills et al. (1971) found no evidence that 20 patients who were hospitalized for 22 hours of bed rest for 4 weeks followed by 18 hours of bed rest for 6 weeks showed superior or inferior results to 22 hospitalized patients who were allowed ad lib activity and encouraged to ambulate.

When the rheumatoid joint is completely immobilized, as is the case when rheumatoid arthritis occurs with hemiplegia (Bland & Eddy, 1968; Thompson & Bywaters, 1962), poliomyelitis (Glick, 1967), or a traumatic peripheral nerve lesion (Kamermann, 1966), rheumatoid activity is generally markedly decreased. Neurological effects on rheumatoid disease, however, may explain these observed correlations between complete immobilization and disease reduction.

The efficacy of a resting or immobilizing splint in an acutely inflamed joint, therefore, may ultimately depend on the causal relationships among immobility, intra-articular temperature, and inflammation; the relative importance of biomechanical stress and positional factors to joint pain and deformity; local versus general effects on disease activity; possible neurological effects on inflammation; and clinical consideration such as the severity and duration of symptoms and patient compliance with wearing the splint. Published estimates of compliance with splints vary from approximately one third (Moon, Moon, & Black, 1976) to two thirds (Feinberg & Brandt, 1981) of patients, although compliant patients may self-regulate the wearing of splints in response to variation in symptoms (Feinberg & Brandt, 1981).

CHRONIC RHEUMATOID JOINT

Compared with splinting the acute rheumatoid joint, the rationale for splinting a chronic rheumatoid joint rests primarily on biomechanical factors. Theoretically, by realigning and redistributing the damaging internal and external forces acting on the joint, the splint may help to prevent deformity, correct deformity, or improve joint function and functional use of the extremity.

Prevention of Deformity

Although theoretically possible, there is no empirical evidence that splinting a chronic rheumatoid joint will prevent deformity and some empirical evidence that functional hand splints do not prevent deformity (Convery, Conaty, & Nickel, 1967). The rationale for splinting to prevent deformity in the chronic rheumatoid joint is based on the hypotheses that physical activity increases joint destruction and proper joint usage minimizes joint deformity. However, the relationships between hand use and joint deformity have not been clearly established (Glick, 1966; Hasselkus, Kshehpakaran, & Safrit, 1981). While proper joint positioning enforced by splinting may help to strengthen the muscles surrounding the joint, and thereby prevent a measure of deformity, the increase in strength achievable through splinting is probably minimal.

Prolonged use of a resting splint may also be harmful. The negative effects of immobilization on healthy human and animal systems—such as decreased bone mass and strength (Steinberg, 1980); cartilage degeneration (Ely & Mensor, 1933); proliferation of connective tissue in the joint cavity, which causes adhesions (Donatelli & Owens-Burkhart, 1981); contractures of capsule, ligaments, tendons, and muscle; and muscle weakness and atrophy (Steinberg, 1980; Lavigne & Watkins, 1972)—are well known and thought to occur with prolonged immobilization of a rheumatoid joint. Criteria for discontinuing a resting splint for an acute joint are important to include in the splint prescription. Training in joint protection combined with an exercise program may be a more efficient approach for maintaining joint integrity and function in the chronic rheumatoid joint.

Correction of Deformity

Splints that apply force to the chronic rheumatoid joint may, however, help to correct contractures caused by connective tissue shortening. Prolonged passive stretch at moderate tension on a contracted joint may elongate tight soft tissues (Kottke, Pauley, & Ptak, 1966). A splint may be used either to hold soft tissues on stretch (for example, serial cylindrical casts) or to apply stretch to the soft tissues (for instance, dynamic spring-loaded splints). For example, three-point pressure, dynamic, extension, and flexion splints are designed to reduce joint contractures by applying maximal stretch to the PIP joint in either flexion or extension by exerting a force on the joint through a figure-of-eight wire. However, since contractures occurring with rheumatoid arthritis are the consequences of partially or completely limited joint mobility, conditions that reduce mobility, such as chronic synovitis, pain, or muscle weakness, promote contractures. Corrective splinting by prolonged stretch does not directly address the predisposing conditions, nor can it correct deformity caused by joint derangement, cartilage, or bony impingements.

Improve Joint Function and Prevent Pain

Splints for chronic rheumatoid joints may also be applied to improve function. Functional splints stabilize, align, increase, or decrease the action of a joint and are designed to facilitate the patient's use of the joint for specific hand functions (for example, grasp or pinch) or tasks (for instance, writing or lifting) and to relieve pain associated with performance of functional activities. Functional splints are designed to enable joints and muscles to function in a mechanically advantageous position in the presence of joint damage. For example, the PIP double-ring flexion splint prevents hyperextension of the PIP joint, which is commonly seen in the swan-neck deformity. By promoting fingertip prehension, the splint may improve grasp and prehensile strength and stability, thumb and digit opposition, fine- and gross-motor activities of daily living, and the appearance of the joint (Noaker, Garty, & Kwoh, 1988). Perhaps the most common functional splint is the static wrist working splint, which stabilizes the wrist in slight extension and allows full opposition of the thumb with the digits. The splint appears to reduce pain and to increase hand strength during functional activities, but may interfere with fine-motor tasks (Backman & Dietz, 1988).

Although a variety of splints may be justified on functional criteria, hand function is complex and often difficult to improve by splints. Splints usually can control only a few joints in a single plane of motion, and many hand functions involve multijoint, multiplanar, coordinated motion. Splints may improve the mechanical components, but impair the sensory components of function. Hands also serve important symbolic, cosmetic, and communicative functions that a splint may hinder. The influence of any one of these nonmechanical factors may alter the splint's intended effects. The remarkable ability of a patient to adapt and compensate for hand impairments also limits the opportunities for splints to improve hand function.

SOME SUGGESTIONS FOR FUTURE DIRECTIONS

A successful splinting program involves complex decision making and requires expert knowledge, skills, and clinical judgment. The apparent simplicity of a well-designed and constructed splint does not diminish the need to apply the same rigorous theoretical, empirical, and clinical standards applied to other treatment modalities. Effective use of patient and professional time will be enhanced and opportunities to advance the conservative treatment of rheumatoid pain and dysfunction will be enlarged through continued analysis and evaluation of both splinting practices and theory.

A splint is only a modality that operates primarily on the mechanical stress component of the complex equation for pain and deformity; therefore, a splint is prescribed within the context of a total program designed to reduce all factors in the equation—inflammation, muscle imbalance, mechanical alteration, and pain. Splinting programs are most effective when combined with medical management of inflammation, training in joint protection and functional use of the joint, strengthening of muscles supporting the joint, maintenance of range of motion, and pain-reduction techniques. Splints therefore probably should not be evaluated outside of this context.

New splint designs, materials, protocols, construction techniques, prescription and evaluation criteria, and program recommendations continue to be revised and improved and regularly appear in the literature on arthritis and related clinical disciplines. Case reports, single-subject designs, and clinical trials of the efficacy of, and compliance with, current splint regimens also produce incremental improvements in practice and are needed. There are so many different kinds of splints, protocols, and presenting conditions, however, that realistically clinical trials could only be used to test the more common and conventional uses of splints. To increase the rate and scope of new therapeutic directions, studies of the theoretical issues underlying splinting principles may need to be conducted. Comparable growth and development in the literature on the theoretical rationale for splinting have not occurred.

Research designed to expand our knowledge about these theoretical issues—such as the etiology and natural history of rheumatoid hand pain and deformity; the effects of rest and activity on inflammation, impairment, and disability; the differential effects on function of joint soft-tissue, cartilage, and bone damage; and the influence of pathophysiological, mechanical, neural, and behavioral factors to rheumatoid joint dysfunction—may have broad generalizability. The relative contribution of pathological, mechanical, and activity effects on joint pain and deformity probably cannot be isolated. Alternatively, an integrated model of hand function may have potential to advance the practice of splinting.

We have the clinical incentives as well as the basic theoretical framework and statistical tools to develop and test an integrated model of hand dysfunction in rheumatoid arthritis. What we appear to need are cross-sectional and longitudinal correlational studies designed to develop and test a hypothesis-driven, multifactorial, causal model of hand function in rheumatoid arthritis. The model needs to incorporate pathological, biomechanical, neural, behavioral, and treatment variables as predictor variables, and valid and reliable quantitative constructs of hand function as criterion variables. Recent developments in video and other computerized motion analyses and assessment technologies enhance our ability to quantitate hand function and offer promising new directions for this purpose. Additional clues to variables that predict or explain hand dysfunction may be best found through careful study of the noncompliant or nonresponding patient. A better theoretical understanding of hand function would allow for diagnostic and prognostic specificity in determining which treatments under which conditions are likely to be superior.

CONCLUSION

The general issues underlying splinting cross the basic sciences of physiology, biomechanics, and pathology and the clinical sciences and disciplines of occupational therapy, physical therapy, orthotics, rheumatology, surgery, and physical medicine. Future improvements may develop from continued and enhanced cross-disciplinary perspectives on the problem. Many of the issues underlying splinting also underlie other nonpharmacological and nonsurgical treatments such as exercise and joint protection training. Although splinting per se may never receive extensive study, splinting may serve as one approach to understanding conservative therapy for hand dysfunction in rheumatoid arthritis.

REFERENCES

Askari, A., Moskowitz, R.W., & Ryan, C. (1974). Stretch gloves: A study of objective and subjective effectiveness in arthritis of the hands. *Arthritis and Rheumatism*, *17*, 263–265.

Backman, C.L., & Dietz, J.C. (1988). Static wrist splint: Its effect on hand functions in three women with rheumatoid arthritis. *Arthritis Care Research*, *3*, 151–160.

Bland, J.H., & Eddy, W.M. (1968). Hemiplegia and rheumatoid hemiarthritis. *Arthritis and Rheumatism*, *11*, 72–78.

Convery, F.R., Conaty, J.P., & Nickel, V.L. (1967). Dynamic splinting of the rheumatoid hand. *Orthotics and Prosthetics*, *21*, 249–254.

Culic, D.D., Battaglis, M.C., Wichman, C., & Schmid, F.R. (1979). Efficacy of compression gloves in rheumatoid arthritis. *American Journal of Physical Medicine*, *58*, 278–284.

Donatelli, R., & Owens-Burkhart, H. (1981). Effects of immobilization on the extensibility of periarticular connective tissue. *Journal of Orthopaedic Sports Physical Therapy*, *3*, 67–72.

Ely, L.W., & Mensor, M.C. (1933). Studies on the immobilization of normal joints. *Surgery, Gynecology and Obstetrics*, *57*, 212–215.

Eyring, E.J., & Murray, W.R. (1964). The effect of joint position on the pressure of intraarticular effusion. *Journal of Bone and Joint Surgery [Am]*, *46*, 1235–1241.

Favreau, J.C., & Laurin, C.A. (1963). Joint effusions and flexion deformities. *Canadian Medical Association Journal*, *88*, 575–576.

Feinberg, J., & Brandt, K.D. (1981). Use of resting splints by patients with rheumatoid arthritis. *American Journal of Occupational Therapy*, *35*, 173–178.

Gault, S.J., & Spyker, J.M. (1969). Beneficial effect of immobilization of joints in rheumatoid and related arthritides: A splint study using sequential analysis. *Arthritis and Rheumatism*, *12*, 34–44.

Glick, E.N. (1966). Influence of mechanical factors on the rheumatoid wrist. *Proceedings of the Royal Society of Medicine*, *59*, 15–18.

Glick, E.N. (1967). Asymmetrical rheumatoid arthritis after poliomyelitis. *British Medical Journal*, *3*, 26–28.

Harris, E.D. (1990). Rheumatoid arthritis: Pathophysiology and implications for therapy. *New England Journal of Medicine*, *322*, 1277–1289.

Harris, R., & Copp, E.P. (1962). Immobilization of the knee joint in rheumatoid arthritis. *Annals of the Rheumatic Diseases*, *21*, 353–359.

Hasselkus, B.R., Kshehpakaran, K.K., & Safrit, M.J. (1981). Handedness and hand joint changes in rheumatoid arthritis. *American Journal of Occupational Therapy*, *35*, 705–710.

Hollander, J.L., & Horvath, S.M. (1949). The influence of physical therapy procedures on the intraarticular temperature of normal and arthritic subjects. *American Journal of the Medical Sciences*, *218*, 543–548.

Kamermann, J.S. (1966). Protective effect of traumatic lesions on rheumatoid arthritis. *Annals of the Rheumatic Diseases*, *25*, 361–363.

Kottke, F.J., Pauley, D.L., & Ptak, R.A. (1966). The rationale for prolonged stretching for correction of shortening of connective tissue. *Archives of Physical Medicine and Rehabilitation*, *47*, 345–352.

Lavigne, A.B., & Watkins, R.P. (1972). Preliminary results on immobilization induced stiffness of monkey knee joints and posterior capsule. In *Perspectives in Biomedical Engineering: Proceedings of a symposium, Biomedical Engineering Society, University of Strathclyde, Glasgow* (pp. 177 179). Baltimore: University Park Press.

Lee, P., Kennedy, A.C., Anderson, J., & Buchanan, W.W. (1974). Benefits of hospitalization in rheumatoid arthritis. *Quarterly Journal of Medicine*, *43*, 205–214.

McKnight, P.T., & Schomburg, F.L. (1982). Air pressure splint effects on hand symptoms of patients with rheumatoid arthritis. *Archives of Physical Medicine and Rehabilitation*, *63*, 560–564.

Mills, J.A., Pinals, R.S., Ropes, M.W., Short, C.L., & Sutcliffe, J. (1971). Value of bed rest in patients with rheumatoid arthritis. *New England Journal of Medicine*, *284*, 453–458.

Moon, M.H., Moon, B.A.M., & Black, W.A.M. (1976). Compliancy in splint-wearing behaviour of patients with rheumatoid arthritis. *New Zealand Medical Journal*, *83*, 360–365.

Nalebuff, E.A. (1963). Diagnosis, classification, and management of rheumatoid thumb deformities. *Bulletin of the Hospital for Joint Diseases*, *29*, 119–137.

Noaker, J., Garty, M.K., & Kwoh, C.K. (1988). A follow-up evaluation of silver ring splints. *Arthritis and Rheumatism*, *31*, S160.

Partridge, R.E.H., & Duthie, J.J.R. (1963). Controlled trial of the effect of complete immobilization of the joints in rheumatoid arthritis. *Annals of the Rheumatic Diseases*, *22*, 91–99.

Steinberg, F.U. (1980). *The immobilized patient.* New York: Plenum.

Swezey, R.L. (1971). Dynamic factors in deformity of the rheumatoid arthritic hand. *Bulletin on the Rheumatic Diseases*, *22*, 649–656.

Swezey, R.L., Spiegel, T.M., Cretin, S., & Clements, P. (1979). Arthritic hand response to pressure gradient gloves. *Archives of Physical Medicine and Rehabilitation*, *60*, 375–377.

Thompson, M., & Bywaters, E.G.L. (1962). Unilateral rheumatoid arthritis following hemiplegia. *Annals of the Rheumatic Diseases*, *21*, 370–377.

CHAPTER 10

Orthotic Management of Rheumatoid Arthritis in the Foot and Ankle

Jane E. Marlor, CO, CPed, LPTA

This chapter exposes the reader to many of the fundamental issues confronting orthotists as they treat patients with rheumatoid arthritis in conjunction with the prescribing physicians.

NORMAL FOOT AND ANKLE FUNCTION

The joints of the ankle and those of the foot should be considered as one functional unit. The foot cannot function properly without the ankle and the ankle cannot be stable without proper foot alignment. Think of the foot as a loose adapter composed of 26 bones held together by soft tissue, which depends on joint congruency upon heel strike to maintain alignment, reduce stress, and prohibit deformity. The definition of a normal foot is best described by Cailliet (1968) in his criteria for normalcy: absence of pain, normal muscle balance, central heel, and straight and mobile toes. These criteria are affected by the external forces delivered to the foot during the cycle of gait (Figure 10–1). When

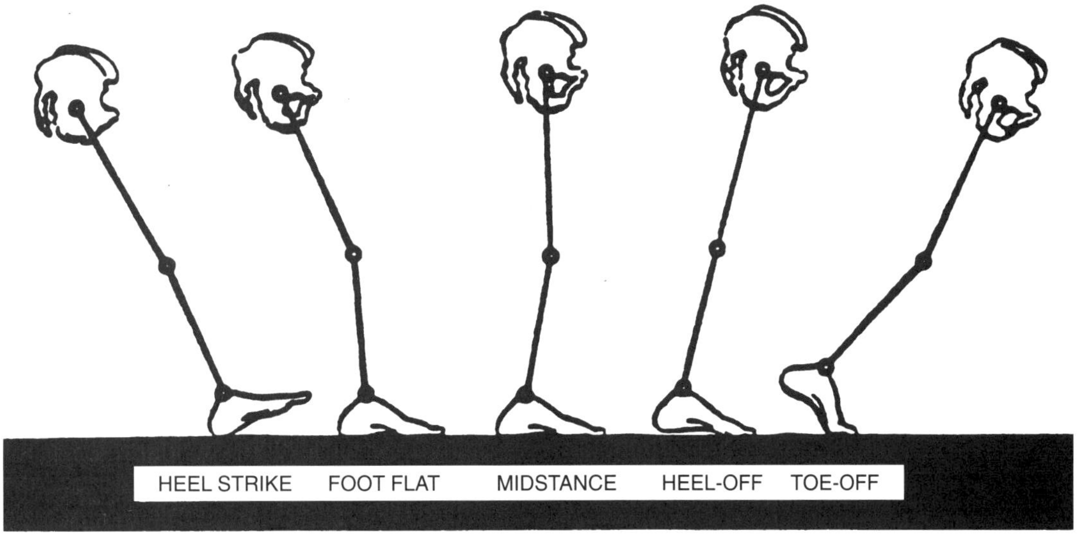

Figure 10–1 Graphic representation of the cycle of gait. *Source:* Reprinted with permission from *Limb Orthotics for Orthotists: Didactic Manual*, Prosthetic-Orthotic Center, © 1995, Northwestern University Medical School.

muscle balance is impaired, proper heel strike may be altered, which may cause the foot to become imbalanced, producing joint incongruency. The foot is designed to accept the shear forces placed upon the lower extremity. At heel strike, torsional forces are exerted on the lower limb. The foot must adapt to these forces. Improper adaptation to the forces may put excessive stress on the lower extremity. Because this motion is repetitive, undue stress is placed on the other joints of the limb, resulting in breakdown of soft tissue and causing overuse of the musculature. This then may produce joint deformity.

When examining the foot, divide it into three mechanical parts: the hindfoot (composed of the talus and calcaneus), the midfoot (navicular, cuboid, and cuneiforms), and the forefoot (metatarsals and phalanges; Netter, 1987; Figure 10–2). The primary function of the hindfoot is to convert torque, which will have a direct effect on the alignment of the midfoot and forefoot. The midfoot should be considered the transmitter. It transmits the forces from the hindfoot to the forefoot during the stance phase. The forefoot should be considered the accommodator. It receives all the input from the forces exerted and accommodates the bony structure to that force. The forefoot is totally dependent on proper hindfoot function. When a valgus or varus stress is placed on the hindfoot at heel strike, the midfoot transmits the alignment to the forefoot and accommodations are made to provide a stable base of support. Treat the foot as a complete unit with component parts working together to provide structural support. When one section works improperly the entire unit is affected (Hicks, 1953).

Ligamentous laxity results from the stress of improper alignment. The primary stabilizers of the hindfoot are the calcaneofibular ligament and the anterior talofibular ligament, which resist inversion, and the deltoid ligament, which resists eversion. The best way to visualize the importance of these ligaments is in a non–weight-bearing or unloaded position. In the unloaded position, the foot-ankle complex may be mobilized in order to palpate the ligaments. When these primary ligaments become lax, joint congruency is compromised and the end result is undue stress on the limb. The combination of weakness in the musculature and ligamentous laxity results in joint breakdown,

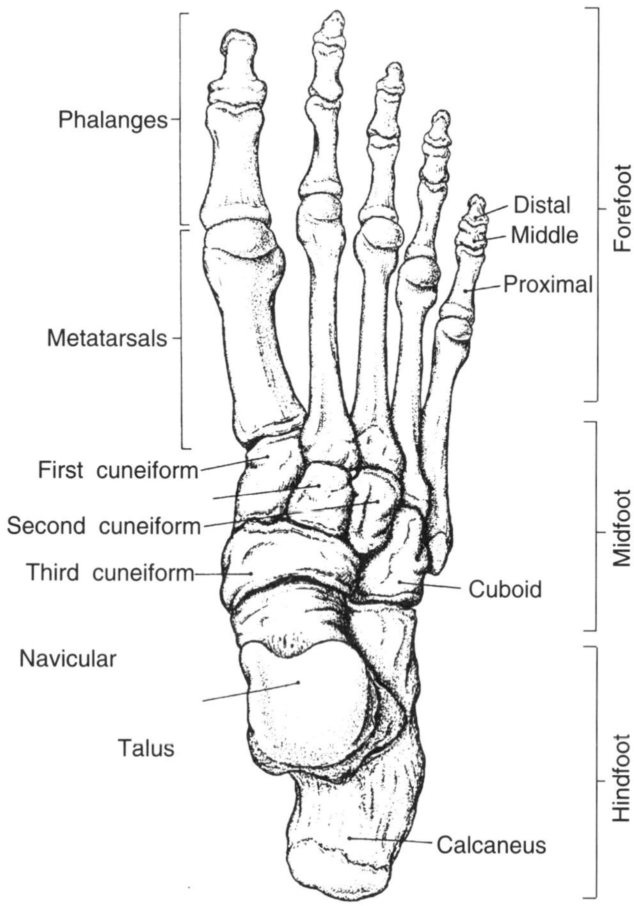

Figure 10–2 Dorsal view of the bones of the foot, showing hindfoot, midfoot, and forefoot. *Source:* From Ruthstein, J.M. et al.: *The Rehabilitation Specialist's Handbook.* F.A. Davis, Philadelphia, 1981, p. 40, with permission.

malalignment, and undue stress upon the knee and hip which may also become improperly stressed.

During the cycle of gait, movement of the joint axis of the foot depends on the torsional forces accepted by the lower limb. The talus and calcaneus form the subtalar joint in the hindfoot (Root, Orien, & Weed, 1977). This joint transmits the rotational forces to the midfoot and the forefoot. When ankle dorsiflexion, forefoot abduction, and hindfoot eversion occur at this joint, the end result is *pronation*. When ankle plantarflexion, forefoot adduction, and hindfoot inversion occur at this joint, the end result is *supination*. To see the positions of pronation and supination, view the foot from the rear while the patient is standing with equal weight on both feet. Pronation is best seen when the calcaneus is in a valgus position. Conversely, when the calcaneus is in a varus position it is considered to be in supination (Stormont et al., 1985; Figures 10–3 and 10–4).

The position of the calcaneus will have a direct effect on the entire limb. When the calcaneus is in valgus the knee will be in valgus also. Conversely, when the calcaneus is in varus the knee will be in varus. When these motions are excessive, the problems begin. The total cycle of gait is heel strike, foot flat, midstance, heel-off, toe-off, and swing. During heel strike, the calcaneus is in inversion with the tibia externally rotated. Pronation occurs during the transition of heel strike to foot flat with the tibia internally rotating. This is when the midfoot joint alignment allows the forefoot to adapt to uneven terrain. At foot flat, the foot is in the maximum position of pronation, which allows the axis of the midtarsal joints to be congruent. Reversal of pronation begins in early midstance. Supination then begins during late midstance. Supination of the subtalar joint

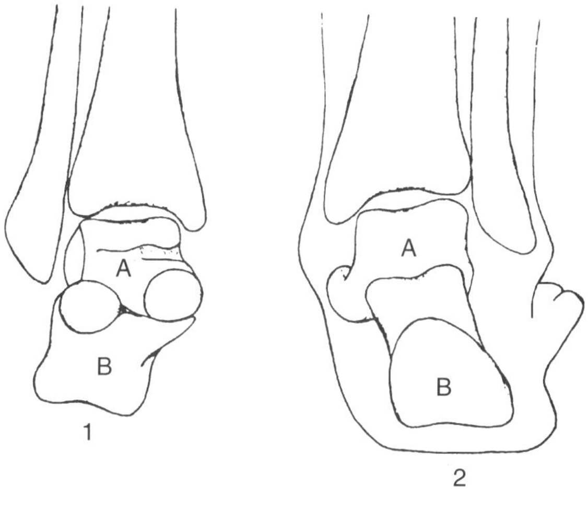

Figure 10–3 Anterior (*1*) and posterior (*2*) views of closed kinetic chain pronation. *A*, Talus; *B*, calcaneus. *Source:* From Donatelli, Robert: *The Biomechanics of the Foot and Ankle*, 2nd Ed. F.A. Davis, Philadelphia, 1996, p. 17, with permission.

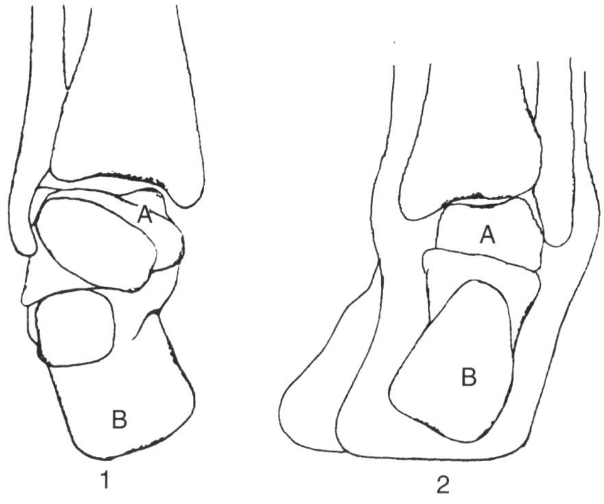

Figure 10–4 Anterior (*1*) and posterior (*2*) views of closed kinetic chain supination. *A*, Talus; *B*, calcaneus. *Source:* From Donatelli, Robert: *The Biomechanics of the Foot and Ankle*, 2nd Ed. F.A. Davis, Philadelphia, 1996, p. 17, with permission.

causes the midtarsal joint axis to become incongruent, which creates a more rigid structure in preparation for heel-off. The calcaneus is inverted, the tibia is rotating externally, and the forefoot is adducted. Now the foot and the lower limb are a rigid lever working as one unit (Donatelli, 1990). Keeping the cycle of gait in mind, it will become easy to determine when there is abnormal alignment. Evaluate the foot's response to the normal forces experienced during the stance phase, then consider which orthotic intervention will be needed. The forces that are exerted on the body begin when the foot meets the ground.

PATHOLOGICAL GAIT

When structural insufficiency is present, the loose adapter remains loose and breakdown of the structure is unavoidable. When this breakdown occurs, a predictable chain of events follows. There will be a valgus condition of the hindfoot, which in turn may yield a valgus condition of the knee, which can produce a leg length discrepancy affecting the hips and low back. Varus insufficiency occurs as a result of the structural deficits due to the overpowering valgus moments. Joint breakdown is unavoidable without orthotic intervention. Joint wear and tear occurs over time and results in breakdown of articular cartilage. Orthotic intervention is required to mediate the effects of this degenerative disorder. This may be achieved in numerous ways, however; the technique of starting at the bottom and working up to the top is key.

COMMON PROBLEMS WITH RHEUMATOID ARTHRITIS

The hindfoot-midfoot complex or the forefoot is usually affected by rheumatoid arthritis. Curiously, one or the other usually predominates. The subtalar and the talonavicular joints are the most commonly involved with rheumatoid arthritis. Because of their common joint axes, hypermobility of one affects the other. Subtalar joint hypermobility occurs when ligamentous laxity begins. This is often followed by lateral deviation of the forefoot secondary to instability. Pain and joint stiffness are the patients' most frequent complaints. The lateral compartment of the foot may also be painful because of the "pinching" that occurs secondary to the deviation. This progresses into valgus instability of the hindfoot and degeneration of the longitudinal area, resulting in the navicular bone becoming displaced and in extreme cases locating under the longitudinal area. Joint fusion may occur over time due to progression of the disease. When synovitis is present, splinting of the joint or protective spasming occurs, which is the body's natural way of reacting to the pain. Immobilization may aid in decreasing the progression of the joint breakdown.

The midtarsal joints are commonly affected by rheumatoid arthritis, leading to a collapse of the medial arch and a rigid, flat foot. This makes walking on uneven surfaces extremely difficult. The forefoot is the most common site of rheumatoid arthritis involvement of the foot. The metatarsal-phalangeal (MTP) joints are usually involved. Because of the synovitis in the MTP joints, the foot flattens and spreads at the forefoot. This is followed by foreward migration of the soft tissue cushion under the MTP joints and dorsal subluxation of the proximal phalanges. This results in the metatarsal heads becoming major sites of weight bearing during the stance phase of gait. Callus formation commonly occurs. A secondary flexion deformity of the proximal interphalangeal joints often occurs, which then creates a clawing of the toes. A hallus valgus deformity can also occur in patients with rheumatoid arthritis because of instability at the first MTP joint. The deformity of the toes can produce a variety of pressure areas on the skin of the foot, which may result in ulcers. Large bursal swelling can also develop under the forefoot, and occasionally these may ulcerate.

Tenosynovitis of the hindfoot occurs primarily on the medial side of the ankle near the tibialis posterior tendon and flexor digitorum longus. When this occurs, uncontrolled edema persists that will interfere with movements of the joint and may result in further lack of motion. In the hindfoot, heel pain often accompanies other types of foot pain. It is addressed after treatment of the forefoot. Patients unload the heel without thought because they speed the cycle of gait to avoid weight bearing on the heel. The result is excessive weight bearing on the forefoot. Heel pain is the result of a tight plantar fascia, which can pull on its insertion at the base of the heel, causing a spur. Typically the patients' chief complaint is that when they get out of bed and walk they experience extreme pain. After walking a few feet this sensation may subside slightly. The combination of weight bearing, which will stretch this area slightly, and wearing a shoe with at least a 1-inch heel will help.

EVALUATION OF FOOT AND ANKLE FUNCTION

The orthotic evaluation of a patient begins with the introduction, the moment the orthotist observes the patient. The orthotist should observe patients rising from their chairs and note the effort for them in transition from sit to stand. Observe any assistive devices that they may use, as well as any shoe modifications that they require. Also note any gait deviations, and pay especially close attention to the time spent on one limb versus another.

Evaluation of range of motion and muscle strength are important considerations; however, functional limitations are paramount. A static standing evaluation should include observing the patient's base of support, any noticeable leg length discrepancy, varus or valgus at the knees, pelvic obliquity, trunk malalignment, and asymmetry of the shoulders and the cervical region. An informal dynamic evaluation was performed as the patient entered the examination room; however, it is useful to ask the patient to take a few strides because patients often find it easiest to ambulate and explain their troubles at the same time. Footwear should be checked for wear patterns that result from the gait pattern as well as the foot's adapting to the shoe. The counter of the shoe should be evaluated for abnormal wear patterns, and any deformation of the counter in relation to the heel base should be noted.

GENERAL ORTHOTIC INTERVENTION FOR THE FOOT, ANKLE, AND KNEE

When constructing an orthosis for a painful arthritic foot in which joint deterioration and skin thinning has occurred, careful attention must be paid to the Three C's: correction, comfort, and compliance. The use of rigid materials may affect the gait pattern of the patient; thus shoe modifications should be made that would assist a smoother gait pattern. The foot orthosis should support the entire foot. Often, the forefoot is overlooked when a foot orthosis is fabricated. When the forefoot is left unaddressed, lateral drifting may occur over the edge of the orthosis. A firm, thermal, moldable, closed-cell foam is best suited for foot orthoses because the firmness is forgiving during the gait cycle. Rollover is not impeded by rigidity; however, it may be enhanced by proper alignment of the foot. A soft top cover may be applied to the orthosis to provide a forgiving surface, which is more comfortable.

Ankle-foot orthoses (AFOs) are used in severe instances. When a foot exhibits severe deformities, stabilization will occur only when the ankle joint is supported and in some instances immobilized. The foot is provided increased support when the ankle is fixed. The design of the AFO should encompass the ankle and the midfoot, providing rigidity with complete support (Figure 10–5). This will deter the progression of forefoot deformity that may occur without total support. A stable foot will be the end result, with a decrease in pain due to the immobilization and total contact that renders the foot fixed. The AFO should be set up by positioning the anatomical articulations as close to normal congruency as possible. When joint congruency is achieved, the bony structure is properly aligned and better able to transmit the forces that are experienced throughout gait.

Knee orthoses are used in many forms, ranging from a simple neoprene sleeve to a custom-made derotational orthosis. Neoprene sleeves provide minimal support and a general thermal effect, maintaining the body heat in the localized area. They may include spiral stays for light support or side bars that provide slight structural support. The patella may be exposed with a buttress to aid in alignment or it may be covered. Derotational orthoses are custom-made from an impression of the patient's knee. An orthosis designed to unload the medial or lateral compartments of the knee is also available. Many patients with severe valgus or varus at the knee who are fit with this orthosis require an AFO to accompany the knee orthosis, providing optimal support and relief for the patient.

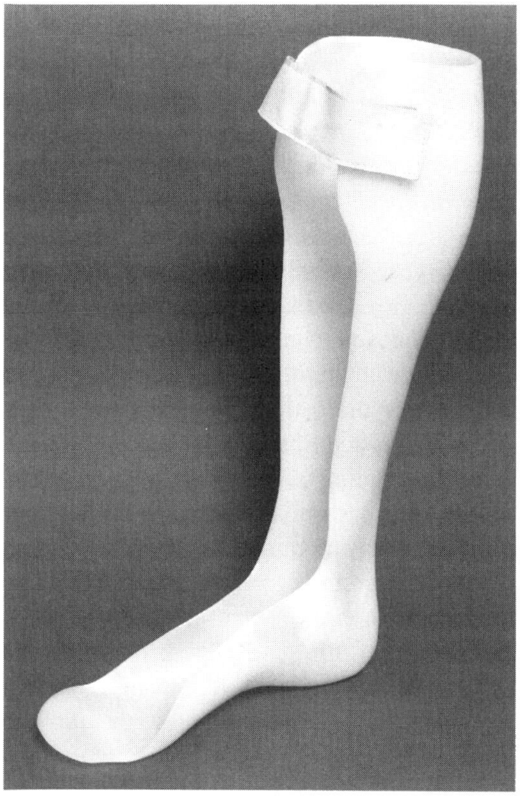

Figure 10–5 An adult ankle-foot orthosis.

PREVENTIVE ORTHOTIC INTERVENTION

Preventive orthotic management should be considered to prevent the long-term effects and disabilities that occur with arthritic changes. When arthritic changes begin, corrective measures may be taken to preserve the joint structures. A simple foot orthosis designed to align the lower limb provides the foundation needed to counteract the ground forces. This early approach to treatment allows the clinician to place corrective forces on the lower limb when the joints are mobile and therefore are able to attain joint congruency. When a foot is supple, it will accept change and correction. Correction may be achieved by decreasing the valgus or varus deformities of the ankle complex. Correction leads to support. By supporting the entire structures of the foot, support to the lower limb is also achieved. This process of support and correction provides the protection that the joints need from the wear and tear they receive daily.

A handy formula used in determining the degree of support needed is based on the patient's age. Treatment for the young arthritic foot differs greatly from treatment given to a more mature foot. For example, the feet of a 65-year-old patient have matured over many years into the condition that they are in. If the orthotist tries to move the feet into "anatomical" position, the patient will return in 3 weeks with back or hip pain. If the patient is a 27-year-old with flexible feet, however, the possibility of correction is greater.

When the decision to correct, accommodate, or support needs to be made, think of the triple-decade approach. Consider the patient's age. A patient younger than 30 years has feet that are young and supple and will be more accepting of change. In general, the structures of the lower limbs and back can accept the changes necessary to become structurally aligned. Thus, in this age group, correction can take place with minimal risks. When the patient is between 30 and 60 years old, however, the structures have already begun to change. If the patient is active, this necessitates partial correction with accommodation to the early stages of deformity. By combining partial correction and accommodation, the results will be comfortable feet with correction when possible and accommodation when needed to provide a stable base of support. Between the ages of 60 and 90, the patient activity level tends to decline, and structural changes are evident. Remember that the patients' bodies have slowly adjusted to whatever the deformities are, yet many times the patients have not changed their shoe size to accommodate the deformities. Accommodation needs to be addressed by using a shoe with a soft top cover and a soft cushion underneath the foot. This will help prevent the risk of increasing pain in the hip, knee, or low back.

TREATMENT FOR SPECIAL RHEUMATOID ARTHRITIS PROBLEMS

The orthotist should be involved during the early stages of disease to help prevent further deformity. If the foot is still supple, the hindfoot may be placed vertically to prevent further deformity. Having the patient accept an AFO in the early stages of deformity is difficult, however, because of its appearance. The AFO should provide a solid ankle so that motion can be avoided. This will preserve the remaining function of the foot. This positioning will also take the pressure off the lateral border of the foot.

When the forefoot is involved because of hammer toes and MTP deformities, the orthotist's main goal should be to recommend appropriate footwear, such as the fashionable deerskin shoe with a deep, wide toe box. The wide toe box allows mobility of the toes and avoids pressure. The suppleness of the shoe's leather allows breathability and provides a soft surface to the hypersensitive foot. When synovitis is present, proper footwear is particularly important. Because of the thickening of the tissue, more room is needed inside the shoe.

Another complication of rheumatoid arthritis of the forefoot is involvement of the plantar fascia–aponeurosis. The constriction of these structures correlates directly to the position of the foot. As the structures constrict, the metatarsal heads are pulled toward the insertion of the structures, causing the metatarsal heads to drop. This dropping effect causes considerable pressure on the heads and, when combined with the thinning of the skin on the ball of the foot, can result in great pain (Gordon, 1986).

To avoid the pain that occurs especially during rollover, or what is also commonly called push-off, patients with rheumatoid arthritis commonly unload the foot quickly. The pain is due to the forefoot involvement, which may include a rigid first ray, the main lever for push-off. When the first ray is immobile the entire gait cycle is interrupted by the lack of mobility. Shoe modification is necessary to encourage the smooth transition of the gait cycle. A rocker-bottom sole is indicated in this case. The shoe should have an extended steel shank that is contoured to the rocker shape and extends from the heel past the ball of the foot with the rocker incorporated. The extended steel shank will help to decrease MTP extension in late stance. A rocker bottom must be incorporated with the extended steel shank to allow a smooth rollover gait.

A crepe sole is placed over the shank and shaped accordingly (Figure 10–6). If rocker bottoms are not indicated for the shoes of both feet, careful attention must be paid to the thickness of the sole and rocker combination. The shoe for the noninvolved side must have the same sole thickness so that a leg length discrepancy is not created. Whenever shoes are being constructed, measurements of the patient's legs taken when the patient is supine as well as measurements taken when the patient is standing should be recorded. When degenerative changes have occurred and if the navicular bone has dropped out of place, a functional leg length discrepancy may be evident and should be addressed. By correcting skeletal alignment as much as possible, trauma to other joints and the back may be avoided. When valgus is present in the hindfoot, valgus of the

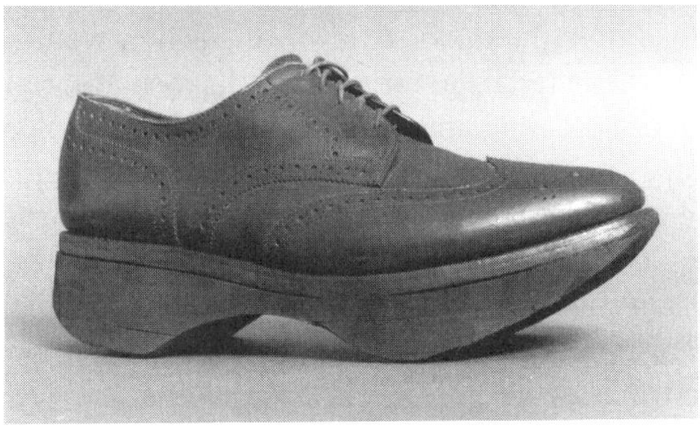

Figure 10–6 An adult shoe with a rocker-bottom sole.

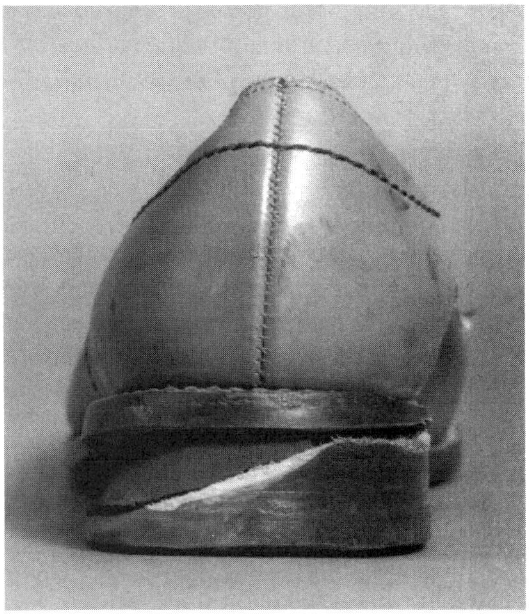

Figure 10–7 An adult shoe with an external medial wedge.

knee may be anticipated. When the valgus is present in the hindfoot, only a foot orthosis is needed to post the foot into alignment. This is accomplished by custom fabricating a full-length foot orthosis, with an increased longitudinal support and an extrinsic post placed on the bottom of the orthosis. The orthosis will wedge the calcaneus medially into a vertical position upon weight bearing. When only the foot is involved, the correction needs to be placed in the shoe to provide the necessary support and begin the joint correction immediately (Figure 10–7).

When valgus of the knee is present, medial wedging provides alignment to the limb. The wedge is placed externally on the shoe. This then shifts the ground reaction, thus counteracting the valgus moment, and aligns the limb during early stance. These valgus forces combine to move the forefoot in the opposite direction, yielding a lateral deviation. The second through fifth toes are most involved because the first toe is usually fixed or lacking mobility. When this lateral deviation occurs, the metatarsal heads may also become involved and sublux, resulting in extreme callus formation on the sole of the foot. The sole needs to be cushioned to help in pain relief. Occasionally a knee orthosis is used if varus-valgus instability is present at the knee.

FOOT EXERCISE

Patients must be taught the proper way to exercise their feet. Passive stretching of the toes in both flexion and extension is important. Teaching proper holding techniques will ensure patient mobility. Soft tissue mobilization should be taught to loosen the plantar fascia. Teaching the patient to perform this simple procedure and follow it with icing helps with pain relief.

ORTHOTIST/PHYSICIAN RELATIONS

A certified orthotist works in conjunction with a physician. The orthotist receives the written order from the physician, fills the prescription, and delivers the prescribed orthosis. What seems a simple procedure may prove to be complicated if the orthotist and the physician do not perceive that the same prescription is required. For example, there are at least three different types of metal double-bar AFOs (free ankle, single-action ankle, and double-action ankle), and thermoplastic AFOs may be fabricated in as many ways as the orthotist's creativity allows. A close professional relationship between the physician and the orthotist will prove to be best for the patient.

Optimal service for the patient is possible when orthotic clinics are established within the hospital or in the physician's office. A smoothly running clinic may include the physician, the orthotist, a physical therapist, occupational therapist, and a nurse clinician. Laboratory and radiology department personnel should be available as needed, and a consulting dietician and psychologist may be needed as well. When a team approach is used in the care of the patient, all professionals are included in the evaluation process. This leads to a comprehensive evaluation performed in one location in an organized way. The patients typically are pleased to receive evaluations and services all in the same day and in the same building. Continuity of care within the team yields optimal results because all team members are involved in the care plan developed for the patient.

When a team approach is unavailable, direct referral to the orthotist by a written prescription is optimal. The prescription should include diagnosis, joint(s) involved, goals for the patient, and type of orthosis desired. Specific styles, control desired, and materials to be used may be determined by the orthotist and discussed with the prescribing physician.

ORTHOTIC MATERIAL USAGE

When working with the foot, it is important to allow the freedom of movement that is natural during the gait cycle. This allows the foot to function as it should in a supported fashion. In this instance, semirigid closed-cell material should be used. When a rigid material such as plastic or carbon fiber is used, the foot becomes a rigid lever arm that may have adverse effects on the gait cycle. If the desire is to make the foot rigid, the ankle should be fixed so that the ankle-foot complex acts as one complete unit. Many materials are available today. One factor to consider is the shear forces that are put on the foot. In the rheumatoid foot, the bony structure changes and can thin the natural cushioning of the foot because of the destruction that occurs to the joint cavities. Thus the replacement of the cushion in conjunction with the appropriate orthoses ensures a more comfortable foot. By combining materials with different characteristics a better product can be achieved. A base of closed-cell material, such as Microcel Puff, is a shock absorber that will not bottom out, is heat moldable to a positive mold, and grindable for accommodating the varus/valgus posting that is needed. An extra-firm molding (EFM) material is used for reinforcing the Microcel Puff. This gives the Puff the rigidity it needs, yet it is still flexible. These two materials combine to yield a good base of support when vacuum formed over the mold. A layer of cushion would then top these materials to provide good shock absorption.

Isopro SR is an open-cell foam that has excellent recovery from compression. It may also be used to provide relief to painful areas of the foot that need increased softening for relief. The layer that lies next to the skin should be composed of a material that imprints as a result of compression. This enables the orthotist to "read" the top cover of the orthosis after a few weeks of use and adjust the orthosis for pressure relief and structural alignment. Plastazote is an excellent material for this. After two weeks of wear the Plastazote will conform to the foot and with the heat of the foot and the weight of the body upon it, it then becomes the road map needed for good follow-up care. The patient should be advised that the top cover will compress and is designed to be used as a diagnostic tool. When structural alignment is needed the degree of valgus/varus needs to be addressed. The orthosis should then be finished to accommodate or correct the problem area using the formula previously given for the age of the foot.

ABOUT SHOES

When the finished product is ready, it should then fit the shoe. Shoes are the most difficult part of orthotic intervention. Most of the population wear shoes that are too small. The foot needs adequate room for proper mobility. During rollover, the foot elongates slightly and the great toe usually ends up fighting to get out of the shoe. Many people conclude that the end of their shoe becomes discolored or the seam at the end of the walking shoe becomes loose as a result of being scuffed on the stairs or curbs, when in reality it is the great toe pulling on the material to make room during rollover. Many times this can be explained to patients by having them feel the inside of their shoe in the area where the ridges are very evident. In a properly fitting shoe the longest toe of the foot should be behind the stitching of the walking shoe. Leaving a thumb nail width between the end of the shoe and the longest toe will yield adequate room for the foot and the orthosis. Many walking shoes have a cushioned innersole that should be removed and replaced with the orthosis. Keep in mind that the orthosis should be full length to treat the entire foot. It should mock the innersole that was removed from the shoe. This decreases slippage of the orthosis within the shoe and fills the shoe, avoiding edge pressure from the orthosis upon the foot. When the foot is deformed, a soft accommodative shoe may be needed, such as a deerskin shoe. Deerskin shoes may be stretched to relieve problem areas and to accommodate existing deformities. Most importantly, patient comfort should not be compromised. When the orthosis fits and functions well, the shoe fits the foot, and the combination of the foot and the orthosis fit the shoe, successful orthotic intervention has been achieved.

REFERENCES

Cailliet, R. (1968). *Foot and ankle pain* (3rd ed.). Philadelphia: F.A. Davis.

Donatelli, R. (1990). *The biomechanics of the foot and ankle*. Philadelphia: F.A. Davis.

Gordon, D. (Ed.) (1986). *Discussions in patient management: Rheumatoid arthritis*. Toronto: Medical Examination Publishing Co.

Hicks, T.H. (1953). The mechanics of the joints. *The Foot Journal of Anatomy*, *87*, 345.

Netter, F.H. (1987). *The Ciba collection of medical illustrations: Vol. 8. Musculoskeletal system. Part I. Anatomy, physiology, and metabolic disorders.* Summit, NJ: Ciba-Geigy.

Root, M.L., Orien W.P., & Weed, J.H. (1977). Normal and abnormal function of the foot. Los Angeles: Clinical Biomechanics.

Stormont, D.M. et al. (1985). Stability of the loaded ankle. *American Journal of Sports Medicine*, *37*, 295.

SUGGESTED READING

Helal, B., & Wilson, D. (1988). *The foot*. New York: Churchill Livingstone.

Inman, V., Ralston, H., & Too, F. (1981). *Human walking*. Baltimore: Williams & Wilkins.

Jahss, M.H. (1991). *Disorders of the foot and ankle: Medical and surgical management* (2nd ed.). Philadelphia: Saunders.

Sheon, R.P., Moskowitz, R.W., & Goldberg, V.M. (1987). *Soft tissue rheumatic pain* (2nd ed.). Philadelphia: Lea & Febiger.

Tillman, K. (1979). *The rheumatoid foot: Diagnosis, pathomechanics, and treatment*. Stuttgart: Georg Thieme Verlag.

Utsinger, P.D., Zvaifler, N.J., & Erlich, G.E. (1987). *Rheumatoid arthritis: Etiology, diagnosis, and management*. Philadelphia: Lippincott.

CHAPTER 11

Psychological Components in the Understanding and Treatment of Patients with Rheumatoid Arthritis

Kenneth A. Lefebvre, PhD

This chapter opens with a section about the experiences of people with rheumatoid arthritis (RA). It discusses loss, grief, and emotional reactions as well as sexuality and self-image issues. The next section provides information about the psychological issues treatment team members may encounter. The last section reviews relevant psychological literature and presents an overview of theoretical and treatment implications for those with RA.

UNDERSTANDING PATIENT PERCEPTIONS

Loss, Grief, and Emotional Reactions

The prognosis for RA and other rheumatic conditions is often uncertain. While this represents a very real problem for the medical practitioner, it is also a complex psychological problem for patients and their family members. From the time the first signs of RA begin to appear, the view that patients have of the world begins to change.

Previously the world may have been seen as a place that provided opportunities for pleasure, success, adventure, and comfort. After diagnosis it is often seen as a dangerous place in which each movement and each desire become a potential opportunity for harm and problems. Instead of being a place in which to exercise options the world becomes a place with increased potential for danger, pain, and loss.

This changed perception of the world is accompanied by a similar change in how patients see themselves and others around them. Frequently, a growing sense of distrust and confusion emerges. Some patients ask a variety of questions, such as: Am I somehow punishing myself or am I being punished for something that I have or have not done? Do I have some evilness or weakness within me? Have I done something that has brought on this disease? If I am causing so much pain and suffering for myself and those around me, does treatment make sense?

This general sense of distrust can appear in other ways as well. It is very common for someone with RA to go from practitioner to practitioner, seeking the ultimate cure and never finding it. This futile search can serve an important psychological function. It allows the individual the feeling that no one really knows what to do. If that is the case, the patient has the opportunity to become as competent as any physician or therapist. In facing these feelings of self-doubt and self-punishment this way, a patient can develop a false sense of competency that essentially says, "To hell with you all. I must know as much or more because you can't seem to agree and somehow you don't seem to care."

This is a significant outcome in the patient's attempt at mastery. At this time, the patient is especially vulnerable to quack cures, inappropriate treatment, or simple neglect. It is also a developmental time during which the patient's need to be in charge can be directed toward sanctioned disease management. However, there will be times when patients are perceived as more difficult to treat because of their lack of compliance. Issues of competency and control exist within the larger framework of self-image, which may be in a state of flux. The more chronic the disease the more important it is to consider the characterological and psychosocial issues that may influence symptom reporting and compliance.

Staff are frequently asked to consult on patients who appear to have difficulty with compliance. Instead of identifying the patient as the root of the problem, staff will often benefit by becoming more flexible in their treatment as well as being sensitive to transference and countertransference issues that may be detracting from the therapeutic relationship.

There are some issues and feelings that chronic disease is likely to generate. Recognizing some of these will help treatment team members experience the phenomenological world of the patient. For instance, adjusting to chronic disease may involve experiencing feelings of rejection and abandonment. Sometimes these feeling come from the external world or from the actions of others. Although it is disappointing to acknowledge, most of us have friends, lovers, and family members who would have a difficult time adjusting to a chronic disease such as RA in themselves or others. Fear of the disabled is common. While nearly everyone will acknowledge death, many fewer will acknowledge the prospect of becoming disabled. More research needs to be done on how reaction to disability can produce fear, confusion, and sometimes the very behaviors that result in increased disability.

The rejection that comes from others is often augmented by the rejection that comes from within. Such feelings occur as people feel disqualified or disenfranchised from certain activities because of their medical condition. Treatment team members need to know about major changes that have occurred since disease onset or exacerbation. Family roles and responsibilities may have been affected. Recreational activities probably have changed. Also, the person's sexual self-image, sexual behaviors, and sexual limitations imposed by the disease need to be examined. This will help staff better address comprehensive patient needs.

Sexuality and Self-Image Issues

Thorn-Gray and Kern (1983) have defined sex as "the verbal, visual, tactual and olfactory communication which expresses love and intimacy between two people" (p. 142). However, sexuality has different meanings for different people. In medical settings, the focus on sexuality is too often entirely on function—how to have an erection or what drugs, procedures, or devices can be offered to enhance sexual function.

The rate of sexual dysfunction is high in the general population, higher still in those with medical problems, and even higher in certain disabled populations. In some cases, a spouse or partner will take the opportunity at the onset of a disability to withdraw sexually or emotionally from an interpersonal situation that was perceived as unrewarding or problematic for some time. Special problems such as alcoholism, drug abuse, a history of physical and sexual abuse, or a history of irresponsible sexual behavior all contribute to sexual dysfunction apart from the disability. It is often these factors more than the disability that cause dysfunction.

Sexual problems that are most likely to occur fall into three categories: (1) sex role changes; (2) physical changes affecting sexual functioning, such as pain, range limitations, positioning, decreased libido, and impaired sexual response cycle; and (3) psychological factors associated with change in body image, sexual infantilization, or sexual deprivation.

Sometimes staff may become physically and emotionally interested in patients. Staff may dress in ways that can be perceived as provocative, especially if the patient has not had the opportunity to be sexually active for some time. Treatment team members may be reluctant to pursue routinely issues of sexuality for fear of aggravating a problem they feel unable to solve. It may be hard to conceptualize what constitutes a good evaluation or intervention. Sometimes staff feel that there is a danger of depressing the patient by making sexual adjustment issues seem too complex or by confronting the patient's denial around this issue. Most patients, however, are willing and relieved to have these topics incorporated into their health care assessment. Of course there are patients and staff who are not comfortable discussing sexuality. Often the professional is most uncomfortable, and more training should be offered to staff in this area.

Generally, an individual's premorbid level of functioning is the goal used to guide rehabilitation. However, in the area of sexuality, the premorbid level itself may have had a narrowly defined performance focus or have been dysfunctional in some way. Therefore, a better goal would be to have the patient reconsider the definition of sexuality and desirable social behavior. This is difficult because usually people are not flexible in changing sexual behavior. The difficulty increases if patients have cognitive dysfunction or limitation, have impaired social skills, or have been in a situation where they have been treated as if they have no sexual interest or potential.

Thorn-Gray and Kern (1983) have outlined important guidelines for the rehabilitation practitioner. Their approach is predicated on the assumption that the success of a patient's postdisability adaptation has more to do with predisability adjustment than with the particular nature of the disability. They also point out that practitioners are often unwilling to probe the accuracy of patient beliefs and may agree on inaccurate assessments of sexual dysfunction. Finally, the practitioner needs to know what limits are imposed on treatment or education by patient values and belief systems (Thorn-Gray & Kern, 1983).

ADDRESSING PSYCHOLOGICAL ISSUES ENCOUNTERED BY STAFF

Prejudice and the Patient Experience

The identification and awareness of a disease state can affect self-image. While some would object to equating disease with disability, clearly most people with acquired disabilities feel this way. The psychological position this puts the person in is interesting. A person who has never known a disabled individual may have some prejudices based on ignorance or fear. When that same person becomes disabled those feelings and attitudes do not disappear simply because the person's state of health has changed. What develops is a curious psychological dilemma in which the newly disabled person has prejudiced feelings about disability and issues in his or her own life. In effect, these patients have become prejudiced against themselves. It is common to hear patients express the feeling that they are a burden on others. Sometimes patients state that only a fool or a saint would become involved with someone with a disability. Such feelings affect work, recreational activities, most social activities, and the potential for happiness. These statements are characteristic of people who are being too hard on themselves and are eliminating opportunities for growth and self-worth in the process.

Status, the power a person enjoys, is a crucial consideration in looking at the health care system. For the person who is healthy, status has many elements beyond body image. With the onset of a chronic medical condition, the interaction of body image and function with self-image increases significantly. Those who feel the limitations and discomfort of arthritis may place disproportionate importance on what they cannot do and the accommodation they must make in their activities of daily living.

Labeling Patients with Rheumatoid Arthritis

Labels are useful when they accurately identify and convey information. Too often they are used to criticize or accuse. Communication theory states that each bit of communication has two components—the "report" and the "command." The "command" aspect addresses the relationship between the communicating parties. Descriptors such as "depressed, manipulative, and inappropriate" when applied to patients put them in inferior positions. Maladaptive behavior does not exist only in the patient population. "Inappropriate" behavior is often described as colorful or eccentric in those we admire. A "manipulative" nonpatient might be seen as someone with great skills in sales or group process. We rarely talk of depressed colleagues. It may even be seen as disloyal or inappropriate to think in terms of psychological process unless we are talking about a patient. It is probably better to avoid using such terms until we are able to describe behaviorally what is happening. Staff should realize that not every complaint a patient has is due to a psychological process. Sometimes patients have legitimate, reality-based concerns or complaints about how service is being provided.

Denial is a well-used defense mechanism. For the treatment team member, denial becomes a problem when the patient acts self-destructively. However, there are other times when denial is a manifestation of goal incongruence between patient and therapist. Not every patient who comes for treatment is there to get better. Some are coming under duress, others are coming to satisfy someone else, and others are coming to confirm their disability. The last thing that patients in this category want is to be "helped" with their problem. Do not take it for granted that you and the patient are working toward the same goal. It is helpful to clarify the patient's goals and needs and explain the treatment approach, treatment alternatives and costs in terms of time and discomfort, and behavior change required or expected.

Almost every person loses something with disease onset and progression, so issues of loss and grief are frequent problems. As losses increase and work and relationships are affected negatively, being depressed is understandable. Depression that is interfering with rehabilitation therapy needs to be addressed. It is not unusual to find that patients have felt depressed prior to admission. In many instances they have had to cope with problems such as pain, restricted activity levels, decreased socialization, and significantly decreased quality of life. For some, the experience of deteriorating health has precipitated other concerns and fears, especially about issues such as aging and mortality. The experience of hospitalization, treatment, and rehabilitation can make age and disability major concerns. Patients may never have thought of themselves as old or disabled until they became "sick" or were hospitalized. Such issues and realizations can seem overwhelming to patients and to those around them. Because of this, many patients experience their feelings of depression as justified and may be skeptical or suspicious of antidepressant medication.

Depressive feelings are not to be discouraged because they may reflect an appropriate appreciation of loss and be quite realistic. However, such feelings may result in or strengthen feelings of helplessness, incompetence, or passive coping styles such as wish-fulfilling fantasy or withdrawal; both clinical and theoretical research has shown that this combination of feelings and attitudes results in increased pain, more impaired activities of daily living, and decreased life satisfaction. This has been a general finding in both Young's review (1992) of the psychological literature and Smith and Wallston's research (1992) on adaptation to arthritis.

Sometimes staff members are more concerned with the patient's affect than the patient is. They need to develop a flexible tolerance for patients' distress. If medications are to be used it is ideal to consult a psychiatrist who is sensitive to the special drug sensitivities and interactions that can occur with the chronically ill or elderly. Many patients have chronic stressors in their lives that will not be helped by medicine per se but require some kind of behavioral intervention or attitudinal change on the part of the patient or family members. Sometimes the better approach is to work with the patient on achieving short-term rehabilitation or medical goals rather than focus on chronic psychological issues. Success in the short term can have a very powerful positive effect in improving mood. Working jointly with team members can be very effective. Some patient problems are so complex that treatment attempts would probably cause the patient and family more distress than benefit. Under these conditions, the best therapeutic approach may be not to treat.

Physicians and other health care providers may overemphasize pain relief as a treatment goal and inadvertently place too much focus on pain and pain experiences. Pain may then become a means to an end, and that end is medical services, attention, and confirmation of the patient as someone with the entitlement for treatment until relief is obtained. Continued pain is perceived as treatment failure. For many patients, achievement of a pain-free life may not be possible.

Patients with RA come to us with long and complicated histories. Most of what is in these histories will never be known but they may greatly affect compliance and discharge planning. Many goals or dispositions may be unknown. Sensitive and aware staff try to balance the good that can be done in the present with the complicating factors of the unknown past and the unknown future of the patient with RA. As we treat we may discover information that is unpleasant. The goal must be to balance the unpleasant and uncertain with hope and motivation. Our tasks are to observe, to motivate, and to persevere.

Working in a rehabilitation setting requires special skills, tolerances, and maturity. Patients can be quite difficult and unrewarding at times. The setting itself can provoke personal feelings and fears of disability for oneself or family members. A humanitarian balance with the goal of confirming the patient's experiences while offering help, understanding, and support should be the ultimate goal.

In summary, many patients with RA have not only joint limitation and inflammation in common but have a constellation of psychological issues and characteristics that may accompany the disease. These are increased feelings of depression and increased psychosocial impairment as measured by global health status and current functional status. Patients with RA may exhibit decreased adherence to medical or rehabilitation therapies. They may have increased perceptions of pain and decreased life satisfaction. Such problems occur frequently in the arthritis literature, and for the past 20 years psychologists have been more systematically studying both good and poor "copers." They hope to better their understanding of how to provide psychological services in a way that is more effective and efficient than a psychotherapy model that emphasizes expression of negative feelings and focuses on the historical past.

OVERVIEW OF THE PSYCHOLOGICAL LITERATURE ON PATIENTS WITH RHEUMATOID ARTHRITIS

In his review of psychological factors in RA, Young (1992) stated that there was remarkable consensus that passive, avoidant, emotion-focused coping strategies such as wish-fulfilling fantasy, self-blame, emotional expressiveness, and catastrophization are associated with poorer adjustment, negative affect, lower self-esteem, and greater depression. In contrast, active, problem-focused coping styles such as information seeking, cognitive restructuring, pain control, and rational thinking were associated with positive affect, better adjustment, and decreased depression. These findings are consistent with the theoretical model of Smith and Wallston (1992), which is discussed later in detail.

Young (1992) also reported a review by Bradley (1989) that noted that compliance was quite variable. Compliance ranged from 33% to 78% for medication and from 38% to 66% for participation in physical therapy exercises. These were self-report measures, and therefore assumed to be higher than the actual levels of behavior. Young also pointed out that few enhancing interventions for compliance have been reported and that empirical research on strategies of enhancing adherence and compliance is especially needed. He suggested guidelines for future research and noted the ones he felt were required for quality work in this area. They were adequate sample size, descriptive patient characteristics, and outcome measures from several response domains. Future studies need to ensure that treatment interventions are comparable/credible and that patients actually implement the new behaviors or coping strategies that are being studied. Attention should be devoted to the assessment and statistical control of disease activity and of medication effects. Future studies must be attentive to the potential biasing factors in patient selection and recruitment. Patients may be more likely to enter a study during intervals of high disease activity with improvement related to natural fluctuating aspects of the disease rather than to specific interventions.

Young's review (1992) reflected a major change that has taken place in the psychological literature in the past 20 years. Much previous psychological research had been devoted to the notion that there were certain psychological characteristics that predisposed an individual to developing arthritis. This line of thinking and research has fallen out of favor with the conclusion that many of the studies that proposed such a link were either poorly designed or poorly controlled (Achterberg-Lawlis, 1982).

In addition, when psychological tests are used to assess the adjustment of people coping with a chronic medical condition, care has to be taken not to overinterpret the results. Tests designed for a psychiatric population will misidentify normal distress as signs of a possible psychiatric disorder (Crown & Crown, 1973). Instead of using the imprecise terms *coping* and *adjustment*, better-designed studies have used standardized measures to describe these concepts in behavioral terms. This approach allows for interventions and duplication of the research approach by others. For example, the active coping and passive coping subscales of the Vanderbilt Pain Management Inventory (Brown & Nicassio, 1987) can be used. Active coping refers to attempts to continue to function despite one's pain, such as staying busy and attempting to ignore the pain.

Passive coping includes bed rest, restricting social activities, and so on. Adjustment is a complex system and may include such factors as current life satisfaction, depressive symptomatology, pain, and psychosocial impairment.

Clearly the process of coping with chronic illness has a psychological price (Gardiner, 1980). A number of researchers have concluded that there are personality variables that are associated with coping with chronic diseases but no personality factors associated with the development of a specific disease. In addition, research has found that there are features of the treatment process that contribute to the negative behavioral styles that develop. Negative patient behaviors may be reduced or eliminated by changes in the behaviors of the health care team as well as programs designed to better educate and empower patients in disease management. There is essentially little or no support for the existence of an arthritis or any other disease-specific personality that predates disease or leads to disease onset (Anderson, Bradley, Young, McDaniel, & Wise, 1985; Friedman & Booth-Kewley, 1987). Other negative characteristics of studies included poor design, poor or absent controls, and designs that had relied too heavily on negative characteristics. Studies of successful copers were few and also poorly designed and poorly controlled (Creed, Murphy, & Jayson, 1990; Polley, Swenson, & Steinhilper, 1970).

Recent research has been much better designed and better controlled, and driven by better theory. Wallston (1993) has written an excellent book chapter on psychological control and the management of rheumatic disorders. He notes that control is a concept that has a number of different aspects and goes by a number of different names but that it generally means either objective or perceived influence over the outcome of an event. He had previously defined perceived control as the belief that a person can determine his or her own internal states and behavior and can influence the environment and/or bring about desired outcomes. There was a variety of psychological terms that referred to control but had different possible meanings and implications. Locus of control (Rotter, 1966) referred to generalized beliefs that were developed over time and that were based on an individual's experiences in a variety of settings. Those with an internal locus of control were felt to perceive more control over important aspects of their lives than those with an external locus of control. When Wallston began to study this concept with health-related behaviors, however, he found that internality and externality were not two opposite ends of a single dimension. He discovered that it was possible for people to hold both internal and external beliefs about health status at the same time. Externality was multidimensional: control by powerful others and control by chance. Believing that other people's actions play a significant role in whether a person becomes well or ill does not necessarily imply a loss of control if the patients believe that these powerful others can be influences to act in their best interest. Contrarily, a strong belief in control by chance in the absence of moderately strong internal feelings of control is fairly indicative of lack of control.

A related concept of self-efficacy is important in the development of cognitive behavioral approaches to medical problems. Self-efficacy refers to a person's belief in his or her ability to use cognitive resources, maintain a motivation level, and carry out behaviors that are necessary under specific situations. Wallston feels that is it appropriate to broaden the work of Bandura (1982) and Lorig, Chastain, Ung, Shoor, and Holman (1989) on self-efficacy into a concept he calls "perceived competence." He feels that as perceived competence increases, the potential stress of a new situation decreases. Successful adaptation is proportional to the perceived competence the individual feels, independent of the level of stress of the complexity of the situation.

Cognitive behavioral therapies can be defined as therapies that have the intention of teaching the patient a new skill or set of skills or changing the ways that person thinks about a particular problem. The underlying principle is that if you can change underlying thought processes, you will change the emotions that accompany certain behaviors. O'Leary, Shoor, Lorig, and Holman (1988) reported on a variety of cognitive behavioral approaches used successfully with some patients with RA. They included electromyographic biofeedback, relaxation training, and specific educational packages designed to give patients more knowledge and a better understanding about RA and better active coping strategies. Many of the studies combine several techniques. This is especially true for studies using relaxation techniques, and for that reason it is sometimes difficult to identify the specific effects of any one approach. Parker et al. (1988) designed a treatment approach using relaxation and pain-management techniques. Although participants reported increased use of coping strategies, outcome variables were unaffected by treatment. The high-adherence subgroup demonstrated reduced pain.

Other studies have found that in general there are positive correlations between internal locus of control and quality of life (Laborde & Powers, 1985). Design and methodological problems, however, make it difficult to know whether feelings of well-being or feelings of control are the critical variables. A number of other researchers have found positive correlations between mood and control in studies that had better design and control characteristics (Affleck, Pfeiffer, Tennen, & Fifield, 1987; Affleck, Tennen, Pfeiffer, & Fifield, 1987; Tennen et al., 1992).

Increasing patients' perceived control and ability to participate in health care seems to be a worthwhile goal. Gonzalez, Goeppinger, and Lorig (1990), Lorig, Seleznick, et al. (1989), and others have suggested ways to increase patients' self-management skills. Gonzalez et al. (1990) described four specific strategies to help patients restructure and correct negative thought and behaviors. They include helping patients understand that certain "self-statements" mediate emotional arousal. Examples are the thoughts, "Everything always happens to me" and "I am always sick." Patients need to know that they have irrational beliefs about health, control, and quality of life. They have to learn to evaluate critically their beliefs and acknowledge that irrational beliefs restrict thinking and coping strategies.

DeVellis and Blalock (1992) reviewed a number of educational and psychological interventions, including hypnosis and biofeedback interventions. They found that such interventions are often bundled so that any individual patient may receive a variety of treatments and that factors that help or exacerbate a condition may be difficult to isolate unless studies are carefully designed and controlled to evaluate outcome.

The process of coping with RA and other chronic medical conditions is very complex and too often has been studied in a fragmented and idiosyncratic fashion. Zautra and Manne (1992) reviewed the research on coping and arthritis. They pointed out that two separate literatures have developed. There is a general literature that uses a stress and coping paradigm and a more specific focus that uses measures based on specific conceptual models of pain or arthritis coping. Progress in understanding the process of effective coping is limited because of theoretical, methodological, and measurement issues.

In a 1992 article Smith and Wallston reported on a line of research they have been involved with that addresses many of the methodological and design problems that have been characteristic of previous studies. This is a model of appraisal, coping, and adaptation in patients with RA. The general model is based on the stress and coping theory of Lazarus and Folkman (1984). The general model of Lazarus and Folkman (see Figure 11–1) has as its fundamental premise the idea that beyond the direct effects of disease activity, how one copes with a disease is an important determinant of adjustment. This model attempts to identify both the consequences of coping and the antecedents that promote particular coping styles. Health is conceptualized as a broad, relatively stable variable that summarizes one's overall functional abilities, or specific abilities and limitations at particular times. These include life satisfaction, depressive symptoms, disease-related pain, and psychosocial impairment. Coping attempts are primarily determined by appraisals of the disease and its associated limitations. Appraisals are determined by three general factors. The central feature is the person's functional status with respect to the disease. The additional factors are generalized beliefs and expectations regarding one's abilities and internal resources and perceived availability of external resources, including social support. Appraisal is the primary influence on coping and it is strongly influenced by both beliefs and perceptions of external resources.

The theoretical position is that there are clearly adaptive and maladaptive styles of coping and that habitually responding to illness and associated limitation with passive behaviors, such as taking to bed or restructuring one's social activities, will result in relatively poor long-term coping (Brown, Nicassio, & Wallston 1989). Two cycles of behavior and coping factors were identified. The first involved perceived competence,

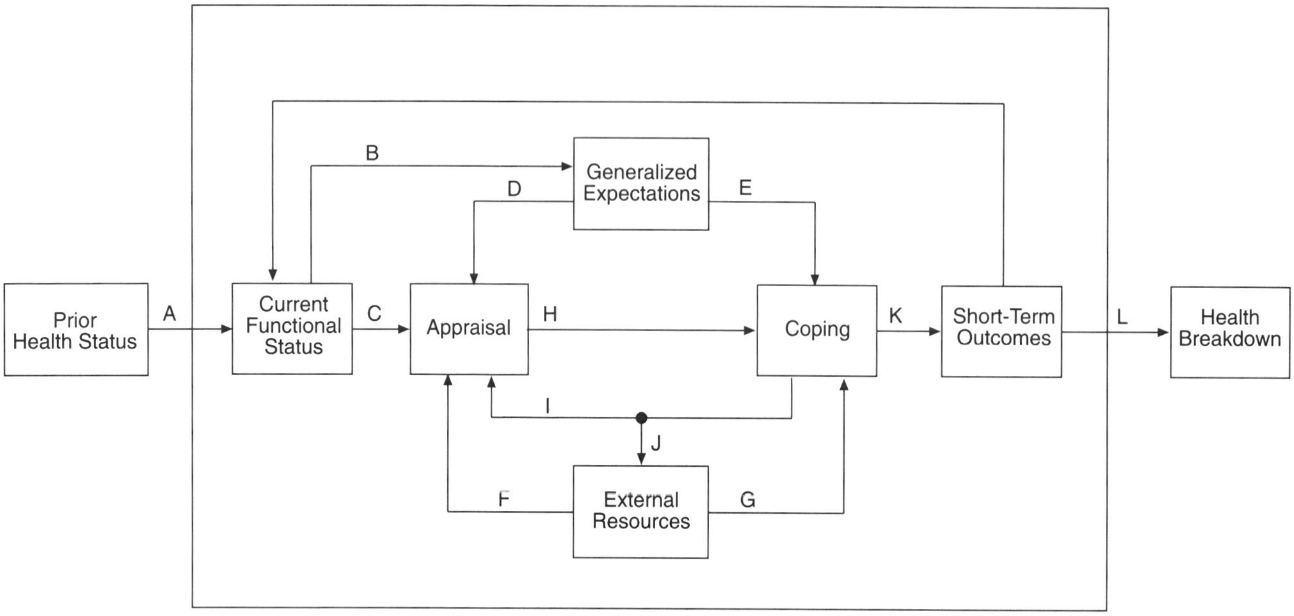

Figure 11–1 Depiction of the theoretical model representing the general variables involved in adjustment to RA, derived from the stress and coping model developed by Lazarus and Folkman (1984). The letters used to label the hypothesized causal paths correspond to the letters used to label the paths involving specific variables. *Source:* Reprinted with permission from C.A. Smith and K.A. Wallston, Adaptation in Patients with Chronic Rheumatoid Arthritis: Application of a General Model, *Health Psychology Journal*, Vol. 11, No. 3, p. 152, Lawrence Earlbaum Associates, Inc.

life satisfaction, and depression. The second included helplessness appraisals and passive coping with pain. These behaviors seem to feed on one another so that the presence of one contributes to an increase in the other. Passive coping with pain appears to produce increases in psychosocial impairment both directly and indirectly through its influence on the perceived quality of emotional support. Psychosocial impairment appears to reduce perceived competence and to increase depression, thereby contributing to the cycle involving perceived competence. It also contributes directly to increases in helplessness appraisals. As a short-term outcome, psychosocial impairment contributes directly to declines in long-term health status. This study supported the utility of the stress and coping model for understanding coping. It did have limitations, which the authors clearly pointed out. Chief among these are that the final data analysis relied on a patient population that might not have been truly representative and the fact that the study provided theoretical areas of intervention but did not study any actual interventions. The model is quite complex (see Figure 11–2) and therefore takes some time and care to understand, but it is a more realistic attempt to understand this complex process.

Interventions

The stress and coping theory of Lazarus and Folkman (1984) conceptualizes coping as being influenced by three factors: (1) generalized expectancies, which can be thought of as a kind of map of experience influenced by personality characteristics and personal history, (2) perceptions of external resources, and (3) the process of appraisal, which in turn is influenced by individual expectations. Historically, psychotherapeutic approaches have been ineffective in part because the focus was on expression of negative affect or resistances characterized by statements that change was not possible. Psychotherapy within a behavioral model is directed to teaching skills that will enhance patients' sense of control; identify irrational statements that individuals make about the world, themselves, or their disease state; and demonstrate the effectiveness and psychological benefit of task- or skill-oriented therapy

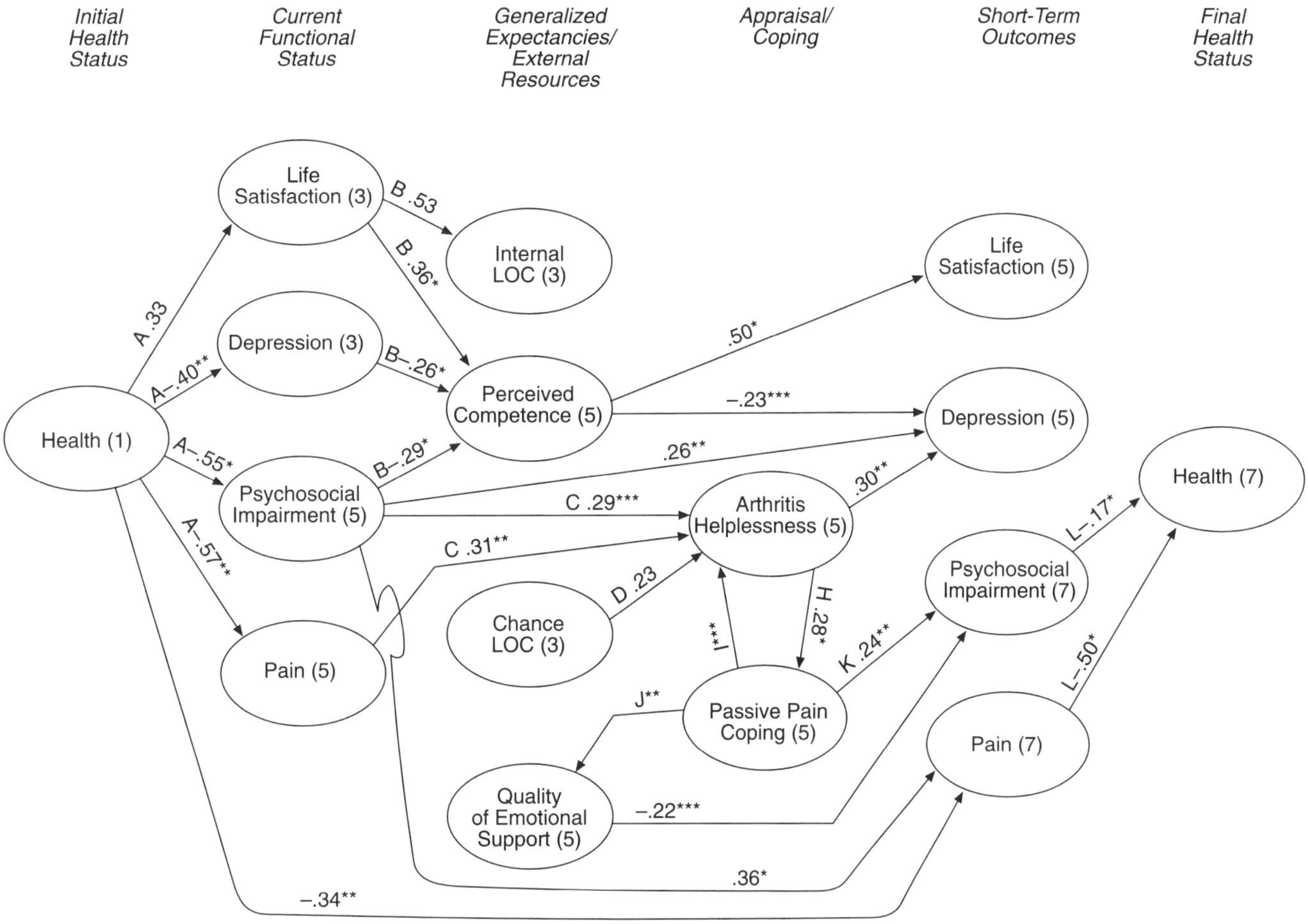

Figure 11–2 Results of the comprehensive path analysis. Only paths significantly different from 0 at $p < .01$ are depicted. The letters labeling the paths correspond to the path in the labels in Figure 11–1. Unlabeled paths were not predicted by the theoretical model. The coefficients are standardized regression coefficients, and the asterisks represent the number of times each path was replicated in the prospective dynamic analyses. LOC, locus of control. *Source:* Reprinted with permission from L.A. Smith and K.A. Wallston, Adaptation in Patients with Chronic Rheumatoid Arthritis: Application of a General Model, *Health Psychology Journal*, Vol. 11, No. 3, p. 158, Lawrence Earlbaum Associates, Inc.

techniques. The presence of a more effective psychotherapy model, however, does not mean that patients or the health care provider will accept the implications of this theoretical approach. The medical community has a long history of seeing disease as something that happens to an individual rather than something influenced by an individual. Medical events and other trauma are still called accidents, when most can alternatively be seen as the predictable end point of a series of health-related behaviors, easily predicted in some cases, not so easily predicted in others. An epidemiological approach to such problems is focused on behaviors and antecedent events rather than internal states that may be difficult to identify or measure.

Although Smith and Wallston's model (1992) holds promise, they noted that future work was necessary to better understand their findings. They found that those variables the model assumed to be important in the adaptation process were related to functioning and health in ways that were consistent with predictions. The model identified two vicious cycles that promote maladjustment. Many of the individual components of these cycles replicate previous findings of intervention-based research. Much recent research has taken a narrower focus and has looked at the connection among affect—usually depressed affect—pain, life satisfaction, perceived control, and outcome. Affective states have been conceptualized as reactions to good or bad behavioral coping strategies, and proposals have been made to improve these strategies. Finally, affect can be seen as a phenomenon that is directly influenced by a person's opportunity for pleasurable or recreational activities. Increasing leisure or pleasurable activities may be the quickest and easiest way to improve affect. The emotional energy that is required to cope with a chronic disease is considerable.

Revenson and Felton (1989) looked at how self-reported functional disability and coping efforts contributed to psychological adjustment in patients with RA. Increases in disability were related to decreased acceptance of illness and increased negative affect. Keefe et al. (1990) studied 93 patients with knee pain and compared those receiving pain-coping skills training with arthritis education and standard care. Those receiving pain-coping skill training had significantly lower levels of psychological and physical disability than patients receiving the educational program, and marginally lower levels than those in the standard care control. Katon and Sullivan (1990) reviewed placebo-controlled, double-blind treatment studies to illustrate that major depression accompanying chronic medical illness, chronic pain, and co-morbidity is amenable to treatment with antidepressants. Epidemiological studies indicate that 15% to 33% of medical inpatients suffer from affective disorders, compared with 2% to 5% of the general population. A community study indicated that patients with one or more chronic medical illnesses had a 41% increase in the relative risk of having any recent psychiatric disorder. Other studies found a high prevalence of major depression in patients with cancer, neurological illnesses, cardiac disease, and rheumatoid arthritis.

Pain Distress and Quality of Life

Kazis, Meenan, and Anderson (1983) studied overall health status. They found that pain was more important than either physical disability or psychological factors in measuring use of medical services. When Rosser (1990) studied treatment goals, the most important were pain relief, relief of psychological distress, and relief of disability. Pain is a phenomenological experience that is influenced by the beliefs and values of both the patient and health care providers. A number of researchers have studied beliefs and how these beliefs affect response to treatment or patients' behaviors with respect to disease (Price, Hillman, Toralt, & Newell, 1983; Lau & Hartman, 1983; Badley & Wood, 1979). Bradley (1993) has reviewed a variety of pain measures that have been used with people with RA. He noted that pain is a complex subjective experience that cannot be measured directly. There are important methodological problems associated with using patient self-reports. Pain measures should be more cost effective, and standardized so that collaborative research and reproducible research are possible goals. Bradley cautions that all pain measurements have limitations and drawbacks. He recommended that at least two measurers of pain, intensity, and affect should be used to determine the consistency of the patients' subjective feelings of distress.

Effectiveness of Cognitive Behavioral Approaches

Research has identified a variety of techniques that are classified as "cognitive behavioral" and that have been found useful with other psychological problems and medical conditions, including arthritis. These approaches assume that factors such as coping strategies and beliefs and expectations have a major impact on disease, pain, and disability. The link between self-efficacy and cognitive behavioral approaches is strong, since such approaches are the most efficient and effective techniques to bolster self-efficacy. Self-efficacy is the belief that one has the ability to act effectively on problems now and in the future. Self-efficacy theory (Bandura, 1977) provides a conceptual framework within which to study how psychosocial factors affect health functioning generally (O'Leary, 1985; O'Leary et al., 1988). The theory postulates that people's perceptions of their capabilities affect their behavior, their thought patterns, and their emotional reactions.

It is felt that an increased sense of self-efficacy will decrease pain and decrease psychological distress. Studies indicate that these approaches demonstrate a short-term decrease in pain and improvement in measures that are designed to assess coping, but that these improvements do not last (Shearn & Fireman, 1985;

Bradley et al., 1987; Bradley et al., 1988; Applebaum, Blanchard, Hickling, & Alfonso, 1988). Pain tolerance and treatment outcomes are both influenced by strength of self-efficacy (Lorig, Chastain, et al., 1989; Lorig, Seleznick, et al., 1989; Keefe et al., 1987; Keefe et al., 1991; Parker et al., 1989). The relapse prevention model of Marlatt and Gordon (1985) can help patients develop skills to recover from treatment failures by classifying relapse as a natural occurrence, not as a failure. By studying relapse, reasons for relapse as well as strategies to recover from relapse can be developed. The relapse prevention model identifies two categories of events that tax coping skills: interpersonal events, such as interactions with friends or relatives, and intrapersonal events, such as feelings, moods, and attitudes. The model states that it is the decision to stop coping, not the amount or severity of external events, that results in a significant relapse. Behavioral techniques that can be used to help recover from relapse include behavioral rehearsal, self-reinforcement techniques, and decision matrix analysis, which allows the patient to see clearly the consequences of a decision to cope compared with a decision to relapse. Unfortunately, the area of maintenance using behavioral techniques is poorly studied and poorly understood (Turk & Rudy, 1991).

Gil, Williams, Keefe, and Beckham (1990) looked at the relationship of negative thoughts to pain and psychological distress. Those patients scoring higher on scales measuring negative self-statements and negative "social cognition" reported more severe pain and psychological distress. Brown (1990) wanted to explore the relationship between pain and depression because there is considerable controversy over the extent to which chronic pain and depression are associated and the causal link between them. His study measured pain in six waves of 6 months each. He found that there was strong support for a causal model in which pain predicted depression during the last 12 months of his study. In an earlier well-controlled study Brown et al. (1989) studied the independent effects of pain and pain-coping strategies as well as the interaction effects between pain and pain-coping strategies on depression. The analysis revealed that pain, passive coping, and the interaction between pain and passive coping contributed independent variance, and all accounted for higher depression. Frequent use of passive pain-coping strategies in the face of high pain contributed to the most severe levels of depression over time. Keefe, Brown, Wallston, and Caldwell (1989) looked at catastrophizing as a maladaptive coping mechanism. Correlational analysis found that catastrophizing was related to pain intensity, depression, and functional impairment as measured on the Arthritis Impact Measurement Scale. A 1991 study by Keefe et al. involved a group of "active copers" who had knee pain. Those who rated their ability to control and decrease pain high and who rarely engaged in catastrophizing had much lower levels of pain and psychological disability than those who did not. Affleck, Urrows, Tennen, and Higgins (1992) reported a study of 75 patients with RA who reported on their pain-coping strategies, mood, and joint pain for 75 consecutive days. Strategies used most often were taking direct action to reduce the pain and using relaxation strategies. Those used less often were expressing emotions about the pain and redefining the pain to make it more bearable. Findings were that those who used relaxation more frequently as part of their coping strategies had less daily pain during the course of the study, and those who reported more overall coping efforts were most likely to display decreasing levels of pain across time.

Kinney and Coyle (1992) studied the perception of life satisfaction among adults with physical disabilities. Results from 790 interviews were evaluated through a stepwise multiple regression analysis and indicated that leisure satisfaction was the most significant predictor of life satisfaction, explaining 42% of the variance. An additional 11% was explained by scores on financial status, self-esteem, health satisfaction, religious satisfaction, and marital status. Satisfaction was also influenced by employment status and whether the disability was developmental or acquired.

CONCLUSION

Affect has been directly associated with a number of different factors, including pain, style of coping, and work and leisure activities. Freud has written that the goal of psychotherapy is *lieben und arbeiten* (love and work); this is so too with this population or any population forced to cope with the problems associated with chronic disease. Affect is both a way of expressing one's satisfaction with life and a message to the world about what one wants from the other. Positive affect is associated with individuals who have taken steps to increase their active coping skills and who have learned how to develop confidence about their own ability to make decisions about health care and to make sense of the goals of their lives within the context of a disease that may be unpredictable. This may result in a process of coping and adjusting to loss that is ongoing. Clearly, when the work of adjustment allows time, it is important to have paid work and leisure activities that allow for individual pleasure and a psychological identification with the good things in life. Empowerment, increased self-reliance, and increased ability to enjoy social and vocational opportunities can lead to better adjustment and better life satisfaction.

REFERENCES

Achterberg-Lawlis, J. (1982). The psychological dimensions of arthritis. *Journal of Consulting and Clinical Psychology, 50*, 984–992.

Affleck, G., Pfeiffer, C., Tennen, H., & Fifield J. (1987). Attributional processes in rheumatoid arthritis patients. *Arthritis and Rheumatism, 30*, 927–931.

Affleck, G., Tennen, H., Pfeiffer, C., & Fifield, J. (1987). Appraisals of control and predictability in adapting to a chronic disease. *Journal of Personality and Social Psychology, 53*, 273–279.

Affleck, G., Urrows, S., Tennen, H., & Higgins, P. (1992). Daily coping with pain from rheumatoid arthritis: Patterns and correlates. *Pain, 51*, 221–230.

Anderson, K., Bradley, L., Young, L., McDaniel, L., & Wise, C. (1985). Rheumatoid arthritis: Review of psychological factors related to etiology, effects and treatment. *Psychological Bulletin, 98*, 358–387.

Appelbaum, K.A., Blanchard, E.B., Hickling, E.J., & Alfonso, M. (1988). Cognitive behavioral treatment of a veteran population with moderate to severe rheumatoid arthritis. *Behavior Therapy, 19*, 489–502.

Badley, E., & Wood, P. (1979). Attitudes of the public to arthritis. *Annals of the Rheumatic Diseases, 58*, 97–100.

Bandura, A. (1977). Self-efficacy: Toward a unifying theory of behavior change. *Psychological Review, 84*, 191–215.

Bandura, A. (1982). Self-efficacy mechanisms in human agency. *American Psychologist, 37*, 122–147.

Bradley, L. (1993). Pain measurement in arthritis. *Arthritis Care and Research* (Vol. 6) *4*, 178–186.

Bradley, L.A. (1989). Adherence with treatment regimens among adult rheumatoid arthritis patients: Current status and future directions. *Arthritis Care and Research, 2*, S33–S39.

Bradley, L.A., Young, L.D., Anderson, K.O., Turner, P.A., Agudelo, C.A., McDaniel, L.K., Pisko, E.J., Semble, E.L., & Morgan, T.M. (1987). Effects of psychological therapy on pain behavior of rheumatoid arthritis patients: Treatment outcome and six-month follow-up. *Arthritis and Rheumatism, 30*, 1105–1114.

Bradley, L.A., Young, L.D., Anderson, K.O., Turner, R.A., Agudelo, C.A., McDaniel, L.K., & Semble, E. (1988). Effects of cognitive behavior therapy on rheumatoid arthritis pain behavior: One year follow-up. In R. Dubner, G. Gebhart, & M. Bond (Eds.), *Pain Research and Clinical Management*, 3 (Proceedings of the Vth World Congress on Pain; pp. 310–314). Amsterdam: Elsevier.

Brown, G.K. (1990). A causal analysis of chronic pain and depression. *Journal of Abnormal Psychology, 99*, 127–137.

Brown, G.K., & Nicassio, P.M. (1987). Development of a questionnaire for the assessment of active and passive coping strategies in chronic pain patients. *Pain, 31*, 53–63.

Brown, G.K., Nicassio, P.M., & Wallston, K.A. (1989). Pain coping strategies and depression in rheumatoid arthritis. *Journal of Consulting and Clinical Psychology, 57*, 652–657.

Creed, F., Murphy, S., & Jayson, M. (1990). Measurement of psychiatric disorder in rheumatoid arthritis. *Journal of Psychosomatic Research, 34*, 79–87.

Crown, S., & Crown, J. (1973). Personality in early rheumatoid diseases. *Journal of Psychosomatic Research, 17*, 189–196.

DeVellis, B.M., & Blalock, S.J. (1992). Illness attributions and hopelessness depression: The role of hopelessness expectancy. *Journal of Abnormal Psychology, 101*, 257–269.

Friedman, H.S., & Booth-Kewley, S. (1987). The disease-prone personality: A metaanalytic view of the construct. *American Psychologist, 42*, 539–555.

Gardiner, B.M. (1980). Psychological aspects of rheumatoid arthritis. *Psychology, 10*, 159–163.

Gil, K., Williams, D., Keefe, F., & Beckham, J. (1990). The relationship of negative thoughts to pain and psychological distress. *Behavior Therapy, 21*, 349–362.

Gonzalez, V.M., Goeppinger, J., & Lorig, K. (1990). Four psychological theories and their application to patient education and clinical practice. *Arthritis Care and Research, 3*, 132–143.

Katon, W., & Sullivan, M.D. (1990). Depression and chronic medical illness. *Journal of Clinical Psychiatry, 51* (Suppl. 6), 3–11.

Kazis, L.E., Meenan, R.F., & Anderson, J.J. (1983). Pain in the rheumatic diseases: Investigation of a key health status component. *Arthritis and Rheumatism, 26*, 1017–1022.

Keefe, F.J., Brown, G.K., Wallston, K.A., & Caldwell, D.S. (1989). Coping with rheumatoid arthritis pain: Catastrophizing as a maladaptive strategy. *Pain, 37*, 51–56.

Keefe, F.J., Caldwell, D.S., Williams, D.A., Gil, K.M., Mitchell, D., Robertson, C., Martinez, S., Nunley, J., Beckham, J.C., Crisson, J.E., & Helms, M. (1990). Pain coping skills training in the management of osteoarthritic knee pain: A comparative study. *Behavior Therapy, 21*, 49–62.

Keefe, F.J., Caldwell, D.S., Queen, K.T., Gil, K.M., Martinez, S., Crisson, J.E., Ogden, W., & Nunley, J. (1987). Pain coping strategies in osteoarthritis patients. *Journal of Consulting & Clinical Psychology, 55*, 208–212.

Keefe, F.J., Caldwell, D.S., Martinez, S., Nunley, J., Beckham, J., & Williams, D.A. (1991). Analyzing pain in rheumatoid arthritis patients: Pain coping strategies in patients who have had knee replacement surgery. *Pain*, *46*, 153–160.

Kinney, W.B., & Coyle, C.P. (1992). Predicting life satisfaction among adults with physical disabilities. *Archives of Physical Medicine and Rehabilitation*, *73*, 863–869.

Laborde, J.M., & Powers, M.J. (1985). Life satisfaction, health control orientation, and illness-related factors in persons with osteoarthritis. *Research in Nursing and Health*, *8*, 183–190.

Lau, R.R., & Hartman, K.A. (1983). Common-sense representations of common illness. *Health Psychology*, *2*, 167–185.

Lazarus, R.S., & Folkman, S. (1984). *Stress, appraisal and coping.* New York: Springer.

Lorig, K., Chastain, R.L., Ung, E., Shoor, S., & Holman H.R. (1989). Development and evaluation of a scale to measure perceived self-efficacy in people with arthritis. *Arthritis and Rheumatism*, *32*, 37–44.

Lorig, K., Seleznick, M., Lubeck, D., Ung, E., Chastain, R.L., & Holman, H.R. (1989). The beneficial outcomes of the arthritis self-management course are not adequately explained by behavior change. *Arthritis and Rheumatism*, *32*, 91–95.

Marlatt, G.A., & Gordon, J.R. (1985). *Relapse prevention.* New York: Guilford.

O'Leary, A. (1985). Self-efficacy and health. *Behavior Research and Therapy*, *23*, 437–451.

O'Leary, A., Shoor, S., Lorig, K., & Holman, H. (1988). A cognitive-behavioral treatment for rheumatoid arthritis. *Health Psychology*, *7*, 527–544.

Parker, J., Frank, R., Beck, N., Smarr, K., Buescher, K., Phillips, L., Smith E., Anderson, S., & Walker, S. (1988). Pain management in rheumatoid arthritis: A cognitive-behavioral approach. *Arthritis and Rheumatism*, *31*, 593–601.

Parker, J.C., Smarr, K.L., Buescher, K.L., Phillips, L.R., Frank, R.G., Beck, N.C., Anderson, S.K., & Walker, S.E. (1989). Pain control and rational thinking. Implications for rheumatoid arthritis. *Arthritis and Rheumatism*, *32* , 984–990.

Polley, H.F., Swenson, W.M., & Steinhilper, R.M. (1970). Personality characteristics of patients with rheumatoid arthritis. *Psychosomatics*, 45–49.

Price, J.H., Hillman, K.S., Toralt, M.E., & Newell, S. (1983). The public's perception and misperception of arthritis. *Arthritis and Rheumatism*, *26*, 1023–1028.

Revenson, T.A., & Felton, B.J. (1989). Disability and coping as predictors of psychological adjustment to rheumatoid arthritis. *Journal of Consulting and Clinical Psychology*, *57*, 344–348.

Rosser, R. (1990). From health indicators to quality adjusted life years: Technical and ethical issues. In A. Hopkins & D. Costain (Eds.), *Measuring the outcome of medical care* (pp. 1–17). London: Royal College of Physicians.

Rotter, J.B. (1966). Generalized expectancies for internal vs. external control of reinforcement. *Psychological Monographs*, *80*.

Shearn, M.A., & Fireman, B.H. (1985). Stress management and mutual support groups in rheumatoid arthritis. *American Journal of Medicine*, *78*, 771–775.

Smith, C.A., & Wallston, K.A. (1992). Adaptation in patients with chronic rheumatoid arthritis: Application of a general model. *Health Psychology*, *11*, 151–162.

Tennen, H., Affleck, G., Urrows, S., et al. (1992). Perceiving control, construing benefits, and daily processes in rheumatoid arthritis. *Canadian Journal of Behavioral Science*, *24*, 186–203.

Thorn-Gray B., & Kern, L. (1983). Sexual dysfunction associated with physical disability: A treatment guide for the rehabilitation practitioner. *Rehabilitation Literature*, *44* (5–6), 138–144.

Turk, D.C., & Rudy, T.E. (1991). Neglected topics in the treatment of chronic pain—Relapse, noncompliance, and adherence enhancement. *Pain*, *44*, 5–28.

Wallston, K.A. (1993). Psychological control and its impact in the management of rheumatological disorders. In M. Shipley & S. Newman (Eds.), *Bailliere's clinical rheumatology: Psychological aspects of rheumatic disease* (pp. 281–295). London: Bailliere Tindall.

Young, L.D. (1992). Psychological factors in rheumatoid arthritis. *Journal of Consulting Clinical Psychologists*, *60*, 619–627.

Zautra, A.J., & Manne, S.L. (1992). Coping with rheumatoid arthritis: A review of a decade of research. *Annals of Behavioral Medicine*, *14*, 31–39.

SUGGESTED READING

Crown, S., Crown, J., & Fleming, A. (1975). Aspects of the psychology and epidemiology of rheumatic disease. *Psychology and Medicine*, *5*, 291–299.

Spergal, P., Ehrlich, G.E., & Glass, D. (1978). The rheumatoid arthritic personality—A diagnostic myth. *Psychosomatics*, *19* (2), 79–86.

CHAPTER 12

Nutrition and Rheumatoid Arthritis

John T. Schousboe, MD

The interaction among diet, nutritional status, and rheumatoid arthritis (RA) has long been a source of great controversy and emotional debate. Despite this, until the last 15 years very little controlled data had been collected in this area. Today, available information is still fragmentary, and few definite conclusions about the relationship between diet and RA can be drawn. However, accumulated data over the past 15 years have highlighted the frequent presence of malnutrition in chronically ill patients, and the possibility that dietary substances may influence the activity of RA.

This chapter explores the potential benefits of nutritional intervention in RA. First the process of nutritional assessment is reviewed briefly. Then the nutritional status of patients with RA is explored. Finally, the effects of both dietary supplementation and dietary elimination on the inflammatory activity of RA are examined.

ASSESSMENT OF DIET HISTORY AND NUTRITIONAL STATUS

Current techniques of assessing a patient's nutritional status involve taking anthropometric measurements, measuring serum proteins, and conducting a history and physical examination to look for signs and symptoms of nutritional deficiency.

Anthropometric measurements are designed to measure body protein and fat stores. These include evaluating body weight for height (body mass index, equal to body weight divided by the square of height) and recent change in body weight. The latter may be more significant clinically because differences in body build can influence the former independent of nutritional status (Grant, Custer, & Thurlow, 1981). Fat stores are estimated by measuring triceps and/or subscapular skinfold thickness with a caliper. Muscle bulk (static protein reserve) in the proximal upper extremity can also be gauged by measuring the circumference of the upper arm and subtracting the contribution of fat as estimated by triceps skinfold thickness (Buzby & Mulein, 1984; Grant et al., 1981).

Serum albumin, transferrin, prealbumin, and retinol-binding protein all reflect visceral protein stores and hence dietary protein. All of these can also be lowered by inflammation, trauma, or infection, and none is specific for inadequate dietary protein. Prealbumin and retinol-binding protein are particularly sensitive to these conditions and have short half-lives (Helliwell, Coombes, Moody, & Batstone, 1984; Shetty, Jung, Watrasiewicz, & James, 1979). Serum albumin is the protein most commonly utilized in clinical practice. Hypoalbuminemia is a relatively more specific indicator of protein malnutrition than abnormal levels of the other serum proteins mentioned above (Anderson, Moxness, Meister, & Burritt, 1984).

Total lymphocyte count and the extent of delayed cutaneous hypersensitivity to a battery of skin test antigens also reflect nutritional status, and are reduced by protein-calorie malnutrition. These are easily measured in clinical practice. Delayed cutaneous hypersensitivity is also reduced by deficiencies of pyridoxine, folic acid, vitamin A, and zinc (Corman, 1985).

The nutritional adequacy of a patient's diet can be assessed by food-frequency interview, 24-hour recall method, and prospective diet record (Esvelt & Dehoog, 1984; Roberge, Sevigny, Leoane, & Richard, 1984). Each of these methods has shortcomings. The food frequency method is imprecise in calculating nutrient intake. The 24-hour recall method may not reflect an individual's habitual intake because of day-to-day variability in nutrient intake. The diet record is appropriate for use with cooperative, highly motivated individuals who nonetheless may alter their eating habits when tediously weighing and measuring portion sizes (Kim, Kelsay, Judd, Marshall, & Mertz, 1984; Roberge et al., 1984).

More detailed reviews of diet and nutritional status assessment are available elsewhere (Blackburn & Thornton, 1979; Buzby & Mullen, 1984; Esvelt & Dehoog, 1984; Grant et al., 1981; Roberge et al., 1984).

NUTRITIONAL STATUS OF PATIENTS WITH RHEUMATOID ARTHRITIS

Using the above-mentioned assessment tools, several studies thus far have suggested that a significant percentage of patients with RA are malnourished.

Helliwell, Coombes, Moody, Batstone, and Robertson (1984) obtained standard anthropometric data and measures of serum proteins, zinc, folic acid, C-reactive protein (CRP), and erythrocyte sedimentation rate (ESR) in 50 patients with RA. These were compared with measurements obtained in 50 control patients with various noninflammatory diseases. Body mass index and triceps skinfold thickness were significantly lower for both male and female RA patients, while midarm muscle circumference was lower in male RA patients compared with controls. Of those with RA, 14% had low serum albumin, 24% had low prealbumin, and 20% had low serum folic acid. Of the 50 RA patients, 13 had significant anthropometric and/or biochemical indices of malnutrition. Dietary protein and calorie intake were judged to be adequate in all these patients. In contrast, the ESR and CRP showed strong negative correlations with the biochemical indices of malnutrition, suggesting that increased protein catabolism from the inflammatory disease itself was responsible for the patients' nutritional state, rather than dietary insufficiency. Unfortunately, the authors did not describe their methods of dietary assessment, and hence these conclusions are open to question.

Kowsari et al. (1983) evaluated food intake over a 3-day period with diet diaries in 24 RA patients and 12 patients with osteoarthritis. All patients in both groups were judged to have adequate protein intake, but 33% of the patients with RA had inadequate calorie intake, and the majority had diets deficient in magnesium, zinc, folic acid, and vitamin B_6. Eising (1963) found fewer patients with RA with diets deficient in calories, and no patients with dietary protein insufficiency.

Collins, Dunn, Walthow, Harrell, and Alarcon (1987) found evidence of malnutrition in 71% of 38 hospitalized patients with RA. Low levels of serum folate, vitamin C, and especially albumin were noted, as were reduced total lymphocyte counts, triceps skinfold thickness, and arm muscle area. The extent of malnutrition in the whole RA population, however, is likely to be substantially lower than this study suggests because only hospitalized patients were evaluated.

A subset of patients with RA may also have malnutrition from malabsorption. Pettersson, Wegelius, & Skrifvors (1970) performed detailed tests of small intestinal function in 22 patients with "definite classical severe rheumatoid arthritis" and 2 patients with ankylosing spondylitis. D-Xylose absorption and lactose intolerance tests were abnormal in one third, and 4 of 9 patients who had a small bowel biopsy showed amyloidosis in the lamina propria. The prevalence of these abnormalities in the entire rheumatoid population is probably quite low; the authors selected patients with very severe disease of long duration for their study.

The data collected thus far suggests that a significant minority of those with rheumatoid disease have mild to moderate protein-calorie malnutrition, principally due to excess protein-calorie catabolism induced by the inflammatory process. Dietary insufficiency may contribute to malnutrition in some patients. Reasons for inadequate dietary intake in RA include anorexia and restricted food preparation due to fatigue and joint pain. Malabsorption may play a role in a small minority of patients as well.

Consequences of Protein-Calorie Malnutrition

Protein-calorie malnutrition may have significant deleterious consequences in patients with RA. Data in several studies of surgical patients have shown that those who are malnourished have an increased risk of perioperative sepsis and death (Mullen, 1981), and prolonged postoperative recovery and hospital stay (Anderson, Collins, Davis, & Bivins, 1985). These poor outcomes are probably due in part to the fact that protein-calorie malnutrition reduces T-cell function, delayed hypersensitivity, and neutrophil chemotaxis (Meakins et al., 1977). Improvement of malnutrition with aggressive enteral and parenteral nutrition has been shown to reduce mortality and the incidence of postoperative complications (Daly, Dudrick, & Copeland, 1980; Mullen, 1981).

Rheumatoid arthritis is a risk factor for joint sepsis (Rosenthal, Bole, & Robinson, 1980), and patients with RA are twice as likely to develop infection of a prosthetic joint than patients with osteoarthritis (Poss et al., 1984). Although non-nutritional factors may be largely responsible for the increased incidence of joint infection in patients with RA, the above-cited data suggest that malnutrition is responsible for some of the incremental risk.

Studies in rehabilitation patients suggest the possibility that malnutrition in patients with RA may contribute to disability, particularly if muscle function and power are affected. Glenn, Carfi, and Belle (1985) followed patients with a variety of primary diagnoses in a rehabilitation setting and found that improvement in mobility during rehabilitation was reduced in patients who remained hypoalbuminemic despite nutritional supplements. Specific effects of malnutrition on muscle function were not evaluated in these patients. However, Brough, Horne, Blount, Irving, and Jeejeebhoy (1986) have postulated that malnutrition also has a direct effect on muscle function. They studied the force of adductor pollicis contraction in response to ulnar nerve stimulation, as described by Edwards, Young, Hoshing, and Jones (1977), in patients with protein-calorie malnutrition. With submaximal ulnar nerve stimulation, the force of muscle contraction and the speed of muscle relaxation were decreased in malnourished patients compared with controls, and improved with nutritional repletion. These abnormalities correlated better with protein and calorie dietary inadequacy than the usual standard measures of malnutrition, such as serum albumin. Chan, McLaughlin, Ponting, Biglin, and Dudley (1986), however, found that these abnormalities of adductor pollicis function could be reversed quickly with intravenous glucose and potassium, casting doubt that the muscle dysfunction noted in the above studies was specifically due to protein-calorie malnutrition. Harrell, Waltham, Collins, Dunn, and Alarcon (1987) identified RA patients with laboratory or anthropometric indices of malnutrition, and prospectively followed them for a mean of 2 years. Malnourished patients were twice as likely to require arthritis-related hospitalization and/or suffer from persistently active disease as well-nourished RA patients. These same authors found in hospitalized RA patients that grip strength was reduced in malnourished patients compared with well-nourished patients (Collins et al., 1987). Although inconclusive, these studies suggest the possibility that protein-calorie malnutrition may increase muscle weakness and disability in RA.

Unfortunately, there are large gaps in the data as they stand. Detailed dietary intake studies need to be done on larger numbers of RA patients. The risk of perioperative infection, especially of joint prostheses, needs to be directly evaluated in malnourished RA patients undergoing orthopaedic surgery. Descriptive studies of malnutrition in RA and its relationship to disability and muscle bulk, power, and function need to be done. In future investigations of these outcomes, the role of malnutrition compared with that of non-nutritional factors needs to be delineated.

Finally, no interventional studies of nutritional supplementation in adult rheumatoid disease have been done. Even if the disease process itself is responsible for most of the malnutrition we see, extra dietary supplements conceivably could reverse negative protein-calorie balance. The effects of such supplementation in malnourished RA patients on anthropometric and biochemical parameters of nutritional status and on muscle function, disability, rates of hospitalization, and mortality need to be evaluated.

Micronutrient Balance

Altered serum levels of minerals, the amino acid histidine, and several vitamins have been described in RA, but attempts to improve disease status by administering micronutrient supplements have been disappointing.

Minerals

Reduced plasma zinc levels have been found in some RA patients (Balough et al., 1980; Helliwell, Coombes, Moody, Batstone, & Robertson, 1984).

Kowsari et al. (1983) found the diet of 24 RA patients to be deficient in zinc. Moderate to severe deficiency can result in loss of cell-mediated immunity (Corman, 1985; McMurray, 1984). Low serum zinc levels in RA appear to be due to inflammatory white blood cell–mediated movement of zinc from serum to the liver, however, rather than true zinc deficiency (Powanda, Cockrell, & Pekarek, 1973). Although Simkin (1976) found zinc supplements to be effective in reducing joint inflammation in RA, two other studies found no benefit from oral zinc therapy in RA (Job, Menkes, & Delbarre, 1980; Mattingly & Mowat, 1982).

Low serum selenium levels have also been described in RA (Tarp, Overvad, Hansen, & Thorling, 1985), but a placebo-controlled trial found no benefit from selenium supplementation in RA, despite raising serum selenium levels to supraphysiologic levels (Tarp, Overvad, Thorling, Grandal, & Hausen, 1985).

Histidine

Gerber (1975) and Kirkham, Lowe, Bird, and Wright (1981) reported low serum levels of histidine in RA, whereas Gerber and Gerber (1977) found normal levels in a variety of other inflammatory and noninflammatory conditions. Histidine levels remained low despite clinical improvement with gold or corticosteroids, suggesting that low histidine levels may not be due to active inflammatory disease. Trang, Furst, Odebach, and Lovgren (1985), however, found normal histidine levels in their RA patients. Protein-calorie malnutrition may cause low levels of histidine, with or without low levels of other amino acids (Smith, Pozefsky, & Chetri, 1974; Swenseid & Kopple, 1973). Histidine supplements were found to be of no benefit for RA in a prospective placebo-controlled trial (Pinals, Harris, Burnett, & Gerber, 1977).

Vitamins

Low Vitamin B_6 levels were found by Schumacher, Bernhart, and Gyorgy (1975) in 32% of RA patients and 7% of control patients. Vitamin B_6 supplements had no beneficial effects on disease activity. D-Penicillamine, used to treat RA, inactivates vitamin B_6 (Jaffe, Altman, & Merryman, 1964), but in the absence of frank or marginal dietary insufficiency this does not appear to be clinically significant.

Folic acid deficiency can be found in a minority of patients. This may be of concern particularly in those treated with methotrexate and/or sulfasalazine; methotrexate is a direct folate antagonist, and sulfasalazine inhibits folic acid absorption and metabolism (Peppercorn, 1984). Folinic acid supplementation has shown promise in reducing toxicity due to methotrexate treatment in RA patients (Shirocky et al., 1993).

Low platelet and/or leukocyte levels of vitamin C have been reported in a minority of RA patients, especially those on high-dose aspirin therapy (Oldryd & Dawes, 1985; Sahud & Cohen, 1971). Scurvy has not been reported in RA, but Oldryd and Dawes (1985) reported cutaneous bruising which was responsive to vitamin C therapy in patients with RA. This has not yet been confirmed by other investigators.

GENERAL NUTRITIONAL THERAPY IN RHEUMATOID ARTHRITIS

What should currently be advised regarding general nutritional therapy in patients with RA? Those undergoing major surgery such as total joint arthroplasty or who are significantly disabled should have a general nutritional evaluation, including assessment of weight for height, history of recent weight loss, serum albumin, total lymphocyte count, and possibly triceps skinfold thickness and arm muscle area. A detailed dietary assessment is a reasonable next step in those with significant abnormalities in these measurements. For those with severe malnutrition, aggressive nutritional therapy is indicated, preferably with enteral supplements or feedings, or with parenteral nutrition if the enteral route cannot be used. For those with mild evidence of malnutrition, enteral supplementation is reasonable, but for many of these patients parenteral nutritional therapy is probably neither appropriate nor cost effective. Folic or folinic acid is appropriate for some patients taking methotrexate, but otherwise vitamin and mineral supplementation appears to be indicated only in those with significantly restricted diets or documented deficiency.

NUTRITIONAL INTERVENTION AS THERAPY FOR RHEUMATOID ARTHRITIS

Many RA patients find the idea of treating their arthritis with dietary changes appealing, and try one or more dietary changes in an attempt to reduce their joint pain (Pullar, Capell, Millar, & Brooks, 1982). Over the past few years, data have accumulated that two particular nutritional therapeutic approaches may have value for some patients with RA.

Altering Fatty Acid Content of the Diet

Eicosanoids (prostaglandins [PGs] and leukotrienes [LTs]) have long been recognized as modulators of inflammation. Dietary fatty acid precursors can influence the amount and type of eicosanoids synthesized by the body (Table 12–1). Specifically, gammalinolenic acid (GLA) is converted into prostaglandins of the PG 1 series, whereas linoleic and arachidonic acids are converted into prostaglandins of the PG 2 series as well as the leukotriene 4 compounds. Eicosapentaenoic acid (EPA), however, an omega-3 fatty acid commonly found in certain fish oils, is converted into prostaglandins of the PG 3 series and LTB_5. Significant immunological and clinical effects of both fish oils containing omega-3 fatty acids and plant oils containing gammalinolenic acid have been demonstrated.

Fish Oil

Prostaglandins of the 3 series derived from EPA are in general less proinflammatory than those of the 2 series, and LTB_5 is a much weaker chemotactic agent than LTB_4 (Lee et al., 1984; Lewis & Austen, 1984). More important, neutrophil synthesis of LTB_4 is inhibited after 3 to 6 weeks of dietary omega-3 fatty acid supplementation (Lee et al., 1985; Sperling, Weinblatt, & Robin, 1987), and to a slight degree the activity of cyclooxygenase is also inhibited (Von Schacky, Fischer, & Weber, 1985). Dietary supplements of omega-3 fatty acids for 6 weeks or more have also been shown to inhibit monocyte production of platelet-activating factor and neutrophil responsiveness to LTB_4 (Lee et al., 1985; Sperling et al., 1987). Additionally, dietary omega-3 fatty acid supplementation reduces monocyte production of interleukin-1 (Kremer, Lawrence, et al., 1990) and tumor necrosis factor-alpha (Endres, et al., 1989). Several investigators have therefore postulated that changes in dietary fatty acid content can alter the relative amounts of these PGs in the body, and hence the inflammatory activity of various diseases.

Fish oils containing omega-3 fatty acids have been demonstrated to have some anti-inflammatory activity in both animal models of autoimmune disease and adult RA. Murine systemic lupus erythematosus has been found to be ameliorated by dietary EPA in both NZB/NZW rats (Robinson, Prickett, Makoul, Steinberg, & Colvin, 1986) and MRL-lpr mice (Kelley, Ferretti, Izui, & Strom, 1985).

Studies in murine models of arthritis have yielded mixed results. The severity and incidence of type II collagen-induced arthritis was reduced by dietary EPA in B10.RIII mice (Leslie et al., 1985), but Prickett, Trentham, and Robinson (1984) found that EPA increased the incidence of collagen-induced arthritis in Srague-Dawley rats. Additionally, McColl, Cleland, Whitehouse, and Vernon-Roberts (1987) found that EPA reduced the severity of adjuvant-induced arthritis in Dark Agouti rats, but enhanced the severity of adjuvant-induced arthritis in Wistar hooded rats. These studies strongly suggest that genetic differences among these strains of rats influence their response to fish oil.

Eight human placebo-controlled, prospective, double-blind studies of fish oil supplementation (containing eicosapentaenoic and docosahexaenoic acids) have been reported thus far (Table 12–2). All of these trials have shown modest improvement in a few clinical parameters after 10 to 14 weeks of fish oil compared with placebo oil, most commonly joint tender-

Table 12–1 Some Eicosanoids and Their Fatty Acid Precursors

	Synthesized	
Fatty Acid Precursor	*Prostaglandins*	*Leukotrienes*
Gammalinolenic acid	PGE_1	—
Arachidonic acid	PGE_2, PGF_{2a}, PGI_2, TXA_2*	LTB_4, LTC_4, LTD_4
Eicosapentaenoic acid	PGE_3, PGI_3	LTB_5

*Thromboxane A_2.

ness and morning stiffness. However, only the 24-week trial of Kremer et al. (1990) showed improvement in multiple clinical parameters, including grip strength and a 20% to 30% reduction in joint swelling count, with fish oil supplementation compared with those treated with olive oil. Slightly better results, including reduced pain, were seen in those treated with fish oil containing 5.4 g of omega-3 fatty acids compared with 2.7 g of omega-3 fatty acids. It is possible that these trials underestimate the potential effects of fish oil: dropouts due to flare of joint disease occurred disproportionately in the control group in the 24-week trial; the other trials were of short duration; and olive oil itself may have slight anti-inflammatory effects (Kremer et al., 1990). Additionally, the two studies with a crossover design (Kremer et al., 1987; Van der Tempel, Tulleken, Limburg, Muskiet, & Van Rijswijk, 1990) may have underestimated the effects of fish oil, because those randomized to receive fish oil first may have had carry-over effects from this treatment after being crossed over to receive the placebo treatment.

Only minor side effects attributable to fish oil occurred in the studies in Table 12–2, notably dyspepsia and eructation. Lippiello, Fienhold, and Grandjean (1990), however, noted a 32% decrease in cartilage proteoglycan synthesis and a 30% to 40% reduction in cartilage hexosamine content in Sprague-Dawley rats fed menhaden oil (rich in omega-3 fatty acids) as their main dietary source of fat. This dietary change was sufficient to reduce substantially the cartilage content of arachidonic acid (an omega-6 fatty acid). Although only minimal, microscopic, cartilaginous defects were noted, this study raises the disconcerting theoretical possibility that long-term, high-dose supplementation of omega-3 fatty acids in humans could have deleterious effects on cartilage.

Before fish oil can be recommended for routine clinical use in RA, further long-term placebo-controlled studies need to be done to document its efficacy and safety. At least some studies should employ low doses of fish oil, which may show more cumulative benefit with long-term administration. Additional animal studies need to be done to examine the effects on cartilage metabolism and integrity of diets containing proportions of omega-3 and omega-6 fatty acids comparable to those that would be used by humans taking supplements of fish oil.

Table 12–2 Studies of Fish Oil Supplementation

Study	*Study Design*	*Duration of Fish Oil Supplementation (wk)*	*No. of Patients Studied*	*Dose of Omega-3 Fatty Acids/Day (g)*	*Control Supplement*
Kremer et al. (1985)	Prospective, double-blind, randomized	12	37 (15 dropouts)	2.7	Paraffin wax
Sperling et al. (1986)	Prospective, randomized	10	19	Not stated	Olive oil
Kremer et al. (1987)	Prospective, randomized, crossover	14	33 (7 dropouts)	4.6	Olive oil
Cleland et al. (1988)	Prospective, randomized, double-blind	12	46 (14 dropouts)	5.2	Olive oil
Van der Tempel et al. (1990)	Prospective, randomized, crossover	12	14 (2 dropouts)	3.36	Coconut oil
Kremer et al. (1990)	Prospective, randomized, double-blind	24	49 (15 dropouts)	5.4 (high dose) 2.7 (low dose)	Olive oil
Kjeldsen-Kraugh et al. (1992)	Prospective, randomized, double-blind	16	67 (12 dropouts)	5.8	Corn oil
Nielsen et al. (1992)	Prospective, randomized, double-blind	12	51 (6 dropouts)	3.6	"Danish diet" (100% omega-6)

Plant Oils

Dietary supplementation of plant oils containing GLA has been tried in experimental animal models of inflammatory disease and in RA. Gammalenolenic acid is metabolized to dihomogammalinolenic acid (DGLA), which inhibits production of inflammatory compounds produced from arachidonic acid via the cyclooxygenase pathway. Another derivative, hydroperoxy-DGLA, also inhibits 5-lipoxygenase (Callegari & Zurier, 1991). Dihomogammalenolenic acid is also converted to PGE_1, a prostaglandin with anti-inflammatory properties. Kunkel, Ogawa, Conran, Ward, & Zurier (1981) found reduced joint swelling in rats with adjuvant arthritis, and reduced vascular permeability in rats with vasculitis treated with a stable analogue of PGE_1, 15-(S)-15-methyl PGE_1. In another study, Kunkel, Ogawa, Ward, and Zurier (1981) treated rats with adjuvant arthritis with dietary supplements of evening primrose oil, a rich source of DGLA, and found reduced joint swelling and neutrophil chemotaxis.

Three placebo-controlled, randomized trials of either evening primrose oil or borage seed oil, both rich in GLA, have been reported in RA (Table 12–3). Belch, Ansell, Madhok, O'Dowd, and Sturrock (1988) compared two active treatment groups with a placebo group, one active group receiving 540 mg of GLA per day and the other receiving 450 mg of GLA plus 240 mg of EPA per day for 12 months. The two groups receiving GLA reported more subjective improvement in pain than those on placebo but did not show any significant improvement in joint swelling, tenderness, morning stiffness, or grip strength. Jantti, Seppala, Vapaatalo, and Isomaki (1989) compared the effects of 20 mL of evening primrose oil (containing approximately 1.5 g of GLA) with those of olive oil in a 12-week trial. Neither group showed significant improvement in joint pain or swelling, morning stiffness, or grip strength. Leventhal, Boyce, and Zurier (1993), however, showed significant improvement in joint tenderness, joint swelling, pain score, and global physician assessment in RA patients randomized to receive 1.4 g of GLA over 24 weeks, compared with those who received cottonseed oil. Only patients not requiring treatment with a disease-modifying drug, however, were allowed in this trial. These results suggest that GLA supplementation may be useful in mild RA, if given in sufficient dosage for 24 weeks or more. Clearly, additional studies better defining the long-term efficacy and safety of GLA supplementation need to be done before routine clinical use can be recommended.

Food-Induced Rheumatoid Arthritis

For years, claims that RA is a disease due to food allergy have provoked emotional debate. Small amounts of potentially antigenic macromolecules can be absorbed intact in the small intestine (Walker & Isselbacher, 1974), and theoretically intestinal absorption of such macromolecules could cause inflammatory arthritis. Several studies have shown that fasting reduces the inflammatory activity of RA (Hafstrom, Ringertz, Gyllenhammar, Palmblad, & Harms-Ringdahl, 1988; Skoldstrom, Larsson, & Lindstrom, 1979; Uden, Trang, Venizelos, & Palmblad, 1983). This could be due to elimination of dietary allergens, but more likely it is the result of a complex series of changes, including the effects of negative protein-calorie balance on leukocyte function and eicosanoid synthesis.

Most published reports of food-induced arthritis have been uncontrolled anecdotal observations, extensively reviewed by Panush (1991). However, many controlled studies of the effects of specific dietary changes on disease activity in RA have been reported. These studies have yielded somewhat conflicting, inconclusive results thus far, but suggest that a minority of those with inflammatory arthritis may have true food-induced flares of joint disease.

Vegetarian Diets

Three studies have evaluated the effectiveness of vegetarian diets in RA. Two studies found that although RA patients improved while fasting, disease activity returned with either a strict vegetarian diet (Skoldstrom, 1986) or a lactovegetarian diet (Skoldstrom, Larsson, & Lindstrom, 1979). On the other hand, Kjeldsen-Kraugh et al. (1991) found that fasting followed by a gluten-free diet for 3 months and then a lactovegetarian diet for 8 months was of benefit in RA. Compared with those who were randomized to a brief

Table 12–3 Studies of Supplemental Plant Oils In RA

Study	*Study Duration*	*No. of Patients Studied*	*Experimental Group(s) Supplement*	*Control Group Supplement*
Belch et al. (1988)	12 mo	49 (13 dropouts)	(1) 540 mg GLA/day (2) 450 mg GLA plus 240 mg EPA/day	Liquid paraffin
Jantti et al. (1989)	12 wk	20	1.5 g GLA/day	Olive oil
Leventhal et al. (1993)	24 wk	27 (10 dropouts)	1.4 g GLA/day	Cottonseed oil

fast followed by a control diet, those on the gluten-free/lactovegetarian diet showed significantly reduced pain, joint tenderness and swelling, and improved grip strength.

Controlled Studies of Other Exclusion Diets

Van der Laar and Van der Korst (1992) randomized 94 patients to receive either an elemental diet supplying all needed nutrients or an elemental diet plus lactoproteins and azo yellow dyes. No differences in joint tenderness or swelling, pain, fatigue score, morning stiffness, or grip strength were noted between the two groups after 12 weeks of diet therapy. Milk allergens and azo dyes, therefore, were not shown to be common causes of RA flare. However, nine participants did note greater than 20% reduction in joint tenderness on an elemental diet and deterioration following resumption of a normal diet.

Darlington, Ramsey, and Mansfield (1986) randomized 53 patients to receive either an exclusion diet or their regular diet with barium sulfate placebo tablets. Patients on the exclusion diet showed improvement in pain, joint count, duration of morning stiffness, and grip strength. Unfortunately, a direct comparison of the outcomes data in the placebo and exclusion diet groups was not provided in their study, and the authors did not state the nature of the exclusion diet. Darlington (1991) has subsequently implicated cereals, especially corn and wheat, as common causes of food-induced arthritis. Similarly, uncontrolled observations by Beri, Malaviya, Shandilya, and Singh (1988) have implicated wheat and rice as causes of flares of RA. Clearly, double-blind, prospective studies have not confirmed these observations as yet.

In one of the best controlled studies to date, Panush and his colleagues (1983) critically examined the effectiveness of the Dong diet (Dong & Banks, 1975) in RA. This widely publicized diet is free of additives, preservatives, fruit, red meats, herbs, and dairy products. Twenty-six patients were randomly assigned to either the Dong diet or a placebo diet proscribing turkey, selected vegetables and cereals, margarine, bananas, and strawberries. No differences between the two groups in patient or examiner global assessment duration of morning stiffness, number of tender or swollen joints, or grip strength were apparent throughout the 10-week study. However, two patients on the experimental diet showed striking improvement in their arthritis and reported exacerbations of symptoms with ingestion of some of the excluded foods.

Double-Blind Food Elimination and Challenge Studies

In all of the studies cited thus far, participants were not blinded to their dietary changes. Changes in diet can have powerful placebo effects, however, and psychological food reactions are common (Lessof, 1984; Pearson, 1991). To prove that a particular food truly is causing flares of arthritis, it needs first to be removed from the diet consistently for an adequate period of time and then reintroduced in a disguised, double-blind fashion. A few investigations have attempted this.

Panush (1990) reported the occurrence of food-induced arthritis in at least 3 of 97 patients with seronegative, palindromic inflammatory arthritis. Of these 97 patients, 29 patients alleged food-related arthritis symptoms, and 19 of this subset subsequently completed double-blind, controlled food challenges after being placed on an elemental diet consisting of Vivonex. One patient had arthritis flares after ingestion of shrimp, along with the appearance of immunoglobulin G (IgG) antishrimp antibodies. One had attacks of arthritis after ingesting nitrites, and one had milk-induced arthritis associated with anti-α-lactalbumin IgG_4 antibodies and delayed skin test reactivity to milk (Panush, Stroud, & Webster, 1986). Parke and Hughes (1981) also reported a patient with seronegative arthritis induced by dairy product ingestion who developed positive radioallergosorbent tests to milk and cheese during these flares.

Van der Laar et al. (1992) studied six seropositive RA patients whose disease activity had improved on an elemental diet with double-blind food elimination and challenges. Four of the six were shown to have true food-induced flares of arthritis, with potatoes, apples, bananas, coriander, and cardamom among those foods implicated. Additionally, three patients had small intestinal and synovial biopsies during flares, and two of these patients demonstrated significantly increased small intestinal and synovial mast cell numbers during food-induced flares. It appears that true food-induced arthritis may indeed occur in a minority of patients with RA. However, in these studies food-induced arthritis could not be confirmed in most of the patients who alleged food-induced symptoms.

These studies may not indicate the true prevalence of food-induced arthritis in the rheumatoid population. In the study by Panush (1990), only 19 of 29 patients completed the food elimination and challenge protocol. Also, presumably patients who did not suspect any relationship of food to their arthritis were not studied with double-blind food elimination trials. If food-induced symptoms are delayed, however, they may be difficult to relate to food ingestion (Lessof, 1984), particularly if the patient ingests the suspected food frequently. Also, the absence of symptoms after food challenge is not conclusive evidence against food allergy; food-induced reactions may occur only in the presence of other potentiating factors, for example, exercise (Lessof, 1984). Finally, it may be difficult to administer the quantity of food in blinded, disguised form that one might ingest as part of a usual diet.

Food elimination and challenge studies can be difficult to perform and interpret. Denman, Mitchell, and Ansell (1983) noted that many of their patients abandoned interest in dietary management of their arthritis when confronted with the demanding protocol of such a study. There is no apparent way of identifying what subset of RA patients may benefit from an investigation of this nature. Perhaps future studies will better define the prevalence of food-induced arthritis in rheumatoid disease and will identify clinical and/or laboratory features that may help distinguish these patients from the rest of the population with RA.

Dietary Elimination Therapy for Rheumatoid Arthritis in Clinical Practice

In the meantime, what should we tell our RA patients who ask whether or not their arthritis may be food-related? A reasonable approach at this time may be for clinicians to acknowledge that a small percentage of their RA patients may have food-induced arthritis. Those patients who feel that certain foods are exacerbating their disease could be offered the opportunity to eliminate those particular foods from their diet empirically. One potential danger, however, of eliminating foods from the diet is nutritional deficiency. Plans for dietary manipulation by the patient and/or physician should be made with the aid of a dietitian to ensure that the patient's diet supplies adequate protein, calories, and micronutrients.

For highly motivated individuals with a history strongly suggestive of food-induced symptoms, a formal food elimination and challenge trial may be warranted, provided the physician has the expertise and resources.

CONCLUSION

The relationship among diet, nutritional status, and RA is a very complex one. At one level, there has been accumulating evidence, although indirect, that mild protein-calorie malnutrition may be present in a large minority of patients with RA, even in Western societies. Further studies are needed to better outline the relationship, if any, of protein-calorie malnutrition to disability and other adverse medical and surgical outcomes.

At another level, better understanding of the role of dietary substances in the inflammatory activity of the disease in at least some individuals with RA may evolve as the relationship between diet and RA is further investigated. Meanwhile, it behooves all of us who care for patients with RA to be aware of our patients' nutritional status and its possible impact.

REFERENCES

Anderson, C.F., Moxness, K., Meister, J., & Burritt, M.F. (1984). The sensitivity and specificity of nutrition-related variables in relationship to the duration of hospital stay and the rate of complications. *Mayo Clinic Proceedings*, 59, 477–483.

Anderson, M.D., Collins, G., Davis, G., & Bivins, B.A. (1985). Malnutrition and length of stay—A relationship? *Henry Ford Hospital Journal*, *33*, 190–193.

Balough, Z., El-Ghobarey, A.F., Fell, G.S., Brown, D.H., Dunlop, J., & Dick, W.C. (1980). Plasma zinc and its relationship to clinical symptoms and drug treatment in rheumatoid arthritis. *Annals of the Rheumatic Diseases*, *39*, 329–332.

Belch, J.J.F., Ansell, D., Madhok, R., O'Dowd, A., & Sturrock, R.D. (1988). Effects of altering dietary essential fatty acids on requirements for non-steroidal anti-inflammatory drugs in patients with rheumatoid arthritis: A double blind placebo controlled study. *Annals of the Rheumatic Diseases*, *47*, 96–104.

Beri, D., Malaviya, A.N., Shandilya, R., & Singh, R.R. (1988). Effect of dietary restrictions on disease activity in rheumatoid arthritis. *Annals of the Rheumatic Diseases*, *47*, 69–72.

Blackburn, G.L., & Thornton, P.A. (1979). Nutritional assessment of the hospitalized patient. *Medical Clinics of North America*, *63*, 1103–1115.

Brough, W., Horne, G., Blount, A., Irving, M.H., & Jeejeebhoy, K.N. (1986). Effects of nutrient intake, surgery, sepsis, and long term administration of steroids on muscle function. *British Medical Journal*, *293*, 983–988.

Buzby, G.P., & Mullen, J.L. (1984). Nutritional assessment. In J.L. Rombeau & M.D. Caldwell (Eds.), *Enteral and tube feedings* (pp. 127–147). Philadelphia: Saunders.

Callegari, P.E., & Zurier, R.B. (1991). Botanical lipids: Potential role in modulation of immunologic responses and inflammatory reactions. *Rheumatic Diseases Clinics of North America*, *17*, 415–425.

Chan, S.T.F., McLaughlin, S.J., Ponting, G.A., Biglin, J., & Dudley, H.A.F. (1986). Muscle power after glucose-potassium loading in undernourished patients. *British Medical Journal*, *293*, 1055–1056.

Cleland, L.G., French, J.K., Betts, W.H., Murphy, G.A., & Elliot, M.J. (1988). Clinical and biochemical effects of dietary fish oil supplements in rheumatoid arthritis. *Journal of Rheumatology*, *15*, 1471–1475.

Collins, R., Dunn, T.L., Walthaw, J., Harrell, P., & Alarcon, G.S. (1987). Malnutrition in rheumatoid arthritis. *Clinical Rheumatology*, *6*, 391–398.

Corman, L.C. (1985). The relationship between nutrition, infection, and immunity. *Medical Clinics of North America*, *69*, 519–531.

Daly, J.M., Dudrick, S.J., & Copeland, E.M. (1980). Intravenous hyperalimentation: Effect on delayed hypersensitivity in cancer patients. *Annals of Surgery*, *192*, 587–592.

Darlington, L.G. (1991). Dietary therapy for rheumatoid arthritis. *Rheumatic Diseases Clinics of North America*, *17*, 273–285.

Darlington, L.G., Ramsey, N.W., & Mansfield, J.R. (1986). Placebo-controlled blind study of dietary manipulation therapy in rheumatoid arthritis. *Lancet*, *1*, 236–238.

Denman, A.M., Mitchell, B., & Ansell, B.M. (1983). Joint complaints and food allergic disorders. *Annals of Allergy*, *51*, 260–263.

Dong, C.H., & Banks, J. (1975). *New Hope for the Arthritic*. New York: Ballantine.

Edwards, R.H.T., Young, A., Hosking, G.P., & Jones, D.A. (1977). Human skeletal muscle function: Description of tests and normal values. *Clinical Science and Molecular Medicine*, *52*, 283–290.

Eising, L. (1963). Dietary intake in patients with arthritis and other chronic diseases. *Journal of Bone and Joint Surgery [Am]*, *45*, 69–81.

Endres, S., Ghorbani, R., Kelley, V.E., Georgilis, K., Lonnemann, G., Van der Meer, J.W.M., Cannon, J.G., Rogers, T.S., Klempner, M.S., & Weber, P.C. (1989). The effect of dietary supplementation with n-3 polyunsaturated fatty acids on the synthesis of interleukin-1 and tumor necrosis factor by mononuclear cells. *New England Journal of Medicine*, *320*, 265–271.

Esvelt, R.M., & Dehoog, S.J. (1984). The role of the clinical dietitian and modified oral diets. In J.L. Rombeau & M.D. Caldwell (Eds.), *Enteral and tube feeding* (pp. 158–170). Philadelphia: Saunders.

Gerber, D.A. (1975). Low free serum histidine concentrations in rheumatoid arthritis. *Journal of Clinical Investigation*, *55*, 1164–1173.

Gerber, D.A., & Gerber, M.G. (1977). Specificity of a low serum histidine concentration for rheumatoid arthritis. *Journal of Chronic Diseases*, *30*, 115–127.

Glenn, M.B., Carfi, J., & Belle, S.E. (1985). Serum albumin as a predictor of course and outcome on a rehabilitation service. *Archives of Physical Medicine and Rehabilitation*, *66*, 294–297.

Grant, J.P., Custer, P.B., & Thurlow, J. (1981). Current techniques of nutritional assessment. *Surgical Clinics of North America*, *61*, 437–463.

Hafstrom, I., Ringertz, B., Gyllenhammar, H., Palmblad, J., & Harms-Ringdahl, M. (1988). Effects of fasting on disease activity, neutrophil function, fatty acid composition, and leukotriene biosynthesis in patients with rheumatoid arthritis. *Arthritis and Rheumatism*, *31*, 585–592.

Harrell, P., Waltham, J., Collins, R.D., Dunn, T.L., & Alarcon, G.S. (1987). Malnutrition in rheumatoid arthritis (RA): A follow-up study. *Arthritis and Rheumatism*, *30 (Suppl. 1)*, S65.

Helliwell, M., Coombes, E.J., Moody, B.J., & Batstone, G.F. (1984). Thyroxine-binding pre-albumin—an index of disease activity or nutritional status in rheumatoid arthritis? *British Journal of Rheumatology*, *23*, 190–194.

Helliwell, M., Coombes, E.J., Moody, B.J., Batstone, G.F., & Robertson, J.C. (1984). Nutritional status in patients with rheumatoid arthritis. *Annals of the Rheumatic Diseases*, *43*, 386–390.

Jaffe, I.A., Altman, K., & Merryman, P. (1964). The anti-pyridoxine effect of penicillamine in man. *Journal of Clinical Investigation*, *43*, 1869–1873.

Jantti, J., Seppala, E., Vapaatalo, H., & Isomaki, H. (1989). Evening primrose oil and olive oil in treatment of rheumatoid arthritis. *Clinical Rheumatology*, *8*, 238–244.

Job, C., Menkes, C.J., & Delbarre, F. (1980). Zinc sulphate in the treatment of rheumatoid arthritis. *Arthritis and Rheumatism, 23*, 1408–1409.

Kelley, V.E., Ferretti, A., Izui, S., & Strom, T.B. (1985). A fish oil diet rich in eicosapentaenoic acid reduces cyclooxygenase metabolites and suppresses lupus in MRL-1pr mice. *Journal of Immunology, 134*, 1914–1919.

Kim, W.W., Kelsay, J.L., Judd, J.T., Marshall, M.W., & Mertz, W. (1984). Evaluation of long-term dietary intakes of adults consuming self-selected diets. *American Journal of Clinical Nutrition, 40*, 1327–1332.

Kirkham, J., Lowe, J., Bird, H.A., & Wright, V. (1981). Serum histidine levels in rheumatoid arthritis: A family study. *Annals of the Rheumatic Diseases, 40*, 501–502.

Kjeldsen-Kraugh, J., Haugen, M., Borchgrevink, C.F., Laerum, E., Eek, M., Mowinkel, P., Hovi, K., & Forre, O. (1991). Controlled trial of fasting and one-year vegetarian diet in rheumatoid arthritis. *Lancet, 338*, 899–902.

Kjeldsen-Kraugh, J., Lund, J.A., Riise, T., Finnager, B., Haaland, K., Finstad, R., Mikkelsen, K., & Oystein, F. (1992). Dietary omega-3 fatty acid supplementation and naproxen treatment in patients with rheumatoid arthritis. *Journal of Rheumatology, 19*, 1531–1536.

Kowsari, B., Finnie, S.K., Carter, R.L., Love, J., Kaltz, P., Longley, S., & Panush, R.S. (1983). Assessment of the diet of patients with rheumatoid arthritis and osteoarthritis. *Journal of the American Dietetic Association, 82*, 657–659.

Kremer, J.M., Jubiz, W., Michalek, A., Rynes, R.I., Bartholomew, L.E., Bigaouette, J., Timchalk, M., Beiler, D., & Lininger, L. (1987). Fish oil fatty acid supplementation in active rheumatoid arthritis. *Annals of Internal Medicine, 106*, 497–502.

Kremer, J.M., Lawrence, D., Jubiz, W., DiGiacomo, R., Rynes, R., Bartholomew, L., & Sherman, M. (1990). Dietary fish oil and olive oil supplementation in patients with rheumatoid arthritis: Clinical and immunological effects. *Arthritis and Rheumatism, 33*, 810–820.

Kremer, J.M., Michalek, A.V., Lininger, L., Huyck, C., Bigauoette, J., Timchalk, M.A., Rynes, R.I., Zieminski, J., & Bartholomew, L.E. (1985). Effects of manipulation of dietary fatty acids on clinical manifestations of rheumatoid arthritis. *Lancet, 1*, 184–187.

Kunkel, S.L., Ogawa, H., Conran, P.B., Ward, P.A., & Zurier, R.B. (1981). Suppression of acute and chronic inflammation by orally administered prostaglandins. *Arthritis and Rheumatism, 24*, 1151–1158.

Kunkel, S.L., Ogawa, H., Ward, P.A., & Zurier, P.B. (1981). Suppression of chronic inflammation by evening primrose oil. *Progress in Lipid Research, 20*, 633–640.

Lee, T.H., Hoover, R.L., Williams, J.D., Sperling, R.I., Ravalese, J., Spur, B.W., Robinson, D.R., Corey, E.V., Lewis, R.A., & Austen, K.F. (1985). Effect of dietary supplementation with eicosapentaenoic acid and docosahexaenoic acid on in vitro neutrophil and monocyte leukotriene generation and neutrophil function. *New England Journal of Medicine, 312*, 1217–1223.

Lee, T.H., Mencia-Huerta, J.M., Shih, C., Corey, E.J., Lewis, R.A., & Austen, K.F. (1984). Characterization and biologic properties of 5, 12-dihydroxy derivatives of eicosapentaenoic acid, including leukotriene B_5 and the double lipoxygenase product. *Journal of Biological Chemistry, 259*, 2383–2389.

Leslie, C.A., Gonnerman, W.A., Ullman, M.D., Hayes, K.C., Franzblau, C., & Cathcart, E.S. (1985). Dietary fish oil modulates macrophage fatty acids and decreases arthritis susceptibility in mice. *Journal of Experimental Medicine, 162*, 1336–1349.

Lessof, M.H. (1984). Food intolerance and food aversion: A joint report of the Royal College of Physicians and British Nutrition Foundation. *Journal of the Royal College of Physicians, 18*, 83–123.

Leventhal, L.J., Boyce, E.G., & Zurier, R.B. (1993). Treatment of rheumatoid arthritis with gammalinolenic acid. *Annals of Internal Medicine, 119*, 867–873.

Lewis, R.A., & Austen, K.F. (1984). The biologically active leukotrienes. *Journal of Clinical Investigation, 73*, 889–897.

Lippiello, L., Fienhold, M., & Grandjean, C. (1990). Metabolic and ultrastructural changes in articular cartilage of rats fed dietary supplements of omega-3 fatty acids. *Arthritis and Rheumatism, 33*, 1029–1036.

Mattingly, P.C., & Mowat, A.G. (1982). Zinc sulphate in rheumatoid arthritis. *Annals of the Rheumatic Diseases, 41*, 456–457.

McColl, S.R., Cleland, L.G., Whitehouse, M.W., & Vernon-Roberts, B. (1987). Effect of polyunsaturated fatty acid (PUFA) supplementation on adjuvant induced polyarthritis in rats. *Journal of Rheumatology, 14*, 197–201.

McMurray, D.N. (1984). Cell-mediated immunity in rheumatoid arthritis. *Progress in Food and Nutrition Science, 8*, 193–228.

Meakins, J.L., Pietsch, J.B., Bubenick, O., Kelly, R., Rode, H., Gordon, J., & MacLean, L.D. (1977). Delayed hypersensitivity: Indication of acquired failure of host defenses in sepsis and trauma. *Annals of Surgery, 186*, 241–249.

Mullen, J.L. (1981). Consequences of malnutrition in the surgical patient. *Surgical Clinics of North America, 61*, 465–487.

Nielsen, G.L., Faarvang, K.L., Thomsen, B.S., Teglbjaerg, K.L., Jensen, L.T., Hansen, T.M., Lervang, H.H., Schmidt, E.B, Dyerberg, J., & Ernst, E. (1992). The effects of dietary supplementation with n-3 polyunsaturated fatty acids in patients with rheumatoid arthritis: A randomized double-blind trial. *European Journal of Clinical Investigation, 22*, 687–691.

Oldryd, K.G., & Dawes, P.T. (1985). Clinically significant vitamin C deficiency in rheumatoid arthritis. *British Journal of Rheumatology, 24*, 362–363.

Panush, R.S. (1990). Food-induced ("allergic") arthritis: Clinical and serologic studies. *Journal of Rheumatology, 17*, 291–294.

Panush, R.S. (1991). Does food cause or cure arthritis? *Rheumatic Diseases Clinics of North America, 17*, 259–272.

Panush, R.S., Carter, R.L., Katz, P., Kowsari, B., Longley, S., & Finnie, S.J. (1983). Diet therapy for rheumatoid arthritis. *Arthritis and Rheumatism, 26*, 462–471.

Panush, R.S., Stroud, R.M., & Webster, E.M. (1986). Food-induced ("allergic") arthritis: Inflammatory arthritis exacerbated by milk. *Arthritis and Rheumatism, 29*, 220–226.

Parke, A.L., & Hughes, G.R.V. (1981). Rheumatoid arthritis and food: A case study. *British Medical Journal, 282*, 2027–2029.

Pearson, D.J. (1991). Pseudo-food allergy. *Rheumatic Diseases Clinics of North America, 17*, 343–349.

Peppercorn, M.A. (1984). Sulfasalazine. *Annals of Internal Medicine, 101*, 377–386.

Pettersson, T., Wegelius, O., & Skrifvors, B. (1970). Gastro-intestinal disturbances in patients with severe rheumatoid arthritis. *Acta Medica Scandinavica, 188*, 139–144.

Pinals, R.S., Harris, E.D., Burnett, J.B., & Gerber, D.A. (1977). Treatment of rheumatoid arthritis with L-histidine: A randomized, double-blind controlled trial. *Journal of Rheumatology, 4*, 414–419.

Poss, R., Thornhill, T.S., Ewald, F.C., Thomas, W.H., Batte, N.J., & Sledge, C.B. (1984). Factors influencing the incidence and outcome of infection following total joint arthroplasty. *Clinical Orthopaedics, 182*, 117–126.

Powanda, M.C., Cockerell, G.L., & Pekarek, R.S. (1973). Amino acid and zinc movement in relation to protein synthesis early in inflammation. *American Journal of Physiology, 225*, 399–401.

Prickett, J.D., Trentham, D.E., & Robinson, D.R. (1984). Dietary fish oil augments the induction of arthritis in rats immunized with type II collagen. *Journal of Immunology, 132*, 725–729.

Pullar, T., Capell, H.A., Millar, A., & Brooks, R.G. (1982). Alternative medicine: Cost and subjective benefit in rheumatoid arthritis. *British Medical Journal, 285*, 1629–1631.

Roberge, A.G., Sevigny, J., Lcoane, N., & Richard, L. (1984). Dietary intake data: Usefulness and limitations. *Progress in Food and Nutrition Science, 8*, 27–42.

Robinson, D.R., Prickett, J.D., Makoul, G.T., Steinberg, A.D., & Colvin, R.B. (1986). Dietary fish oil reduces progression of established renal disease in (NZBxNZW) F1 mice and delays renal disease in BXSB and MRL/1 strains. *Arthritis and Rheumatism, 29*, 539–546.

Rosenthal, J., Bole, G.G., & Robinson, W.D. (1980). Acute nongonococcal infectious arthritis. *Arthritis and Rheumatism, 23*, 889–897.

Sahud, M.A., & Cohen, R.J. (1971). Effect of aspirin ingestion on ascorbic acid levels in rheumatoid arthritis. *Lancet, 1*, 937–938.

Schumacher, H.R., Bernhart, F.W., & Gyorgy, P. (1975). Vitamin B_6 levels in rheumatoid arthritis. *American Journal of Clinical Nutrition, 28*, 1200–1203.

Shetty, P.S., Jung, R.T., Watrasiewicz, K.E., & James, W.P.T. (1979). Rapid-turnover transport proteins: An index of subclinical protein-calorie malnutrition. *Lancet, 2*, 230–232.

Shirocky, J.B., Neville, C., Esdaile, J.M., Choquette, D., Zummer, M., Hazeltine, M., et al. (1993). Low-dose methotrexate with leucovorin (folinic acid) in the management of rheumatoid arthritis: Results of a multicenter, randomized, double-blind, placebo controlled trial. *Arthritis and Rheumatism, 36*, 795–803.

Simpkin, P.A. (1976). Oral zinc sulphate in rheumatoid arthritis. *Lancet, 2*, 539–542.

Skoldstrom, L. (1986). Fasting and vegan diet in rheumatoid arthritis. *Scandinavian Journal of Rheumatology, 15*, 219–225.

Skoldstrom, L., Larsson, L., & Lindstrom, F.D. (1979). Effects of fasting and lactovegetarian diet on rheumatoid arthritis. *Scandinavian Journal of Rheumatology, 8*, 249–255.

Smith S.R., Pozefsky, T., & Chetri, M.K. (1974). Nitrogen and amino acid metabolism in adults with protein-calorie malnutrition. *Metabolism, 23*, 603–618.

Sperling, R.I., Weinblatt, M., & Robin, J.L. (1986). Effects of dietary fish oil on in vitro leukocyte function, leukotriene generation, and activity of disease in rheumatoid arthritis. *Arthritis and Rheumatism, 29*, (Suppl.), S18.

Sperling, R.I., Weinblatt, M., & Robin, J.L. (1987). Effects of dietary supplementation with marine fish oil on leukocyte lipid mediator generation and function in rheumatoid arthritis. *Arthritis and Rheumatism, 30*, 988–997.

Swenseid, M.E., & Kopple, J.D. (1973). Nitrogen balance, plasma amino acid levels, and amino acid requirements. *Transactions of the New York Academy of Sciences, 35*, 471–479.

Tarp, U., Overvad, K., Hansen, J.C., & Thorling, E.B. (1985). Low selenium levels in severe rheumatoid arthritis. *Scandinavian Journal of Rheumatology, 14*, 97–101.

Tarp, U., Overvad, K., Thorling, E.B., Grandal, H., & Hansen, J.C. (1985). Selenium treatment in rheumatoid arthritis. *Scandinavian Journal of Rheumatology, 14*, 393–402.

Trang, L.E., Furst, P., Odebach, A.C., & Lovgren, O. (1985). Plasma amino acids in rheumatoid arthritis. *Scandinavian Journal of Rheumatology, 14*, 393–402.

Uden, A.M., Trang, L., Venizelos, N., & Palmblad, J. (1983). Neutrophil functions and clinical performance after total fasting in patients with rheumatoid arthritis. *Annals of the Rheumatic Diseases, 42*, 45–51.

Van der Laar, M.A.F., Aalbers, M., Bruins, F.G., Van Dinther-Janssen, A.C.H.M., Van der Korst, J.K., & Meijer, C.J.L.M. (1992). Food intolerance in rheumatoid arthritis, II: Clinical and histological aspects. *Annals of the Rheumatic Diseases, 51*, 303–306.

Van der Laar, M.A.F., & Van der Korst, J.K. (1992). Food intolerance in rheumatoid arthritis, I: A double blind, controlled trial of the clinical effects of elimination of milk allergens and azo dyes. *Annals of the Rheumatic Diseases, 51*, 298–302.

Van der Tempel, H., Tulleken, J.E., Limburg, P.C., Muskiet, F.A.J., & Van Rijswijk, M.H. (1990). Effects of fish oil supplementation in rheumatoid arthritis. *Annals of the Rheumatic Diseases, 49*, 76–80.

Von Schacky, C., Fischer, S., & Weber, P.C. (1985). Long-term effects of dietary omega-3 fatty acids upon plasma and cellular lipids, platelet function, and eicosanoid function in man. *Journal of Clinical Investigation, 76*, 1626–1631.

Walker, W.A., & Isselbacher, K.J. (1974). Uptake and transport of macromolecules by the intestine. *Gastroenterology, 67*, 531–550.

SUGGESTED READING

Emery, P., Panayi, G., Symmons, D., & Brown, G. (1984). Mechanisms of depressed delayed-type hypersensitivity in rheumatoid arthritis: The role of protein energy malnutrition. *Annals of the Rheumatic Diseases*, *43*, 430–434.

Henderson, C.J., & Lovell, D.J. (1989). Assessment of protein-calorie malnutrition in children and adolescents with juvenile rheumatoid arthritis. *Arthritis Care and Research*, *2*, 108–113.

Henderson, C.J., & Lovell, D.J. (1991). Nutritional aspects of juvenile rheumatoid arthritis. *Rheumatoid Diseases Clinics of North America*, *17*, 403–413.

Larheim, T.A., Hoyeraal, H.M., Stalbrun, A.E., & Haanaes, H.R. (1982). The temporomandibular joint in juvenile rheumatoid arthritis: Radiographic changes related to clinical and laboratory parameters in 100 children. *Scandinavian Journal of Rheumatology*, *11*, 5–12.

Lovell, D.J., & White, P.H. (1990). Growth and nutrition in juvenile rheumatoid arthritis. In P. Woo & B. Ansell (Eds.), *Pediatric Rheumatology Update* (pp. 47–56). New York: Oxford University Press.

Miller, M.L., Chacko, J.A., & Young, E.A. (1989). Dietary deficiencies in children with juvenile rheumatoid arthritis. *Arthritis Care and Research*, *2*, 22–24.

Warady, B.D., McCammon, S.P., & Lindsley, C.B. (1980). Anthropometric assessment of patients with juvenile rheumatoid arthritis. *Topics in Clinical Nutrition*, *4*, 7–14.

CHAPTER 13

Speech, Language, and Swallowing Disorders in Rheumatoid Arthritis

Marion J. Mito, MA, CCC-SLP, and Anne V. Sasso, MA, CCC-SLP

Speech, language, and swallowing disorders traditionally have not been addressed in rheumatoid arthritis (RA) patients. Therefore, speech/language pathologists (SLPs) who work with individuals having disorders of articulation, language and cognition, motor speech production, voice and swallowing often have a limited familiarity with rheumatology. This chapter reviews symptoms of RA and those related conditions that are relevant to the SLP and considers patient treatment. Many of these conditions are relatively unexplored, so review of the literature yields only a few studies and especially few large prospective studies.

CONDITIONS ASSOCIATED WITH RHEUMATOID ARTHRITIS

Cricoarytenoid Arthritis

Rheumatoid involvement of the cricoarytenoid joint is well described. Early studies reported the frequency of signs of cricoarytenoid arthritis in 17% to 33% of patients with RA (Bienenstock, Ehrlich, & Freyburg, 1963; Grossman, Martin, & Root, 1961; Lofgren & Montgomery, 1962). The recent development of more accurate diagnostic technology has led to an increase in the reported occurrence, ranging from 52% (Lawrey et al., 1984) to 75% (Brazeau-Lamontagne, Charlin, Levesque, & Lussier, 1986). This disorder is of particular concern because of the variety of speech and swallowing symptoms that can occur.

The rheumatoid process can affect the cricoarytenoid articulation because it is a true synovial joint. The early pathological features of this condition are limited to the synovium and are similar to changes seen in other peripheral small joints (Bridger, Jahn, & Van Nostrand, 1980). Soft tissue swelling and pain are common early manifestations. Later, articular cartilage may be undermined and resorbed with erosion of underlying bone. Finally, arytenoid fixation can result as fibrous tissue connecting the cartilages contracts, causing a bilateral abductor paralysis of the vocal cords (Bridger et al., 1980). Although most authors attribute symptoms directly to articular involvement, Wolman, Darke, and Young (1965) state that symptoms may also result from recurrent laryngeal nerve compression secondary to synovitis, neural degeneration due to fasiculitis, and myositis of the muscles of phonation.

Symptoms of cricoarytenoid arthritis vary with the acuteness of the involvement. Lawry and his co-workers (1984) reported the following symptoms in their study of 45 RA outpatients: sore throat not associated with upper respiratory infections (49%); persistent or intermittent hoarseness (44%); "tension" or "fullness" in the throat when swallowing, speaking, or coughing (31%); a sense of choking or gagging; dysphagia and/or difficulty drawing a full breath during inspiration (29%); throat pain on swallowing (22%); chronic cough (13%); and decreased ability to sing (13%). The incidence of hoarseness perceived by health professionals exceeds that reported by patients alone, suggesting that patients may be less aware of changes in vocal ability because of their concern about other aspects of their condition (Lawry et al., 1984). Studies correlating symptoms with detection of laryngeal abnormalities in adults with RA have revealed that only sore throats and difficulty during inspiration predict abnormalities seen on indirect laryngoscopy (Lawry et al., 1984) and that no symptoms predict abnormalities seen on computed tomography (Brazeau-Lamontagne et al., 1986; Lawry et al., 1984).

Acute inflammation superimposed on chronic cricoarytenoid changes can present life-threatening complications. Although erythema and swelling of the cricoarytenoid joints and vocal cord edema may be signs of early or acute involvement, chronic laryngeal inflammation causes fixation of the arytenoids and airway narrowing. Laryngeal symptoms may be evident in both acute and chronic cases. Acute flare-up involving the vocal cords, already fixed in adduction, can lead to airway obstruction (Hollingsworth, 1978; Tozman & Gottlieb, 1986). Upper respiratory tract infections can precipitate respiratory distress or arrest (Brazeau-Lamontagne et al., 1986). Many authors stress the need for a thorough assessment of laryngeal function in RA patients before surgery because any intubation could significantly damage the already weakened glottic rim (Brazeau-Lamontagne, et al. 1986; Hollingsworth, 1978; Tozman & Gottlieb, 1986).

Local injection of a soluble corticosteroid has been used successfully to treat patients with early symptoms of laryngeal obstruction (Hollingsworth, 1978). There have been reports of improvement in vocal hoarseness, throat pain, stridor, and fear of swallowing in three patients treated with a topical corticosteroid aerosol. Respiratory obstruction due to active cricoarytenoid arthritis may also improve with anti-inflammatory and analgesic drugs, vocal rest, local heat, and humidified air (Jurik, Pedersen, & Norgard, 1985). The role of systemic corticosteroids is controversial (Hollingsworth, 1978). Most cases of cricoarytenoid arthritis are mild and do not require any specific treatment.

Rheumatoid Nodules of the Larynx

Rheumatoid nodules are another manifestation of laryngeal involvement in rheumatoid disease. These granulomas are found subcutaneously in approximately 25% of patients, typically with seropositive RA (Webb & Payne, 1972; Wolman, Darke, & Young, 1965). Rheumatoid nodules have been identified in the subhyoid region (Bridger et al., 1980), epiglottis (Raven, Weber, & Price, 1948), postcricoid region (Bridger et al., 1980), arytenoid cartilages (Abadir & Forster, 1974), and the vocal cords (Bienenstock et al., 1963; Friedman & Rice, 1975; Webb & Payne, 1972). Rheumatoid involvement of the cricoarytenoid joint is not a necessary concomitant of laryngeal nodules (Friedman & Rice, 1975). Diffuse interstitial and infiltrative pulmonary involvement may coexist.

Rheumatoid nodules are usually associated with pressure or chronic trauma in soft tissues around joints and in synovial membranes. On the basis of their findings and a review of the literature, Bridger and his coworkers (1980) concluded that the subhyoid and postcricoid regions are predilective sites for rheumatoid nodule formation. They hypothesize that subhyoid nodules either may be associated with the bursitis occasionally found in this area or may result from recurrent trauma due to laryngeal elevation during phonation and swallowing. These investigations suggest that postcricoid nodules may result from trauma during deglutition and chronic pressure from the tonic cricopharyngeal sphincter.

The frequency of laryngeal nodules in the RA population is not well established. In one study, Lawry and his co-workers (1984) report the occurrence of vocal nodules in 4 of 45 RA outpatients. Various investigators speculate that these lesions may be more common than has been reported because patients may be asymptomatic (Friedman & Rice, 1975), nodules may not be detectable by indirect laryngoscopy (Abadir & Forster, 1974), and these nodules appear similar to vocal abuse nodules (Friedman & Rice, 1975). Direct laryngoscopy, computed tomography scan, and microlaryngoscopy are procedures used for detecting rheumatoid laryngeal nodules.

The presence of a vocal cord nodule adds mass to the affected vocal cord. This can interfere with complete or well-aligned vocal cord closure, obstruct the airway, and/or cause a decrease in the fundamental frequency of vocal cord vibration. Resulting acoustic correlates might include breathiness, diplophonia (two-pitched phonation), reduced loudness, or lower pitch, any combination of which might be perceived as hoarseness.

Indeed, the most commonly reported symptom of rheumatoid nodules of the larynx is vocal hoarseness (Abadir & Forster, 1974; Friedman & Rice, 1975; Webb & Payne, 1972). Loss of voice, approaching complete aphonia, has also been described (Schwartz & Grishman, 1980). Less commonly cited symptoms include throat pain and exertional dyspnea (Abadir & Forster, 1974). Surgical excision is occasionally required for laryngeal nodules (Tozman & Gottlieb, 1986). Calin (1983) reported that these granulomas may shrink during a course of penicillamine or gold therapy that was prescribed for other rheumatoid symptoms.

Atlantoaxial Subluxation

Atlantoaxial subluxation in the cervical spine is another complication of RA. Its frequency has been variously reported in the literature, ranging from 7% (Mathews, 1974) to 37% in patients with 10 or more years of RA (Park, O'Brien, De Forger, & Hollingsworth, 1966). Rothermich and Whisler (1985) report that the typical patient at risk for atlantoaxial subluxation has had seropositive arthritis for several years. Atlantoaxial subluxation can lead to symptoms of brain stem and spinal cord compression.

Articulation of the atlas (C-1) and axis (C-2) allows for head rotation. The odontoid process of the axis normally fits into a tight pocket on the atlas, with a strong transverse ligament holding the anterior ring of the atlas during the swiveling movements of the head. Rheumatoid synovitis can occur in the small synovial joints about the odontoid process. Atlantoaxial subluxation results when the transverse ligament loosens or ruptures, allowing the odontoid process to press in toward the spinal cord (Louis & Gerard, 1986).

There are three types of atlantoaxial subluxation: anterior, posterior, and vertical. Most commonly, C-1 moves anteriorly on C-2. As the bursa and associated ligaments of the odontoid become inflamed, erosions of bone and ligaments can occur and cause protrusion of the odontoid posteriorly into the spinal canal (Louis & Gerard, 1986). Less commonly, C-1 may move posteriorly on C-2, causing the head to compress the spine posteriorly. This occurs only in cases in which the odontoid base is either significantly eroded by the rheumatoid process or fractured in trauma. Posterior subluxation can result in spinal canal stenosis, spinal cord compression, or compression of other vertebral arteries (Louis & Gerard, 1986). Finally, vertical subluxation of the odontoid and body of C-2 occurs due to destruction of bones about the foramen magnum into the posterior fossa. In this way, vertical subluxation can cause compression of the brain stem, medulla, and lower cranial nerves of other vertebral arteries (Louis & Gerard, 1986).

Review of the literature suggests that symptoms of atlantoaxial subluxation are rare, with the majority of patients being asymptomatic or presenting only local symptoms of neck pain or occipital headaches (Davidson, Horn, Herndon, & Grin, 1977). Additional reported symptoms include difficulty in swallowing solids, reduced pharyngeal peristalsis, cricopharyngeal dysfunction and aspiration (Davidson et al., 1977; Gow & Gibson, 1977), coughing and nasal regurgitation of liquids (Davidson et al., 1977), tongue fasciculation (Gow & Gibson, 1977), sensory deficits in the lower face (Louis & Gerard, 1986), vocal hoarseness (Davidson et al., 1977), and nystagmus (Gow & Gibson, 1977). Transient ischemic attacks can also occur due to compression of the vertebral artery (Louis & Gerard, 1986). The most serious complications include quadriparesis caused by pressure on the spinal cord and respiratory arrest secondary to odontoid compression of the medulla (Rothermich & Whisler, 1985).

Intervention is required when there are bulbar and spinal cord symptoms of atlantoaxial subluxation. Various investigators report partial or temporary resolution of dysphagic symptoms when the patient wears a tight-fitting collar (Gow & Gibson, 1977; Hollingsworth, 1978; Sutro, 1967). Surgical stabilization of the cervical spine may be indicated to alleviate symptoms (Davidson et al., 1977; Hollingsworth, 1978).

Vasculitis

"Vasculitis may complicate RA in approximately 1%–2% of patients" (Panush, 1981, p. 163). This condition involves inflammation of blood vessels, with different symptomatology depending on which vessels are affected. One consequence of vasculitis may be laryngeal dysfunction. Several cases have been documented in which rheumatoid vasculitis resulted in impaired blood supply to the recurrent laryngeal and vagus nerves (Lovoy & Hughes, 1980; Wolman et al.,

1965). Indirect laryngoscopy revealed bilateral abductor paresis with inability to adduct the vocal cords to midline for phonation. Patients reportedly displayed hoarseness, whispered speech, and/or loss of voice.

Sensorineural hearing loss occurs in RA patients more often than in the general population. One suspected cause for this is vasculitis neuritis affecting the eighth cranial nerve (Goodwill, Lord, & Jones, 1972; Heyworth & Liyanage, 1972).

In RA patients with widespread or generalized vasculitis, reported complications have included stroke (Hollingsworth, 1978), intracerebral and subarachnoid hemorrhage (Watson, 1979), diffuse cerebritis (Ramos & Mandybur, 1975; Skowronski & Gatter, 1974), and coma (Louis & Gerard, 1986). Patients with generalized vasculitis tend to be those with far-advanced or rapidly progressive disease with high titers of rheumatoid factor and multiple subcutaneous nodules (Hollingsworth, 1978).

The course and prognosis of vasculitic conditions varies. Progressive vasculitis has a poor prognosis. Death may occur in half of affected patients within 5 years secondary to visceral involvement or severe inanition (Sergent, 1981). On the other hand, some symptoms may be transitory, abating over a period of weeks or months in response to treatment or clearing spontaneously. One patient with vasculitic laryngeal dysfunction discussed by Lovoy and Hughes (1980) regained normal voice after a 2-month period of azathioprine and prednisolone treatment. Corticosteroids or cytotoxic drugs commonly are used to treat widespread vasculitis.

Pleuropulmonary Complications

Four major categories of pleuropulmonary involvement associated with RA are identified in the literature. These complications may reduce the patient's vital capacity and, subsequently, phonic breath support. Although not commonly reported in the literature, it is possible that voice problems such as reduced loudness, vocal hoarseness, and shortened phrases may result from pulmonary complications of RA.

Pleural effusion is the most common type of pleuropulmonary involvement, with frequency ranging from 5% of RA patients in clinical studies to 50% of RA patients in postmortem studies (Rothermich & Whisler, 1985). Similar to most other systemic complications of RA, this condition typically occurs in patients with severe chronic arthritis (Tozman & Gottlieb, 1986). The patient may be asymptomatic or may exhibit chest pain. Reduced phonic breath support can result from shallow respirations due to pain during deep inhalation or restricted movement secondary to scarring.

Diffuse interstitial pulmonary fibrosis is clinically apparent in 2% to 5% of RA patients but may be demonstrated in up to 45% of patients on pulmonary function tests (Rothermich & Whisler, 1985; Tozman & Gottlieb, 1986). It typically occurs in men with chronic, nodular, seropositive RA (Tozman & Gottlieb, 1986). Symptoms often include progressive, nonproductive cough, chest rales, and clubbing (Tozman & Gottlieb, 1986). Early changes usually involve the appearance of patchy infiltrates in the lower lobes, which may progress to a honeycomb pattern (Tozman & Gottlieb, 1986).

Pulmonary nodules have been reported in 0.4% to 6% of RA patients, occurring more frequently in men with chronic seropositive disease (Rubin, Gordon, & Thelmo as reported by Tozman & Gottlieb, 1986). Lung nodules are usually multiple and histologically identical with other subcutaneous nodules found in RA. The patient may be asymptomatic or present with cough, hemoptysis, or shortness of breath (Tozman & Gottlieb, 1986). Pulmonary nodules can be associated with diffuse interstitial disease or pleural effusion (Hollingsworth, 1978).

Caplan's syndrome, or rheumatoid pneumoconiosis, is a condition of nodular lung disease in RA patients who have been exposed to occupational dusts that occur from asbestos, silica textiles, granite, and chalk (Rothermich & Whisler, 1985). These nodules are usually multiple and tend to cavitate.

Temporomandibular Joint Involvement

Rheumatoid involvement of the temporomandibular joint (TMJ) is well recognized. A range in the percentages of RA patients affected has been reported, with figures from 5% to 86% (Syrjanen, 1985). This range may be so large because the majority of RA patients come for treatment with mild or transient symptoms, with complaints often elicited only upon direct questioning (Hollingsworth, 1978). Also, the incidence of radiographic abnormality apparently increases the longer the history of RA (Syrjanen, 1985). Syrjanen (1985) found that abnormalities were twice as frequent in patients who had had RA for 15 years or more as in those with a shorter illness duration. The frequency of RA patients demonstrating involvement in one or both TMJs centers between 59% and 86%, according to studies that combined both radiographic and clinical examinations and control subject comparisons (Chalmers & Blair, 1973; Franks, 1969).

Numerous consequences of TMJ involvement have been reported. Syrjanen (1985) found that the most common structural abnormalities observed radiographically included changes in the morphology of the condylar head and articular amentia, marginal irregularities, and an anterior position of the condylar head. Commonly cited functional problems included stiffness and discomfort anterior to the helix of the ear (Rothermich & Whisler, 1985), swelling and tenderness of the joints (Hollingsworth, 1978; Rothermich & Whisler, 1985), acute severe pain aggravated by chewing (Hollingsworth, 1978; Rothermich & Whisler, 1985), reduced joint mobility (Syrjanen, 1985), reduced ability to open the mouth fully (Rothermich & Whisler, 1985; Syrjanen, 1985), and palpable grating and crepitation when the mouth opens or closes (Rothermich & Whisler, 1985). Rarely, malocclusion from TMJ erosion can cause sleep disturbances such as apnea, snoring, hypersomnolence, or cardiopulmonary dysfunction during sleep (Davies & Iber, 1983; Tozman & Gottlieb, 1986).

Treatment of TMJ problems in RA patients focuses on reducing pain and inflammation, correcting occlusal and jaw imbalance, restoring function, and eliminating aggravating factors such as excess tension or inappropriate oral habits (Carlson, Kopp & Oberg, 1979; Gelb, 1985). The most common treatment procedures include medication to control inflammation and systemic disease, dental adjustments and appliances, physiotherapeutic modality treatments, and exercise programs. Modifying patients' diets to soft foods and liquids reduces functional demands and stress on inflamed TMJs. Hypnotism and/or biofeedback can help eliminate excess tension and habits such as clenching or grinding the teeth, if these are contributing factors (Friedman & Weisberg, 1985). For severe malocclusion cases with airway obstruction during sleep, tracheostomy may be required (Tozman & Gottlieb, 1986). A multidisciplinary approach with collaboration among professionals in rheumatology, dentistry, physical therapy, psychology, and any other appropriate areas will be most effective.

CONDITIONS CO-OCCURRING WITH RHEUMATOID ARTHRITIS

Sjögren's Syndrome

Xerostomia (dry mouth) and xerophthalmia (dry eyes) are common manifestations of Sjögren's syndrome (SS). The syndrome is a chronic autoimmune disorder involving lymphocytic infiltration of secretory gland tissue. Most frequently, the associated connective tissue disease is RA in approximately 50% of cases, and the affected structures are the salivary and lacrimal glands (Anderson & Talal, 1972; Cummings, Schall, Asofsky, Anderson, & Talal, 1971). Less commonly, SS may involve other exocrine glands, affecting the skin and respiratory, gastrointestinal, and/or genital mucosa, or there may be extraglandular lymphoproliferation affecting sites such as the lungs, kidneys, liver, or lymph nodes (Barrs, McDonald, & Duffy, 1979). Xerostomia is associated with abnormalities in mucosal tissue, dentition, and articulation and with dysphagia. Because salivation is reduced or absent, there may be irritation or fissuring of the buccal mucosa (Rothermich & Whisler, 1985), tongue, and/or lips (Hollingsworth, 1978), and patients may complain of mucosal surfaces adhering to the teeth (Cummings, 1981). Conceivably, this could interfere with speech articulation and patients do report articulation difficulties (Hollingsworth, 1978). No studies are available, however, specifically describing the nature or degree of articulation problems in xerostomia. Problems of dentition reported in xerostomia include gingivitis (Cummings, 1981), loose fillings (Hollingsworth, 1978), extensive dental carries (Hollingsworth, 1978), premature loss of teeth (Rothermich & Whisler, 1985), and discomfort wearing dentures (Hollingsworth, 1978). Certainly, problems in dentition have been known to impair articulation and/or chewing abilities in the general population.

In addition to chewing problems from poor dentition, other factors can contribute to dysphagia in patients with xerostomia. Reduced lubrication in the mouth makes it difficult to manipulate and traffic food orally. Food reportedly adheres to buccal surfaces and is hard to clear from the mouth after the swallow. Reduced salivation also leads to thick, tenacious secretions on the posterior pharyngeal walls, making it difficult for the food bolus to pass through the pharynx (Doig et al., 1971). Patients reportedly find it necessary to alternate food with fluid to facilitate swallowing (Cummings, 1981), have an increased intake of fluid with meals (Collins & Ball, 1986), and have particular difficulty tolerating dry foods (Cummings, 1981). In addition to constant thirst (Hollingsworth, 1978), loss of taste (Henkin, Talal, Larson & Mattern, 1972), and loss of weight (Hollingsworth, 1978) are common findings. As for incidence, Lenoch, Bremova, Kankova, Streda, and Balik (1964) report that 56% to 76% of patients reviewed complained of dysphagia.

There are other consequences of SS. Dysfunction of exocrine glands in the respiratory tract can cause dryness of the nares, pharynx, larynx, trachea, and bronchi (Collins & Ball, 1986). Nasal discomfort can result with symptoms of nasal crusting and epistaxis (nosebleeds; Collins & Ball, 1986; Doig et al., 1971). Infectious sinusitis, chronic cough, bronchitis, and recurrent bacterial pneumonitis are other reported consequences (Bloch, Buchanan, Wohl, & Bunim, 1965; Collins & Ball, 1986; Cummings, 1981; Doig et al., 1971). Conductive hearing loss is another possible complication of SS. With reduced secretions in the middle ear and ear canal, there may be cerumen impaction and/or large crusts covering the eustachian tube (Cummings, 1981; Doig et al., 1971).

Problems of phonation are another complication of SS. Hoarseness, which is frequently cited, is commonly attributed to dryness or tenacious mucus coating the vocal cords (Doig et al., 1971). Prytz (1980) refers to the occurrence of nongranulomatous vocal nodules caused by dryness of laryngeal mucous membranes. The nodules are characteristically symmetrical, localized near the border of the anterior third of the vocal cord. Histologically, they are similar to vocal abuse nodules, but they have a different pathogenesis. In other cases, hoarseness may be caused by extraglandular lymphoproliferation. Grundy (1972) described a patient with nonmalignant lymphoproliferation of the larynx. There was a progressively enlarging smooth mass of the vocal cord with vocal symptoms of hoarseness and stridor. Barrs and colleagues, (1979) reported a case of diffuse swelling, thickening, and scarring of the supraglottic and glottic larynx with narrowing of the glottic airway. There was massive submucosal infiltration of plasma cells and lymphocytes consistent with SS. Vocal symptoms included progressive hoarseness and inspiratory stridor. Exertional dyspnea was also present.

Although SS typically is a benign disease, in 5% of patients the lymphoproliferation may be malignant. Tozman and Gottlieb (1986) reported one such case in which the malignant lymphoproliferation manifested as a laryngeal lesion. The patient had SS associated with RA.

Another problem that may occur with SS is the presence of upper esophageal webs. Incidence figures range from 10% to 20% of patients (Doig et al., 1971; Hradsky, Hybasek, Cernoch, Sazmova, Juran, 1967; Kjellen, Gransson, Lindstrom, Sokjer, & Tibbling, 1986). Studies indicate that in some patients these webs contribute to dysphagia, whereas in other patients there is no related swallowing problem (Eckberg, 1981; Kjellen et al., 1986). Finally, Malinow, Gordon, Selnes, Provost, and Alexander (1985) suggest that neurological and psychiatric disturbances may be complications of primary SS. Of 40 patients studied, they found a significant number with affective disturbances, abnormal personality profiles, and/or defects in memory, attention, and/or concentration.

Treatment for SS is tailored to patients' specific symptoms. Increasing the humidity in the environment and avoiding possible irritants such as hair dryers or cigarette smoke is recommended (Collins & Ball, 1986). Saline sprays can help hydrate nasal passages and break up mucous plaques that may form in the eyes (Collins & Ball, 1986). Artificial tears and, in serious cases, surgery on the lacrimal ducts may be used to increase eye moisture (Collins & Ball, 1986; Cummings, 1981). Ointments and occasionally soft contact lenses may be recommended to protect the eyes (Collins & Ball, 1986; Cummings, 1981). For patients with xerostomia, artificial saliva, special alkaline or methylcellulose preparations, and zinc sulfate supplements are sometimes helpful (Collins & Ball, 1986; Cummings, 1981). Sipping water frequently provides additional relief (Cummings, 1981; Hollingsworth, 1978), and pilocarpine may improve salivary flow (Collins & Ball, 1986). Systemically bromhexine has been used for SS with mixed results (Collins & Ball, 1986). Prytz (1980) described a patient with vocal nodules secondary to SS whose laryngeal examination results and voice improved to normal after treatment with bromhexine and citrus mixture. There was also simultaneous improvement in secretions from the eyes, mouth, and throat. Cyclophosphamide and plasmaphoresis have improved severe extraglandular complications of SS, also with a simultaneous decrease in sicca symptoms and salivary gland pathology (Collins & Ball, 1981). Intravenous bolus methylprednisolone was successful in treating a patient with extraglandular profileration to the larynx (Barrs et al., 1979). The patient's symptoms improved within 2 days and were maintained at the 4-month follow-up. Previous treatment with prednisone had been ineffective.

Drug-Related Communication and Swallowing Disorders in Persons with Rheumatoid Arthritis

Drug therapy in RA treatment has numerous potential side effects. Mental status changes, for example, have been known to occur in some patients after treatment with steroids, nonsteroid anti-inflammatory agents, gold salts, or antimalarial drugs (Rothermich & Whisler, 1985). Myasthenia gravis and Guillain-Barré syndrome can occasionally arise as complications of D-penicillamine (Rothermich & Whisler, 1985) or gold salt therapy. D-Penicillamine can also induce other autoimmune disorders, including SS, polymyositis, and systemic lupus erythematosus (Rothermich & Whisler, 1985). Both D-penicillamine and gold salts have been associated with oral ulcers, changes in taste, and weight loss (Hollingsworth, 1978; Rothermich & Whisler, 1985). Changes in vision are possible complications of ibuprofen and the remittive antimalarial drugs. Reported changes include reduced visual acuity, visual field defects, diplopia, and—for ibuprofen only—visual hallucinations (Louis & Gerard, 1986; Rothermich & Whisler, 1985). Salicylates commonly cause tinnitus and decreased hearing, although these symptoms can be reversed by reducing the drug dosage (Rothermich & Whisler, 1985). Finally, problems in gastrointestinal and pulmonary function such as nausea, vomiting, dyspepsia, and asthmatic symptoms are potential side effects of most categories of RA drugs (Rothermich & Whisler, 1985).

EVALUATION AND TREATMENT OF SPECIFIC DISORDERS

Clearly RA and its associated conditions can be the etiology of various speech, language, voice, and swallowing problems. Assessments need to be tailored to highlight any existing rheumatoid involvement and symptomatology that may be contributing to the presenting problem.

Patients who are referred to an SLP because of chewing or swallowing problems are generally evaluated using a clinical dysphagia assessment that includes observation of eating skills with foods of different textures and consistencies and, if appropriate, videofluoroscopic examination of the swallow. Problems identified in chewing may be due to impaired TMJ mobility or poor dentition secondary to sicca symptomatology. In this case, the SLP can modify patients' diets to a softer consistency and refer patients to other appropriate specialists. Impaired manipulation and oral trafficking of food may be due to muscular weakness caused by myositis or bulbar involvement, or insufficient secretions from the sicca complex. Oral exercises to improve strength and range of movement and diet modifications may help muscle weakness problems. With siccal syndrome, patients should be counseled to avoid dry or sticky foods, alternate liquids with solids, increase fluid intake with meals, use artificial saliva preparations, and maintain scrupulous oral hygiene.

Videofluoroscopy will indicate whether food transit through the pharynx or esophagus is compromised. This might occur in patients with SS, myositis, or C-1 to C-2 subluxation. Patients can be trained to take repeated swallows and to alternate liquids with solids to help clear the pharynx. The Mendelsohn maneuver (voluntarily prolonging the upward and forward movement of the larynx at midswallow) can be taught to improve cricopharyngeal opening and entry of material from the pharynx into the esophagus (Logemann & Kahrilas, 1990). Postural changes such as head turning or tilting may compensate for cases of unilateral pharyngeal weakness. Esophageal problems generally are not amenable to the types of intervention an SLP can provide. For cricopharyngeal dysfunction in myositis, a myotomy may be necessary.

Videofluoroscopy can also confirm whether aspiration is occurring during the swallow. This could be a problem for patients whose RA has contributed to bulbar involvement, vocal cord paresis from recurrent laryngeal nerve damage, or myositis. Glottal adduction exercises and training in the use of the supraglottic swallow technique may be appropriate for these patients.

In the area of voice and RA, the SLP has two roles: (1) identifying problems and assisting in differential diagnosis and (2) providing remediation and counseling. During an initial evaluation, patients who come for treatment with voice problems should be asked whether they have any known rheumatoid involvement, a dry mouth and/or throat as might occur in sicca syndrome, or symptoms associated with cricoarytenoid involvement, such as fullness in the throat, chronic cough, pain on swallowing or speaking, sore throat, and/or impaired singing. In assessing vocal quality, the SLP needs to keep in mind that complications of RA can lead to hoarseness, aphonia, stridor, abnormal or changed vocal resonance, reduced mobility to modify vocal pitch, or inadequate loudness. Whether or not there is known RA, the SLP should determine whether the patient uses abusive vocal behaviors (ie, glottal attack, inappropriate pitch, excessive talking, or yelling) or is subject to allergies or exposure to environmental irritants. Finally, trial treatment techniques should be used and evaluated.

The SLP's findings can provide the physician with data that supports a functional abuse component or a probable organic component to the voice problem. Data from the voice evaluation can lead the physician to assess for rheumatoid involvement by analyzing vocal nodule tissue.

Differential diagnosis has significant implications for treatment. Patients with organic rheumatoid involvement may require surgical or pharmacological intervention rather than voice treatment to change vocal behaviors. On the other hand, glottal adduction exercises, digital pressure to the thyroid cartilage, raising vocal pitch, or changing head position may improve phonation in cases of vocal cord paresis. Vocal cord augmentation may also be recommended. For patients with compromised respiratory function (secondary to C-1 to C-2 subluxation or pulmonary damage), breath support exercises may be beneficial, speech phrasing could be learned as a compensatory measure, or a voice amplifier could be purchased to augment communication. For patients with voice problems induced by abuse, traditional voice therapy measures would apply. Finally, all patients with voice disorders might benefit from counseling on voice conservation techniques.

A final area of concern is hearing. Hearing assessment is a routine component of all speech/language evaluations because impaired hearing adversely affects communication skill. Patients either will be evaluated by the SLP or referred to an audiologist, who can evaluate and, if indicated, perform a range of audiological tests. Assessment of hearing is particularly important in the RA population because a higher incidence of hearing loss is found in these patients that is thought to be associated with toxicity from salicylates, synovitis of the ossicular joints, or neuritis of the eighth nerve.

CONCLUSION

Certain conditions, such as cricoarytenoid arthritis, rheumatoid nodules of the larynx, and atlantoaxial subluxation, are regularly associated with RA. This chapter also addressed other conditions that occur less frequently, such as vasculitis, and the four categories of pleuropulmonary involvement. Although some progress in these specialized areas is occurring, much more research is required to define further specific therapeutic interventions that would improve the speech, language, and swallowing functions of persons with RA.

REFERENCES

Abadir, W.F., & Forster, P.M. (1974). Rheumatoid vocal cord nodules. *Journal of Larynogology and Otolaryngology, 88*, 473–478.

Anderson, L.G., & Talal, N. (1972). The spectrum of benign to malignant tymphoproliferation in Sjogren's syndrome. *Clinical and Experimental Immunology, 10*, 199–221.

Barrs, D.M., McDonald, T.J., & Duffy, J. (1979). Sjogren's syndrome involving the larynx: Report of a case. *Journal of Laryngology and Otology*, *93*, 933–936.

Bienenstock, H., Ehrlich, G.E., & Freyberg, R.N. (1963). Rheumatoid arthritis of the cricoarytenoid joint: A clinico-pathologic study. *Arthritis and Rheumatism*, *6*, 48.

Bloch, K.S., Buchanan, W.W., Wohl, M.S., and Bunim, J.J. (1965). Sjogren's syndrome: A clinical, pathological and serological study of sixty-two cases. *Medicine*, *44*, 187.

Brazeau-Lamontagne, L., Charlin, B., Levesque, R. & Lussier, A. (1986). Cricoarytenoidins: CT assessment in rheumatoid arthritis. *Head and Neck Radiology*, *158*, 463–466.

Bridger, M.W., Jahn, A.F., & Van Nostrand, A.W. (1980). Laryngeal rheumatoid arthritis. *Laryngoscope*, *90*, 296–303.

Calin, A. (1983). *Diagnosis and management of rheumatoid arthritis*. CA: Addison-Wesley.

Carlsson, G.E., Kopp, S., & Oberg, T. (1979). Arthritis and allied diseases of the temporomandibular joint. In G.A. Zarb & G.E. Carlsson (Eds.), *Temporomandibular joint: Function and dysfunction* (pp. 269–320). St. Louis: Mosby.

Chalmers, I.M., & Blair, G.S. (1973). Rheumatoid arthritis of the temporomandibular joint: A clinical and radiological study using circular tomography. *Quarterly Journal of Medicine*, *42*, 369.

Collins, R.D., Jr., & Ball, G.V. (1986). Sjogren's syndrome. In G.V. Ball & W.J. Koopman (Eds.), *Clinical rheumatology* (pp. 157–163). Philadelphia: Saunders.

Cummings, N.A. (1981). Sjogren's syndrome. In R.S. Panush (Ed.), *Principles of rheumatic diseases* (pp. 233-244). New York: Wiley.

Cummings, N.A., Schall, G.L., Asofsky, R., Anderson, L.G., & Talal, N. (1971). Sjogren's syndrome: Newer aspects of research, diagnosis, and therapy. *Annals of Internal Medicine*, *75*, 937.

Davidson, R.C., Horn, J.R., Herndon, J.H., & Grin, O.D. (1977). Brain-stem compression in rheumatoid arthritis. *Journal of the American Medical Association*, *238*, 2633–2634.

Davies, S.F., & Iber, C. (1983). Obstructive sleep apnea associated with adult acquired micrognathia from rheumatoid arthritis. *American Review of Respiratory Disease*, *127*, 245.

Doig, J.A., Whaley, K., Dic, W.C., Nuki, G., Williamson, J., & Buchanan, W.W. (1971). Otolaryngological aspects of Sjogren's syndrome. *British Medical Journal*, *4*, 460–463.

Eckberg, O. (1981). Cervical esophageal webs in patients with dysphagia. *Clinical Radiology*, *32*, 633–641.

Franks, A.S.T. (1969). Temporomandibular joint in adult rheumatoid arthritis: A comparative evaluation of 100 cases. *Annals of the Rheumatic Diseases*, *28*, 139.

Friedman, A., & Rice, D.H. (1975). Rheumatoid nodules of the larynx. *Archives of Otolaryngology*, *101*, 361–363.

Friedman, M.H., & Weisberg, J. (1985). *Temporomandibular joint disorders: Diagnosis and treatment*. Chicago: Quintessence.

Gelb, H. (1985). Effective management and treatment of the craniomandibular syndrome. In H. Gelb (Ed.), *Clinical management of head, neck and TMJ pain and dysfunction: A multidisciplinary approach to diagnosis and treatment* (pp. 277–367). Philadelphia: Saunders.

Goodwill, C.J., Lord, I.J., & Jones, R.P.K. (1972). Hearing in rheumatoid arthritis. *Annals of the Rheumatic Diseases*, *31*, 170.

Gow, P.J., & Gibson, T. (1977). Dysphagia due to vertical subluxation of the axis in rheumatoid arthritis. *Rheumatology and Rehabilitation*, 16, 155–157.

Grossman, A., Martin, J.R., & Root, M.S. (1961). Rheumatoid arthritis of crico-arytenoid joint. *Laryngoscope*, *71*, 530.

Grundy, D.J. (1972). Sjogren's disease with widespread lymphoid deposits. *Proceedings of the Royal Society of Medicine*, *65*, 167–168.

Henkin, R.I., Talal, N., Larson, A.L., & Mattern, C.F.T. (1972). Abnormalities of taste and smell in Sjogren's syndrome. *Annals of Internal Medicine*, *76*, 375.

Heyworth, T., & Liyanage, S.P. (1972). A pilot survey of hearing loss in patients with rheumatoid arthritis. *Scandinavian Journal of Rheumatology*, *1*, 81.

Hollingsworth, J.W. (1978). *Management of rheumatoid arthritis and its complications*, Chicago: Year Book.

Hradsky, M., Hybasek, I., Cernoch, V., Sazmova, V., & Juran, J. (1967). Oesophageal abnormalities in Sjogren's syndrome. *Scandinavian Journal of Gastroenterology*, *2*, 200–203.

Jurik, A., Pedersen, U., & Norgard, A. (1985). Rheumatoid arthritis of the cricoarytenoid joints: A case of laryngeal obstruction due to acute and chronic joint changes. *Laryngoscope*, *93*, 846–848.

Kjellen, G., Gransson, S.G., Lindstrom, F., Sokjer, H., & Tibbling, L. (1986). Esophageal function, radiography, and dysphagia in Sjogren's syndrome. *Digestive Diseases and Sciences*, *31*, 225–229.

Lawry, G.V., Finerman, M.L., Hanafee, W.N., Mancusc, A.A., Fan, P.T., & Bluestone, R. (1984). Laryngeal involvement in rheumatoid arthritis: A clinical, laryngoscopic, and computerized tomographic study. *Arthritis and Rheumatism*, *27*, 873–882.

Lenoch, F., Bremova, A., Kankova, D., Streda, A., & Balik, J. (1964). The relation of Sjogren's syndrome to rheumatoid arthritis. *Acta Rheumatologica Scandinavica*, *10*, 297.

Lofgren, R.H., & Montgomery, W.W. (1962). Incidence of laryngeal involvement in rheumatoid arthritis. *New England Journal of Medicine*, *267*, 193.

Logemann, J.A., & Kahrilas, P.J. (1990). Relearning to swallow after stroke—Application of maneuvers and indirect biofeedback: A case study. *Neurology*, *40*, 1136–1138.

Louis, S., & Gerard, G. (1986). Neurological complications of rheumatoid arthritis. In S.P. Blau (Ed.), *Emergencies in rheumatoid arthritis* (pp. 127–155). Mount Kisco, NY: Futura.

Lovoy, M.R., & Hughes, G.R.V. (1980). Laryngeal dysfunction and rheumatoid arthritis. *Journal of Rheumatology*, *7*, 759–760.

Malinow, K.L.R., Gordon, B., Selnes, O.A., Provost, T.T., & Alexander, E.L. (1985). Neuropsychiatric dysfunction in primary Sjogren's syndrome. *Annals of Internal Medicine*, *103*, 344–349.

Mathews, J.A. (1974). Atlanto-axial subluxation in rheumatoid arthritis: A five year follow-up study. *Annals of the Rheumatic Diseases*, *33*, 526–531.

Panush, R.S. (1981). Rheumatoid arthritis: Clinical aspects. In R.S. Panush (Ed.), *Principles of rheumatic diseases* (pp. 159–173). New York: Wiley.

Park, W.M., O'Brien, W.M., DeForger, G.K., & Hollingsworth, J.W. (1966). Neck involvement in chronic rheumatoid arthritis. *Arthritis and Rheumatism*, *9*, 530.

Prytz, S. (1980). Vocal nodules in Sjogren's syndrome. *Journal of Laryngology and Otology*, *94*, 197–203.

Ramos, M., & Mandybur, T.I. (1975). Cerebral vasculitis in rheumatoid arthritis. *Archives of Neurology*, *32*, 271.

Raven, R., Weber, F., & Price, L. (1948). The necrobiotic nodules of rheumatoid arthritis. *Annals of the Rheumatic Diseases*, *7*, 63–82.

Rothermich, N.O., & Whisler, R.L. (1985). *Rheumatoid arthritis*. Orlando, FL: Grune & Stratton.

Schwartz, I.S., & Grishman, E. (1980). Rheumatoid nodules of the vocal cords as the initial manifestation of systemic lupus erythematosus. *Journal of the American Medical Association*, *244*, 2751–2752.

Sergent, J.S. (1981). Vasculitis. In R.S. Panush (Ed.), *Principles of rheumatic disease* (pp. 287–312). New York: Wiley.

Skowronski, T., & Gatter, R.A. (1974). Cerebral vasculitis associated with rheumatoid arthritis: A case report. *Journal of Rheumatology*, *1*, 473.

Sutro, C. (1967). Calcification of the anterior atlanto-axial ligament as cause for painful swallowing and for painful neck. *Bulletin of the Hospital for Joint Diseases*, *28*, 1–3.

Syrjanen, S.M. (1985). The temporomandibular joint in rheumatoid arthritis. *Acta Radiologica Diagnosis*, *26*, 235–243.

Tozman, E.C.S., & Gottlieb, N.L. (1986). Respiratory emergencies and rheumatoid arthritis. In S.P. Blau (Ed.), *Emergencies in rheumatoid arthritis* (pp. 249–273). Mount Kisco, NY: Futura.

Watson, P. (1979). Intracranial hemorrhage with vasculitis in rheumatoid arthritis. *Archives of Neurology*, *36*, 58.

Webb, J., & Payne, W.H. (1972). Rheumatoid nodules of the vocal folds. *Annals of the Rheumatic Diseases*, *31*, 122–125.

Wolman, L., Darke, C.S., & Young, A. (1965). The larynx in rheumatoid arthritis. *Journal of Laryngology and Otology*, *79*, 403–434.

SUGGESTED READING

Cohen, A.S. (1967). Amyloidosis. *New England Journal of Medicine*, *277*, 522, 574, 628.

Dietz, F., Logemann, J.A., Sangal, V., & Schmid, F. (1980). Cricopharyngeal muscle dysfunction in the differential diagnosis or dysphagia in polymyositis. *Arthritis and Rheumatism*, *23*, 491–495.

Fenster, L.F., Buchanan, W.W., Laster, L., & Bunim, J.J. (1964). Studies of pancreatic function in Sjogren's syndrome. *Annals of Internal Medicine*, *61*, 498.

Goodwill, C.J., & Steggles, B.G. (1966). Destruction of the temporomandibular joints in rheumatoid arthritis. *Annals of the Rheumatic Diseases*, *25*, 133.

Hardin, J.G., Jr. (1986). Rheumatoid arthritis. In G.V. Ball & W.J. Koopman (Eds.), *Clinical rheumatology* (pp. 63–88). Philadelphia: Saunders.

Strimlan, C.V., Rosenow, E.C., III, Divertie, M.B., & Harrison, E.C. (1976). *Chest*, *70*, 354–361.

Spurlock, R.G., & Richman, A.V. (1983). Rheumatoid meningitis. *Archives of Pathology and Laboratory Medicine*, *107*, 129–131.

Symmers, W. (1956). Primary amyloidosis: A review. *Pathology*, *9*, 187–211.

CHAPTER 14

Rehabilitation Following Hip, Knee, and Shoulder Arthroplasty

Victoria Anne Brander, MD

Total joint arthroplasties have revolutionized the care of patients with end-stage joint disease. They offer almost miraculous pain relief and functional improvements for patients who were disabled by pain and deformity. Most studies report good or excellent results in well over 90% of patients who undergo hip or knee replacements regardless of age or level of preoperative impairment (Harris & Sledge, 1990). The early results of shoulder arthroplasties are encouraging. With improvements in surgical experience and technique these procedures are being performed on many different types of patients—younger individuals, the elderly, and those with multiple medical impairments or disabilities—previously not considered candidates for the surgery. It is estimated that approximately 120,000 hip and 120,000 knee replacements are performed annually, and the total physician and hospital costs for each procedure are about $25,000 to $30,000 (Harris & Sledge, 1990; Poss, 1993). These procedures have made an enormous socioeconomic impact, both on health dollars spent and improvements in patients' quality of life. With the aging population increasing and continued improvements in technology, it is reasonable to expect that the numbers of these procedures performed will grow.

TOTAL KNEE ARTHROPLASTY

Total knee arthroplasty (TKA) is considered when patients have substantial pain and loss of function secondary to arthritis that does not respond to conservative management. Conservative management should include rest, anti-inflammatory or other pain-relieving medications, and exercise prescription. Patients with rheumatoid arthritis (RA) are candidates for total knee replacement regardless of their age. In other diagnoses, TKA is generally reserved for patients over age 45 or 50 years. The contraindications to the procedure are relatively clear. If there is the presence of an acute pyogenic infection, gross quadriceps weakness, or a sound, painless arthrodesis, total knee arthroplasty should not be performed. The presence of genu recurvatum associated with significant muscular weakness makes the procedure much more difficult. Age and weight should be considered when total knee arthroplasty is contemplated.

The principle of the knee arthroplasty is to resect the articular surfaces and replace them with prosthetic devices. Fixation may be provided by acrylic bone cement, screws, and/or porous surfaces with bony ingrowth. During the operative procedure the articular surfaces are resected, and implants of appropriate thickness are selected and then fixed to the bone surface. The posterior cruciate ligament may be either retained or resected and substituted for by the design of the prosthesis. The collateral ligaments may be tightened during the operation. If there was a preoperative contracture, soft tissue structures may be released in order to obtain correct limb position. The patella is then either resurfaced or left alone. At present, the patella is replaced only in extreme circumstances.

Preoperative Medical Considerations

Because of the potential for increased intra- and postoperative bleeding, aspirin and other nonsteroidal anti-inflammatory drugs (NSAIDs) are discontinued far enough before surgery such that platelet function (as measured by a bleeding time) is normal. This time may be as much as 10 to 14 days for aspirin, to 7 days for the longer half-life NSAIDs (eg, piroxicam), to 2 days for the short half-life NSAIDs (eg, ibuprofen, naproxen, and indomethacin). If inflammatory symptoms worsen, low-dose oral prednisone or parenteral steroids can be used.

Long-acting antirheumatic agents can be given up to the day of surgery, but commonly are omitted during the hospitalization. This is especially true for all immunosuppressive drugs. Reinstitution of these drugs usually occurs approximately 2 weeks after surgery or sooner if the patient's RA disease activity worsens postoperatively.

Perioperative Considerations

Most patients are admitted to the acute care hospital the morning of surgery. Intravenous antibiotics are usually begun within 2 hours of the surgical incision, a practice that has drastically reduced the incidence of deep wound infections. The perioperative prevention of deep vein thrombosis (DVT) is critical (Bohannon & Cooper, 1993; Craig, 1988). Mechanical measures are almost universally used—pneumatic compression stockings are placed while the patient is still in the operating room. Chemoprophylaxis is obtained using warfarin, heparin, or low-molecular weight heparin. The appropriate doses of these medications are under debate. Commonly, 325 mg of aspirin is given once or twice daily, warfarin is titrated to maintain an INR of 2 to 3 (or 1.5 to 2 times control value), and the only currently available low-molecular-weight heparin (Lovenox) is given as 30 mg subcutaneously twice daily or 40 mg once daily. Regular surveillance for DVT (via noninvasive studies or venograms) is controversial; however, screening blood flows on patients 3 to 5 days postoperatively is justifiable. Pain control helps ensure adequate participation in rehabilitation. Epidural anesthesia is common for the first 48 hours after surgery, followed by acetaminophen with codeine or hydrocodone or other analgesics every 4 to 6 hours afterward.

Therapy begins the afternoon after surgery. On the first day, the nursing staff instructs and supervises the patients in performing deep-breathing exercises, lower extremity isometrics (particularly quadriceps, hamstring, and gluteal sets), active ankle range of motion (ROM) exercises, and in-bed mobility wearing a knee immobilizer. The knee immobilizer is prescribed to assist the quadriceps in providing lower stability and to prevent flexion contracture. When the patient develops active knee extension and exhibits good leg control during ambulation and transfers, the knee immobilizer is discontinued. This usually occurs by the third or fourth postoperative day.

Continuous passive motion (CPM) machines, essentially the *only* rehabilitation intervention rigorously studied after TKA, are widely used. Knees treated with CPM obtain greater early flexion and require fewer inpatient hospital days and manipulations, but no differences in ROM are seen at follow-up (Maloney et al., 1990; McInnes et al., 1993). Continuous passive motion does result in a net cost savings as a consequence of the fewer manipulations (McInnes et al., 1993). Because the knee is primarily in flexion while in the CPM machine, patients with knee flexion contractures, significant extensor lags pre- or postoperatively, or wound drainage are generally not candidates for CPM. Patients are encouraged to use the CPM machine whenever they are resting in bed, for 3 hours to more than 10 hours daily. Continuous passive motion should be discontinued when patients reach 90° of passive or active knee flexion.

By the first postoperative day, physical and occupational therapy begin. The goals of rehabilitation for this in-hospital phase are the achievement of rapid recovery of knee ROM, the development of knee and hip muscle strength, and the obtainment of functional independence. Specifically, rehabilitation in the acute care hospital is prescribed until the patient (1) is independent in transfers and bed mobility, (2) is independent with the basic activities of daily living with adaptive equipment (dressing stick, extended shoehorn, reacher, elevated toilet seat, and tub bench), (3) is able to ambulate independently 150 feet indoors with an assistive device, (4) is able to negotiate stairs with minimal to standby assistance, (5) has at least 75° of active knee flexion and lacks no more than 10° to 15° of active extension, (6) has approximately three-fifths strength of the quadriceps, hamstrings, and hip musculature, and (7) is independent after the home exercise program. Physical therapy is prescribed for 45-minute sessions twice daily and occupational therapy daily until the patient reaches his or her goals.

On the first postoperative day, the patient begins to sit at the side of the bed and transfer to the chair. Isometric knee- and hip-strengthening exercises are performed, focusing primarily on the quadriceps. The patient begins active, assistive, straight leg raises. In addition, we use a self-exercise program to augment the scheduled therapy sessions and actively involve the patients in their recovery. The slings-and-springs apparatus allows active, assisted, gentle ROM and strengthening of the operated extremity to be performed by the patient independently. Patients are given a schedule of exercises to follow throughout their hospitalization (see Figure 14–1). Standing at the bedside begins by postoperative day 2, with the knee immobilizer and partial weight bearing on the operated extremity. The only orthopaedic precaution following a TKA is the weight-bearing restriction, which may be partial or weight bearing as tolerated for the 6 weeks after the TKA, depending on the preference of the surgeon.

Active assisted ROM while sitting is added to the therapeutic regimen by postoperative day 2, and by postoperative day 4 the patient usually begins progressive isotonic and isometric knee and hip muscle strengthening. Again, quadriceps strengthening is the focus, particularly the terminal arc of motion. Patients concentrate on terminal knee extension through active knee extension exercises done supine with the knee over a bolster. Isotonic exercises with small ankle weights (1 to 2 lb) are prescribed for individuals with good leg control, no extensor lag, and good muscle strength. Ambulation now begins in the hallway, and most patients are encouraged to use crutches instead of a walker. Occupational therapy and the nursing staff give instruction in dressing, bathing, and toileting and reinforce equipment use. By postoperative day 4, the patient should be able to walk independently to the bathroom and get into and out of bed. Patients are taught their home program and demonstrate learned exercises to the therapist before discharge (see Figure 14–2). Most patients are discharged home with home services by postoperative day 5. Patients receive home or outpatient physical therapy after discharge.

Often, patients with RA do not progress rapidly or are unable to go home to independent living after a TKA. Multiple medical co-morbidities, multiple impaired joints, severe deconditioning, and preoperative immobility are common reasons for slower recovery. Patients, particularly the elderly, who cannot return home from the acute care hospital because they lack the in-home resources (spouse, family, caregiver) to assist them may require a short-term stay at a skilled nursing or extended care facility where they can receive therapy until they are more safely able to manage on their own.

Postoperative Intensive Rehabilitation Phase: Postoperative Days 5 to 21

By postoperative days 5 to 7, patients exhibit the following common physical impairments: they have a small knee effusion, have limited flexion (to approximately 75°), have a small extensor lag (-10° or -15°), have about three-fifths strength of their quadriceps and hamstring, have 1+ to 2+ pretibial edema, and still have pain requiring narcotic analgesics. The incision is closed and warm (particularly after exercise) and exhibits a redness that blanches with compression. Staples or sutures remain in place for 2 to 3 weeks. Patients should be ambulating independently with a walker or crutches, but frequently exhibit a stiff-knee gait. They can rise from a higher chair with arms, but sit with the operated leg extended. Patients often climb stairs one step at a time using one or two handrails. They need adaptive equipment for dressing and bathing and an elevated toilet seat to facilitate toilet transfers. Generally they are unable to bathe independently. Their lack of endurance usually prohibits any light housekeeping or meal preparation, and thus they need assistance in these tasks.

The goals of rehabilitation during this phase are (1) to achieve rapid increase of knee ROM (to 90° of flexion and -5° of extension both actively and passively); (2) to improve muscle strength to four-fifths (particularly the quadriceps); (3) to improve distance ambulating, cadence, and gait pattern (eliminating the stiff-knee gait); (4) to improve the quality and independence of all transfers; and (5) to show progress with stair

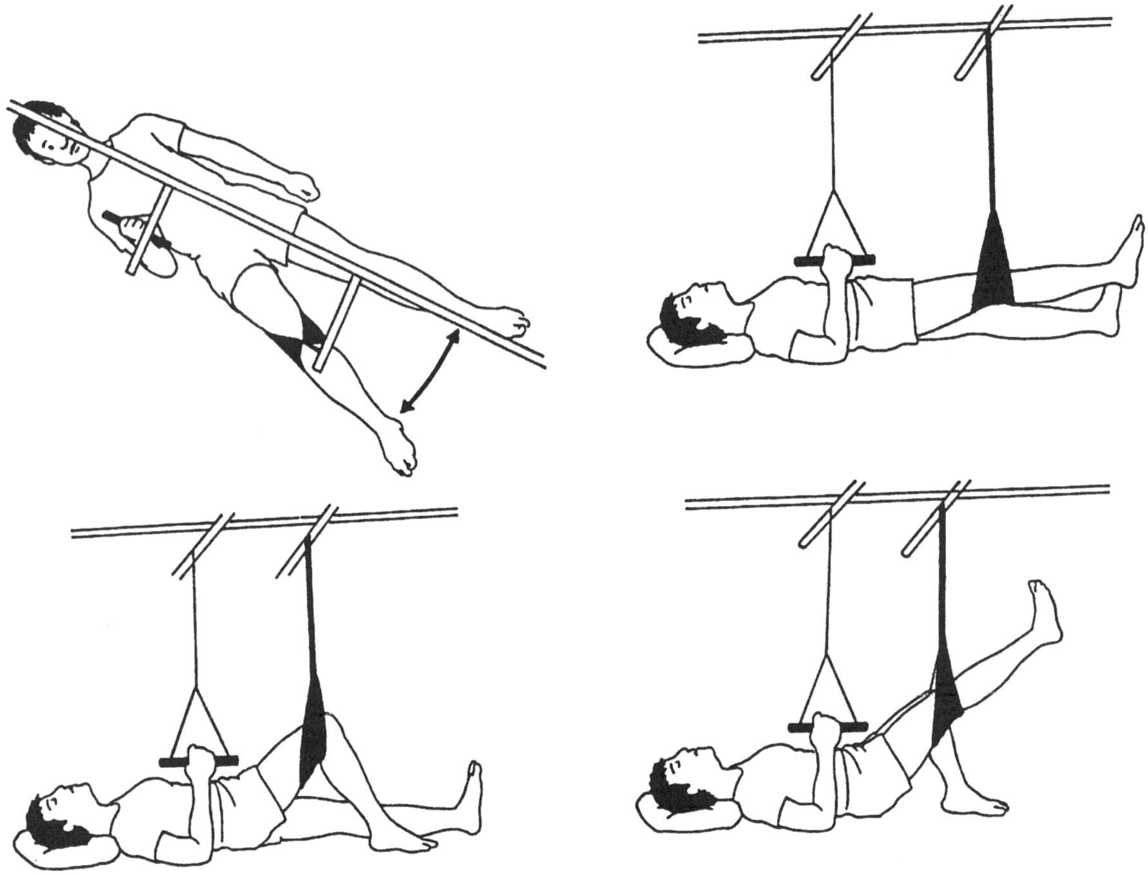

Figure 14–1 Slings and springs.

climbing. If patients exhibit a particularly stiff knee, muscle weakness, substantial impairment in the quality of gait, or have difficulty following a home program, it may be prudent to prescribe physical therapy daily in the home for the first week. Otherwise, most patients can receive physical therapy three times weekly and achieve a good clinical outcome.

Physical therapy progresses to include aggressive isometric and isotonic strengthening exercises adapted to the patient's tolerance and weight-bearing restrictions. Physical therapy may include closed kinetic chain exercises if the patient is fully weight bearing. In theory, closed kinetic chain exercises limit anterior tibial displacement (which stresses the passive knee restraints provided by soft tissue structures) while strengthening muscle groups by a more physiological method than traditional open kinetic chair exercise, (Yack, Collins, & Whieldon, 1993). Because the patellofemoral joint is compromised after a TKA, the need for aggressive knee extensor strengthening must be balanced with limiting stressors about the patellofemoral joint. Some suggest that closed kinetic chain exercise, via leg presses, provides less patellofemoral joint stress in normal subjects than traditional open kinetic chair strengthening exercise via leg extension exercise (Steinkamp et al., 1993). Whether closed kinetic chain exercises provide any "neuromuscular retraining" is debatable. In our experience, however, patients tolerate closed kinetic chair strengthening exercises very well, and they are an efficient method of lower extremity strengthening.

Range of motion exercises should be active or active-assisted. Unless a patient has a significantly stiff knee, passive ROM exercises do not provide any added

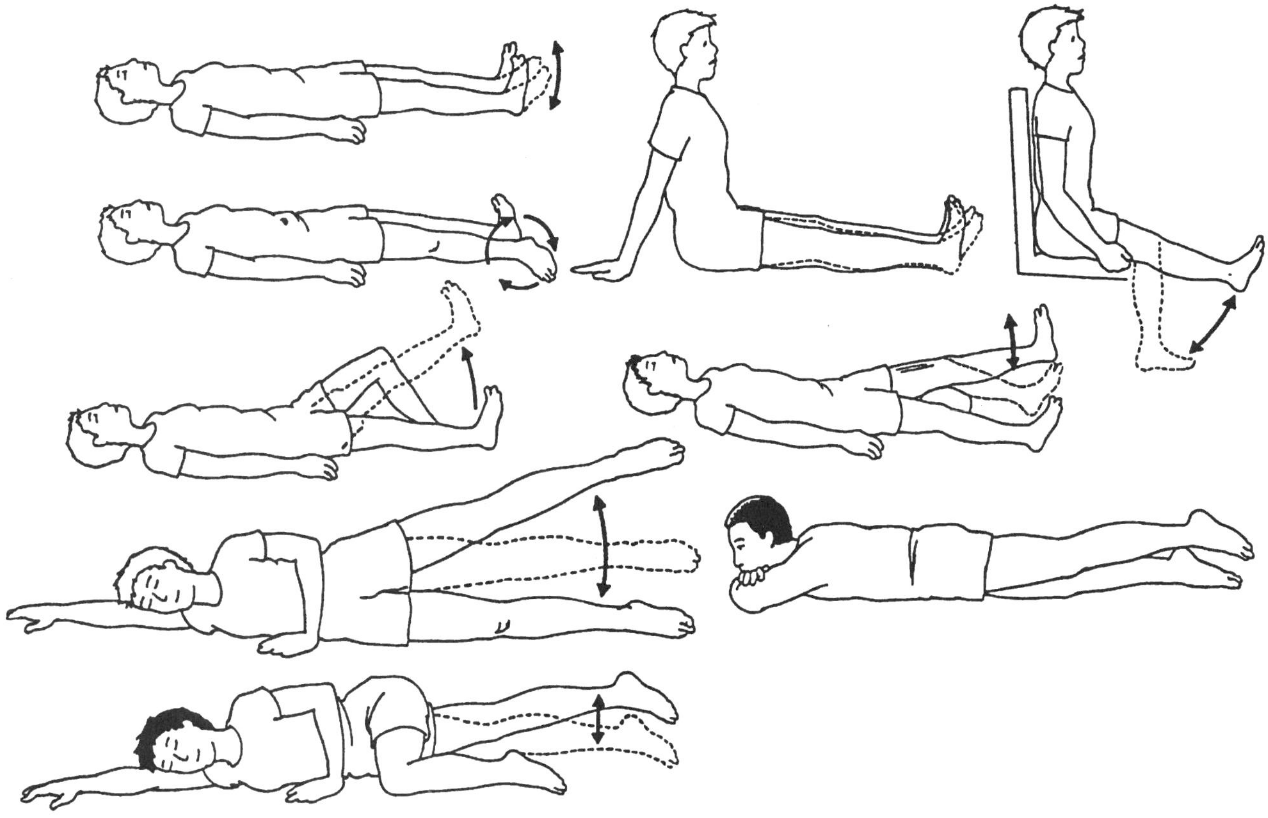

Figure 14–2 Hip and knee home exercise program.

advantage. Patients who have difficulty isolating their hamstrings or quadriceps during knee flexion and extension are at risk for developing a stiff knee. Active assisted and active ROM exercises encourage coordinated motor recovery. The addition of biofeedback techniques, using superficial electrical stimulation to assist in motor contraction, may be a useful adjunct to therapy for patients who have difficulty isolating specific muscle groups. Knee manipulation, performed by the orthopaedic surgeon under general or spinal anesthesia, is considered for patients with postoperative knees that are considered particularly stiff and not improving with therapy. However, whether manipulation improves long-term outcome is not known. If a TKA does not obtain 70° to 75° of knee flexion by postoperative day 14 and has plateaued in therapy, the patient should be evaluated for manipulation.

Stationary bicycle riding is an excellent lower extremity–strengthening, endurance, and ROM exercise following TKA surgery. Patients can be encouraged to begin riding the stationary bike as soon as they have no wound discharge. To maximize comfort, the seat of the bicycle usually is placed in a high position.

Therapeutic pool exercises are another excellent method of rehabilitation following TKA. The goals of pool therapy are to improve gait pattern, increase muscle strength, improve ROM, and decrease pain. Patients may begin pool therapy as early as postoperative day 5 if their incision is closed, is not draining, and is approximated with staples (not sutures). Pool therapy should begin with 5 minutes of warm-up exercises (forward and backward laps), followed by strengthening and ROM exercises (Figure 14–3). Patients should do these exercises for at least 30 minutes to ensure cardiovascular conditioning. Finally, patients end with 10 to 15 minutes of cool-down, again forward, backward, and sidestepping laps.

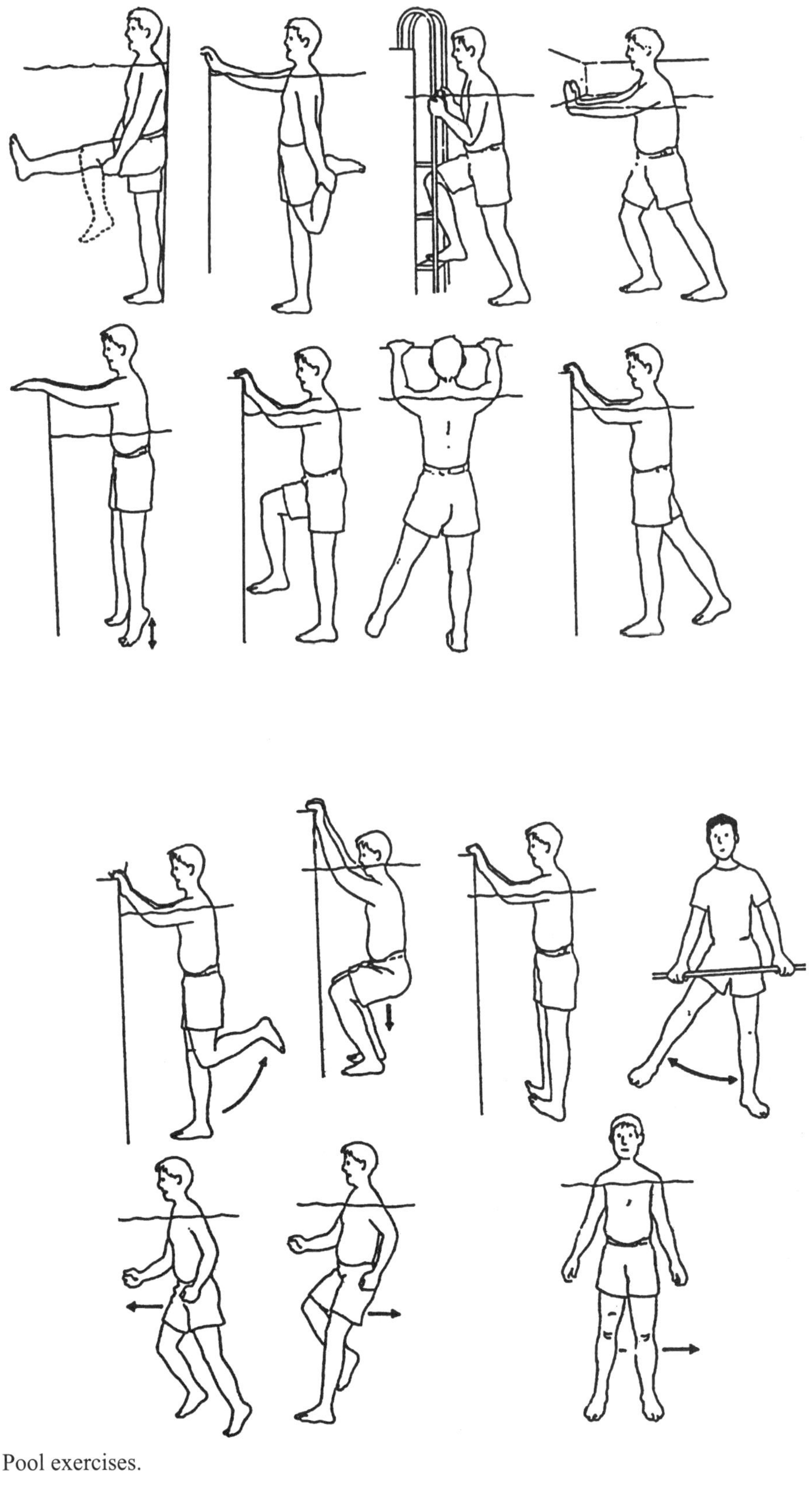

Figure 14–3 Pool exercises.

Gait training is a critical and frequently overlooked component of physical therapy. Patients who are allowed to bear weight as tolerated can progress to ambulation with a straight cane. The quality of ambulation is the guiding criterion to upgrade the assistive device. Patients should focus on ambulation with a smooth heel-to-toe gait pattern, with active knee flexion and extension during gait. If patients exhibit a stiff-knee gait, ambulating with their operated leg held in extension, certain gait-training techniques may be helpful. Patients can practice ambulating with exaggerated knee flexion and extension, walking as if they were stepping over boxes.

Patients who are in rehabilitation settings, either acute comprehensive rehabilitation programs or less intensive "subacute" settings, follow the therapy guidelines described but need more intensive services. Patients in inpatient rehabilitation programs, because of their increased frailty and diverse disabilities, need additional therapy with a greater focus on activities of daily living, upper extremity strengthening, endurance, balance, and education. Many of these patients have significant psychosocial or emotional problems that affect their functional recovery. In a retrospective study of elderly TKA patients, age, sex, diagnosis, Hospital for Special Surgery Knee Score, and co-morbidity score had no predictive value for patient-assessed outcome measured by the SF-36 Health Status Questionnaire. However, study subjects who had higher scores on the SF-36 Mental Health Subscale had a higher likelihood of satisfaction following TKA surgery (Anderson et al., 1994). Mental health may influence interpretation of pain, rehabilitation outcome, and perception of quality of life. Outcome may be improved by addressing the psychological barriers to recovery—depression, anxieties, neuroses, and grief over perceptions of loss (eg, of youth and independence).

Because of their prolonged hospital stays and medical frailty, patients in inpatient rehabilitation programs must be aggressively monitored for complications, particularly DVT and wound infection. The duration of prophylaxis against DVT is controversial. We continue prophylaxis for the entire inpatient rehabilitation stay. If a patient is admitted on no DVT prophylaxis, we begin use of low-molecular-weight heparin (pending publication of the formal studies of low-molecular-weight heparin to prevent DVT in TKA subjects) and obtain venous blood flows on all patients who have not had the procedure. Unless there is a contraindication, patients are discharged with the prescription for one aspirin per day until 6 weeks after surgery.

Preventing wound infection and managing wound drainage are other common postsurgical issues in rehabilitation units. Patients who have RA, are obese, are immunosuppressed, have undergone revision surgery, or have a history of joint infection are at a higher risk for wound complications after joint reconstruction surgery. Wounds may exhibit benign drainage (either serous or serosanguineous) as a consequence of fat necrosis or a seroma under the incision. Alternately, wound drainage may signify a local soft tissue infection or (more unusually) a joint infection. Knee arthroplasty surgical wounds that drain require Gram stain and culture, discontinuation of ROM activities, and aggressive local care. If there is evidence of infection, intravenous antibiotics should be started and consideration given to surgical debridement. *Staphylococcus aureus* is the most common organism causing deep wound infection. These infections require debridement and long-term antibiotics or hardware removal and antibiotics, with ultimate knee revision surgery or knee fusion.

Postoperative Subacute Phase: Postoperative Day 21 to Week 6

By 3 weeks after surgery, patients' functional capacities progress rapidly. Knee strength should improve to more than four fifths, knee flexion should be at least 90°, and there should be no extensor lag or knee flexion contracture. Hip strength should be nearly normal. Patients begin ambulation outdoors, and by 6 weeks postoperatively should be walking outdoors for exercise. Healthy patients may walk up to 30 minutes at a time with their assistive device. Narcotic analgesics are rarely used. Lower extremity edema lessens. Physical therapy should consist of open and closed kinetic chain exercises for strength and endurance (including the addition of weights as tolerated), terminal knee extension strengthening exercises, gait training, and active-assisted and active ROM, pushing knee flexion to more than 90° of flexion. Patients are encouraged to exercise daily and follow their home exercise program.

Intermediate Postoperative Rehabilitation: Postoperative Weeks 6-12

At their 6-week orthopaedic recheck, patients report the extent and location of their pain, the frequency and duration of walking, their ability to climb stairs, and their use of narcotic analgesics. If patients exhibit good leg control, have a normal gait pattern with the assistive device, and do not have substantial pain when walking, they can begin full weight bearing and depend less on the assistive device. Standing alignment of the knee is observed for the presence of varus, vagus, or flexion deformity. Knee joint laxity in the anterior, posteromedial, and lateral planes is assessed. Degrees of ROM, particularly knee flexion and active knee extension, are critical aspects of the evaluation. Patients should reach 110° of knee flexion between 6 and 12 weeks postoperatively. At 110° of knee flexion, most individuals can perform any functional task comfortably, including rising from a chair. Knee extensor strength will have an impact on higher-level functional tasks, such as climbing stairs in the normal foot-over-foot manner and the ability to walk steadily on uneven surfaces. Patients are encouraged to continue and progress in their knee extension exercises. Most patients can discontinue physical therapy during this period as soon as they progress to a cane and can follow a home exercise program.

Long-Term Outcome

Overall, good or excellent results after TKA can be expected in most patients. Individuals with RA, however, have slightly worse recoveries—less pain relief, increased risk of infection, and less function—than individuals with osteoarthritis. Good results still occur in more than 80% of patients with RA who undergo surgery (Harris & Sledge, 1990). Infection may occur in 3% of cases. Although loosening occurs, most frequently of the tibial component, most patients can expect their prostheses to last more than 15 years. The capacity of this surgery to improve ambulation, pain, and consequently quality of life in individuals with RA is remarkable, and despite the specter of potential complications, patients should be wholly encouraged to undergo TKA when it is indicated.

TOTAL HIP ARTHROPLASTY

Total hip arthroplasty (THA) is a widely successful procedure. Preoperative patient selection is an important factor in achieving satisfactory outcome. Indications for THA are pain that is unresponsive to conservative management and decline in function. Relative contraindications to the surgery include profound osteoporosis, recent infection, dementia, and paralysis of an extremity. Although THA is not routinely performed in patients younger than 50 years, individuals with RA and other inflammatory arthropathies are candidates for joint reconstruction at any age. With technological advancements in the design of prostheses, including computed tomography–generated custom fit components, the life span of an implant may be greatly improved. Today's patients can expect more than 15 years of use from their prostheses.

There are several methods of providing implant fixation using cement (methylmethacrylate) or a variety of cementless techniques. The acetabular components are routinely uncemented. Cementless femoral components theoretically have the advantage of improved longevity; they are reserved for use in younger patients, primarily under age 65 years. Other advantages include better bone remodeling and easier revision. These uncemented prostheses may be associated with a period of thigh pain until the implant is firmly adhered to the bone. Older patients and patients with poor bone stock (such as in RA) receive cemented femoral implants. These cemented implants have proven longevity and provide excellent, immediate, pain relief.

Perioperative Considerations

The perioperative surgical procedures to prevent complications following THA are similar to those described for TKA. Aggressive DVT prophylaxis is critical. Patients receive pneumatic compression boots and nearly all receive anticoagulation, usually either warfarin or low-molecular-weight heparin. Selected patients (eg, those with diffuse idiopathic skeletal hyperostosis, ankylosing spondylitis, or a history of ectopic bone formation) who have undergone THA are at risk for heterotopic ossification, which may interfere with recovery. Prophylaxis against the occurrence of heterotopic ossification can be obtained through irradiation in the range of 700 to 800 cGy within the first 2 days after surgery. Alternately, a variety of NSAIDs (particularly indomethacin) may be effective in reducing the incidence of heterotopic ossification (Poss, 1993).

The protocol for rehabilitation after THA is similar to that described after TKA. On the day of surgery, patients are instructed in deep-breathing exercises, active ankle ROM exercises, and lower extremity isometrics (focusing on the hip abductors, extensors, and adductors) while in an abductor brace. By postoperative day 1, patients begin physical therapy. Dangling the lcgs over the bed is encouraged twice that first day, and patients may stand at the bedside with a walker if they feel able. We begin supine hip- and knee-assisted flexion exercises on postoperative day 1, as long as there are no contraindications to this early activity (such as a trochanteric osteotomy or femur fracture).

The orthopaedic precautions following THA depend on a number of factors. These include (1) the method of implant fixation (cemented versus uncemented), (2) the quality of the fixation, (3) the integrity of the patient's bone, (4) the extent of the operative procedure (eg, whether or not a trochanteric osteotomy was performed), (5) the operative approach, (6) the periarticular soft tissue integrity, and (7) the particular preferences of the surgeon. Range of motion precautions are provided to prevent hip dislocation. These precautions depend primarily on the surgical approach. The standard recommendations for a posterolateral incision are to avoid hip flexion over 90° and hip adduction and internal rotation beyond the neutral position. For an anterior incision, hip extension and external rotation must be avoided. The duration of ROM restriction is usually 6 to 12 weeks postoperatively, depending on the strength of the patient's periarticular soft tissues. Patients are asked to wear an abductor splint for the first few days and to sleep with a pillow between the legs for the first 2 months after surgery.

Most dislocations occur during the first few weeks after surgery. They may occur for a number of reasons, including a malpositioned implant, profound soft tissue weakness (as occurs after revision surgery in patients with connective tissue diseases and in hemiplegic patients), inadherence to precautions (sitting on a low surface), or a traumatic event (such as a fall). After the soft tissues are healed and considered strong (usually 12 weeks after surgery) patients may begin working on isolated hip flexion over 90° to assist in their activities of daily living (particularly donning shoes and socks). Patients are cautioned, however, to avoid the combination of extreme flexion with adduction or internal rotation for a prolonged period of time. Weight-bearing restrictions are more variable. The surgeon generally prescribes weight bearing depending on his or her assessment of the quality of implant fixation while in the operating room, but patients with cemented components usually begin weight bearing as tolerated within a few days of surgery. Most surgeons restrict weight bearing for a longer period of time after uncemented THA theoretically to allow the patient's bone stock to grow into and securely fit the femoral component of the prosthesis. If a trochanteric osteotomy was performed during the procedure (which is common in revision hip arthroplasty), independent straight leg raising, active abduction, and adductor stretching are prohibited for up to 12 weeks.

By postoperative day 2, patients begin standing at the bedside with the walker and transfer training. Hip flexor stretching should begin early. One method to stretch the hip flexors safely is through use of a modified Thomas stretch (see Figure 14–4). Active assisted ROM and strengthening exercises are usually postponed until the third postoperative day. The focus is on hip flexors, extensors, abductors, and external rotators as well as knee flexors and extensors at this early stage of rehabilitation. Patients are encouraged to use crutches instead of a walker if they are able. By this time, patients should be sitting in a chair for at least 30 minutes 3 times a day, in addition to their therapy schedule.

By postoperative day 4, patients usually are ambulating much more comfortably and safely. Many pa-

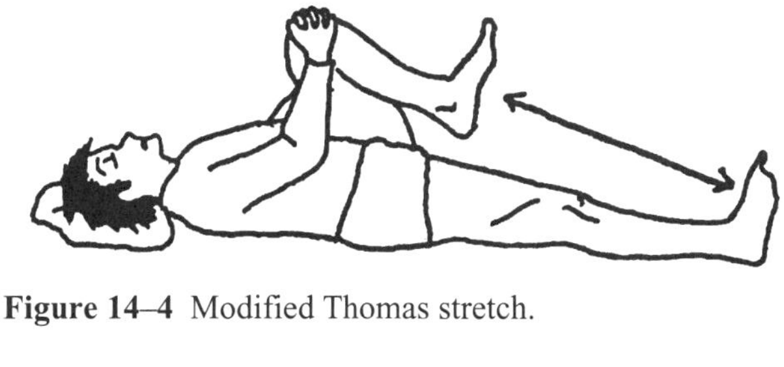

Figure 14–4 Modified Thomas stretch.

tients are able to ambulate independently to the lavatory. Active ROM exercises in standing are begun, emphasizing hip abduction. Active assisted supine abduction exercises using a skateboard are effective and safe abductor-strengthening exercises. Active assisted straight leg raising may begin, but this is quite controversial because it may put undue load on the implanted hip. A group of investigators implanted an instrumented total hip arthroplasty in a subject and reported the forces across the hip during the rehabilitation process (Brenner, Ferlic, Clayton, & Dennise, 1989). Force was directed in the anterosuperior portion of the femoral head, and with each loading cycle, out-to-plane forces increased dramatically. This was particularly apparent with straight leg raising and stair climbing. Thus during early rehabilitation, when muscle weakness is most profound and implant stability at its lowest, there may be reason to limit these activities.

The teaching of adaptive behavior by the occupational therapy staff is particularly important after THA. Patients must learn to don and doff shoes and socks; dress their lower bodies, reach for and attain items from the floor or lower surfaces; and transfer into and out of bed, on and off the toilet, and into and out of the tub without violating their hip precautions. Patients are instructed in the use of adaptive equipment from the second postoperative day, and compliance with equipment use is very high. Adaptive equipment routinely distributed includes a long-handled sponge, a shoehorn, a dressing stick, a reacher, an elevated toilet seat, and a bath bench.

By postoperative day 5, most patients are ambulating independently. There should be an increased focus on the quality and stability of the gait cycle. Patients are taught their home exercise program, and many are able to be discharged between the fifth and sixth postoperative days. Patients are discharged when they are able (1) to perform a straight leg raise to approximately 75°, (2) to abduct the hip actively to 25°, (3) to have approximately three-fifths strength in the operated extremity, (4) to ambulate with an assistive device with a smooth gait pattern indoors for 100 to 150 feet, (5) to be independent with equipment with basic activities of daily living, (6) to climb stairs with minimal assistance, (7) to understand and perform their home program, (8) to follow their orthopaedic precautions, and (9) to contact the necessary community resources. Patients receive outpatient or home physical therapy for the first month after surgery to progress their physical and functional skills.

Postoperative Intensive Rehabilitation Phase: Postoperative Days 5 to 21

By postoperative days 5 to 7, patients often exhibit the following common physical impairments: they have limited active flexion, abduction, and extension of the operated hip; they have some mild weakness of the knee extensors; they may have mild hip and knee flexion contractures; they have 1+ to 2+ lower extremity edema; and they still have some pain in the groin and lateral hip. Staples or sutures generally remain in place for about 10 to 14 days. Patients should be ambulating independently for short distances with an assistive device, but they exhibit a significant abductor lurch when ambulating without contralateral support. They require the use of their arms to rise from a chair and they climb stairs one step at a time, usually using the unoperated leg as the first leg up and the operated leg as the first leg going down. Their shortened endurance and muscle weakness generally prohibit any light housekeeping or meal preparation.

The goals of rehabilitation during this phase are to increase muscle strength and ROM (particular hip abduction, flexion, and extension), to improve gradually the distance and quality of gait with simultaneous progression from two crutches to one crutch or a cane (if precautions allow), and to improve the safety and quality of all transfers. Physical therapy progresses to include aggressive isometric and isotonic strengthening exercises, adapted to the patient's tolerance and orthopaedic restrictions. Closed kinetic chain exercises and bicycling may be included at this point in rehabilitation. Pool therapy is encouraged. The goals of pool therapy are to improve gait pattern, maintaining partial weight bearing using the buoyancy of the water, to strengthen hip and lower trunk stabilizers to improve hip stability and gait pattern, to improve overall endurance, and to achieve independence in a pool exercise program for carry-over in the community.

As described following TKA, patients who are hospitalized for a prolonged period of time after THA are at risk for the same medical and surgical complications. We follow the protocols described for DVT prophylaxis and wound management.

Postoperative Subacute Phase: Postoperative Day 21 to Week 6

During this period, patients commonly exhibit rapid progression of their physical and functional skills. Hip strength should improve to the good range, particularly the hip abductors. Patients should be able to perform active hip flexion to 70° with a strong isometric hold for about 5 seconds. Patients should have at least 30° of active abduction and exhibit no hip flexion contracture during the Thomas test. There may still be a Trendelenburg sign, and there is usually a Trendelenburg lurch when the patient is asked to ambulate without the assistive device. Patients should be walking for exercise, increasing their distance and duration as tolerated.

Many patients complain that the operated leg feels "shorter" than the leg on the unoperated side. Although leg length discrepancies can occur after total hip replacements, they are unusual in primary, elective joint replacement surgery. The cause of this apparent leg length discrepancy is usually pelvic tilt following surgery. The measurement of leg length is an important part of the physical examination at 6 weeks postoperatively. It is critical to measure the true leg length (from the anterosuperior iliac crest to the medial malleolus); a comparison of this value to the apparent leg length (from the umbilicus to the lateral malleolus) may provide some information as to the degree of pelvic tilt. Assessment of the degree of pelvic tilt on radiographs and during gait also provides critical information for prescription of therapy. Prescription of a lift for a patient early after surgery, even if temporary, may only encourage the pelvic tilt to become a permanent impairment. The pelvic tilt generally abates by about 6 months after surgery as long as the patient is correctly ambulating and performing exercises. Thus lifts are not recommended for primary THA patients until at least 6 months after surgery unless the leg length discrepancy appears permanent and is compromising function or causing pain. Patients need to follow their home exercise program to guarantee a good clinical result and so should be encouraged regularly to comply.

Intermediate Postoperative Rehabilitation: Postoperative Weeks 6 to 12

At the 6-week physician recheck the standard physical and functional issues assessed include the level and location of pain, distance walked daily, time able to stand or sit in one location, use of an assistive device, method of stair climbing, use of analgesics, and community reintegration. During physical examination, ROM is assessed in hip flexion, extension (using the Thomas test), abduction, internal and external rotation, and (gentle) adduction. Muscle strength in these motions should be graded. True leg lengths are recorded. The patient is evaluated for the presence of a Trendelenburg sign. Gait is to be observed both with and without an assistive device, and sit-to-stand transfer is evaluated.

Most patients do not need an assistive device at this point after surgery. Gait training should focus on establishing a smooth swing-through gait, normal cadence, and elimination of the abductor lurch. The criteria for advancement off the assistive device are the absence of a limp, minimal pain, and improving endurance with longer-distance ambulation. Patients begin walking without support at home and use their cane when they are walking outdoors or in crowded public places. Physical therapy should focus on progressive isometric and isotonic hip- and knee-strengthening exercise, focusing on hip flexion, extension, abduction, and rotation. In addition, the therapist should focus on pelvic- and trunk-stabilization exercises. We prescribe physical therapy until the patient's impairments can be eliminated with a home exercise program.

Many patients wish to return to driving at this time. We allow patients to return to driving as soon as they have good control of the operated extremity and are comfortable sitting in a car. There is one published study of resumption of driving by patients who had undergone total hip replacement surgery. There were significant differences before and after surgery; most patients showed improvements by 8 weeks postoperatively, but a minority of subjects did not recover their capacity until the 8-month retest. All of these subjects had a right THA. The author concludes that the 8-week delay in driving that is standardly recommended is appropriate for most individuals following THA, but after right limb surgery there is a subgroup of individuals who may need to delay driving further.

Stern et al. (1991) reported the issues related to sexual functioning after THA. As in studies of different patient impairment groups, most patients reported that they wanted more information regarding sexuality after surgery but were reluctant to bring up the subject with their physicians. Many patients wished to be sexually active regardless of age. Forty-six percent of patients reported difficulty with sexual functioning preoperatively, while only 1% felt that their hips precluded sexual activity postoperatively. The most comfortable position for the patient was supine; the next most comfortable position for women was sidelying (on the unoperated limb).

There is debate in the literature regarding return to sporting activities after a THA. Most surgeons routinely counsel their patients to avoid high-impact activities (such as competitive tennis, racquetball, and running) because of the presumed deleterious effect these activities may have on implant longevity. Kilgus et al. (1990) studied the effects of activity on implant survival in patients with cemented hip replacements. Revision rates for aseptic loosening were greatest for the subset of patients with diagnoses other than osteoarthritis. The effects of activity were evident 10 years after surgery. The consequences of high-impact activity on uncemented hip replacements is not known. Patients can be safely encouraged to participate in regular low-impact activities (such as golf, walking, and swimming). Recreational exercise may begin as soon as patients feel physically able, have little pain, and have good control of their operated extremity, usually 12 weeks postoperatively.

Long-Term Outcome

The clinical results of THA surgery are well documented, with "good" or "excellent" results in about 90% of cases. The incidence of infection (about 1% in primary surgeries and 3% in revisions) and loosening, however, is still of concern. Radiographic evidence of loosening may be as high as 30% to 50% at 10 years, but clinically significant loosening, as judged by rates of revision, is much less common. Present data suggest that prosthesis failure rates are actually low in the first 10 years but increase to 13% to 40% in the first 15 years (Harris & Sledge, 1990). With well-prescribed and aggressively pursued exercise, some patients believe they can rehabilitate the THA to approximate a normal hip. In most patients with RA, the magnitude of positive change in quality of life after THA is significant and fully warrants encouragement of surgery when indicated.

TOTAL SHOULDER ARTHROPLASTY

The indication for total shoulder arthroplasty (TSA) is pain from a pathological condition of the glenohumeral joint that has resulted in congruity of joint surfaces. Relief of pain is the primary goal of the procedure; functional improvements in increased active ROM are secondary objectives. Thus severe pain is an absolute prerequisite to surgery. The conditions for which a TSA is indicated include osteoarthritis, posttraumatic arthritis, old fractures and fracture dislocations, avascular necrosis, inflammatory arthropathies (eg, RA and ankylosis spondylitis), proximal humerus neoplasms, complex fractures in which the glenoid is involved, failed previous reconstructive surgery, and old septics (Barret, Franklin, Jackins, Wyss, & Matsen, 1987). The contraindications to an elective TSA are recent joint infection, neuropathic joint, paralysis (with loss of the deltoid and rotator cuff), extreme osteoporosis, and most important, insufficient symptoms.

The most commonly used prothesis is the unconstrained Neer prothesis. It is anatomically similar to the normal shoulder, necessitates only limited resection of bone, allows for maximal functional recovery, and relies heavily on the integrity of the soft tissue structures. Complications with use of constrained prostheses are frequent and substantial, including high rates of fracture, loosening, and infection. Thus constrained prostheses are used only in salvage procedures, when the rotator cuff is entirely irreparable, or in extensive tumor resection during arthroplastic surgery. The semiconstrained designs have some internal stability built into the prosthesis through the biomechanics of the design, but some rotator cuff musculature is necessary (Craig, 1988).

An anterior approach is used most commonly for surgery, through a deltopectoral incision. The articular surface of the humeral head is resected, the joint is debrided, synovectomy is performed if indicated, and marginal osteophytes are excised. The rotator cuff may be repaired. Care is taken to avoid the axillary nerve during surgery. A trial prosthesis is evaluated for "fit" with trial reduction, stability, and ROM assessment. The trial prosthesis is removed and the permanent prosthesis is cemented in place after careful preparation of the humerus and glenoid (Turner, 1991).

Several complications may occur as a consequence of TSA. The axillary and suprascapular nerves may be injured during surgery because of the proximity to the glenohumeral joint. Humeral fractures also occasionally occur intraoperatively in osteoporotic patients or during revision surgery. With the use of intravenous preoperative antibiotics and advanced intraoperative steroid techniques, the incidence of infection is less than 1%. As in hip and knee replacements, *Staphylococcus aureus* is the most common organism for infection. Once an infection has occurred, debridement and intravenous antibiotics may salvage the joint, but removal and revision frequently are necessary. Long-term prophylactics against bacteria are also recommended following total shoulder replacement, as discussed for total knee and hip replacements.

After a total shoulder replacement chronic instability may result from an impaired rotator cuff mechanism or surgical errors in prosthesis positioning. Acute postoperative dislocation is prevented by adherence to the ROM precautions. Patients are prohibited from external rotation of the shoulder past 15° and extension of the shoulder past 0° until the soft tissue structures have healed, approximately 6 to 12 weeks after surgery. Intraoperative repair of the rotator cuff necessitates additional exercise precautions following surgery. During rehabilitation the freshly repaired rotator cuff must be protected against aggressive stretching or strengthening. Rarely, reflex sympathetic dystrophy may follow total shoulder arthroplasty. This is a disastrous complication but can be managed with physical therapy, control of edema, and sympathetic nerve–blocking agents. Loosening of the prosthesis does occur. Clinically significant loosening presents as pain, instability, and progressive inability to use the arm. Radiolucent lines are common as early as 5 years after surgery, but revision rates are only about 3% at 5- to 10-year follow-up in many studies (Brenner et al., 1989).

Postoperative Rehabilitation

Huges and Neer outlined the "standard" rehabilitation program after TSA, a variant of which is used by most rehabilitation centers. Rehabilitation is generally divided into three phases, as outlined in this adaptive protocol.

Phase I

The patient wears a sling at all times except during exercise, and is taught one-handed activities of daily living. The arm remains non–weight-bearing. The hand is used as a stabilizing assist for objects held in the opposite hand.

Approximately the first 2 weeks after surgery, gentle passive and active-assisted ROM exercises are begun, focusing on shoulder flexion to 90°, abduction to 90°, internal rotation to 45°, and external rotation to 15°. Pendulum exercises are prescribed.

At 2 to 3 weeks postoperatively, isometric strengthening exercises begin in shoulder flexion, extension, internal rotation, external rotation, and abduction. Isometric exercises are performed at ROM intervals (for example, 0°, 45° and 90° of abduction).

Phase II

Exercises and precautions are upgraded when adequate motor control, a stable shoulder on examination, and relatively good pain relief are obtained. The patient is allowed to lift objects weighing up to 2 lb with the operated extremity. Vigorous isometric and gentle isotonic exercises, (eg, elastic tubing resistance exercise) are added. Active and active-assisted ROM (past 90° of flexion and abduction) is begun. Wand exercises are particularly helpful. Two-handed activity of daily living techniques are encouraged.

Phase III

Approximately 3 months after surgery, the weight-bearing and ROM precautions are lifted. The focus is stretching and strengthening. Progressive resistance and active ROM exercises are prescribed. Stretching is performed in abduction, flexion, and external rotation.

Long-Term Outcome

The outcome after TSA is critically dependent on well-prescribed rehabilitation and proper patient selection. Studies of Neer prostheses consistently demonstrate about 90% relief of pain, increases in ROM, better functioning, and revision rates of up to 10%. Patients who have undergone TSA for the treatment of osteoarthritis have a much higher success rate than individuals with inflammatory arthropathies or other disorders. For example, osteoarthritic individuals can anticipate average gains in flexion and abduction in the 40° to 80° range, increases in ROM, and good to excellent relief of pain (Barret et al., 1987; Turner, 1991).

TOTAL JOINT ARTHROPLASTY: ISSUES REGARDING LONG-TERM RECOVERY

The rehabilitation process following total joint reconstruction is a long-term process. One study estimated that muscle strength 3 to 6 months after hip replacement is only at 50% and increases to 80% of normal 6 to 12 months after surgery (Poss, 1993). Studies of gait analysis suggest that it may take several years for patients to regain normal gait. Many patients, however, never regain normal functioning. Others find that with aggressive, continued rehabilitation they are able to get the artificial joint to approximate the normal one. All patients, however, need regular follow-up and routine musculoskeletal evaluations. Patients should be carefully assessed at 6 months, 1 year, and 2 years after surgery to identify persistent physical and functional impairments. Intermittent physical therapy or a change in the home exercise program may eliminate the impairment and make a significant positive contribution to the patients' ability to function and quality of life.

REFERENCES

Anderson, J., Wixson, R., Stulberg, S. et al. (1994).

Barret, W.P., Franklin, J.L., Jackins, P.T., Wyss, C.R., & Matsen, F.A. (1987). Total shoulder arthroplasty. *Journal of Bone and Joint Surgery [Am]*, *69*, 865–872.

Brenner, B.C., Ferlic, D.C., Clayton, M.L., & Dennise, D.A. (1989). Survivorship of unconstrained total shoulder arthroplasty. *Journal of Bone and Joint Surgery [Am]*, *71*, 1289–1296.

Bohannon, R.W., & Cooper, J. (1993). Total knee arthroplasty: Evaluation of an acute care rehabilitation program. *Archives of Physical Medicine Rehabilitation*, *74*, 1091–1094.

Craig, E.V. (1988). Total shoulder replacement. *Orthopaedics*, *2*(1), 125–136.

Harris W.H., & Sledge C.B. (1990a). Total hip and total knee replacement: 1. *New England Journal of Medicine*, 323, 725–731.

Harris, W.H., & Sledge, C.B. (1990b). Total hip and total knee replacement (2). *New England Journal of Medicine*, *323*, 801–807.

Kilgus, D.J., Dorey, F.J., Finerman, G.A., et al, (1990). Patient activity, sports participation, and impact loading on the durability of cemented total hip replacements. *Clinical Orthopaedics and Related Research*, *269*, 25–31.

Maloney, W.J., Schurman, D.J., Hangen, D., Goodman, S.B., Edworthy, S., & Bloch, D.A. (1990). The influence of continuous passive motion on outcome in total knee arthroplasty. *Clinical Orthopaedics and Related Research*, *256*. 162–168.

McInnes, J., Larson, M.G., Daltroy, L.H., et al. (1993). A controlled evaluation of continuous passive motion in patients undergoing total knee arthroplasty. *Journal of the American Medical Association*, *268*, 1423–1428.

Poss, R. (1993). Total joint replacement: Optimizing patient expectations. *Journal of the American Academy of Orthopaedics*, *1*, 18–23.

Steinkamp, L.A., Dillingham, M.F., Markel, M.D., et al. (1993). Biomechanical considerations in patellofemoral joint rehabilitation. *American Journal of Sports Medicine*, *21*, 438–444.

Stern, S.H., Fuchs, M.D., Ganz, S.B., et al. (1991). Sexual function after total hip arthroplasty. *Clinical Orthopaedics and Related Research*, *260*, 228–235.

Turner, J.A. (1991). Shoulder replacement arthroplasty. In W. Petty (Ed.), *Total shoulder replacement*. (pp. 601-659). Philadelphia: Saunders.

Yack, H.J., Collins, C.E., & Whieldon, T.J. (1993). Comparison of closed and open kinetic chain exercise in the anterior cruciate ligament-deficient knee. *American Journal of Sports Medicine*, *21*, 49–54.

SUGGESTED READING

Davy, D.T., Kotzar, G.M., & Brown, R.H. (1988). Telemetric force measurements across the hip after total arthroplasty. *Journal of Bone and Joint Surgery [Am]*, *79*, 45–50.

MacDonald, W., & Owen, J.W. (1988). The effect of total hip replacement on driving reactions. *Journal of Bone and Joint Surgery [Br]*, *70*, 202–205.

CHAPTER 15

Adaptive Equipment and Assistive Devices

Holly Yvonne Lusa,, MOT, OTR/L, and Karen Freeman Ortmann, MM, PT

Adaptive equipment and assistive devices assist the patient with rheumatoid arthritis (RA) in achieving a higher level of functional independence. The occupational therapist introduces the patient to adaptive equipment that will assist in activities of daily living (ADLs), with emphasis on self-care, home management, work, and leisure pursuits. The physical therapist introduces the patient to assistive devices that will assist in mobility (transfer of the body from one position to another), posture, and ambulation.

The patient's lifestyle, home environment, vocational pursuits, leisure interests, energy level, and physical or attitudinal tolerance for adaptive equipment and assistive devices are considered when equipment is selected. It is also essential to include joint protection and energy conservation principles in the decision-making process. Consideration of these factors will promote patient compliance.

JOINT PROTECTION

The goal of joint protection with adaptive equipment and assistive devices is to reduce the deforming forces on joint structures that may occur during ADLs, mobility, and ambulation. The movement patterns that cause stress to vulnerable joints are identified. After potentially harmful movements have been isolated, the patient is taught to modify these activities through the use of equipment and/or techniques. Instructions on joint protection (Exhibit 15–1) are given to patients so they can understand why equipment was recommended.

The importance of patient and therapist collaboration can be observed in the problem-solving process of deciding which daily living skills are regularly performed and thus what equipment solutions may exist to protect joints. This collaboration is required so that the patient will understand fully the importance of maintaining joint integrity in daily living skills. Through the use of carefully selected equipment, the value of joint protection can be experienced by the patient as a reduction of pain, inflammation, and stress on joints (Melvin, 1982)

One clinical example incorporating joint protection techniques with adaptive equipment is the use of built-up grips on eating and grooming handles and writing utensils. The built-up grip is constructed from commercially available cylindrical foam padding that is attached to the handle of the utensil. This adaptive equipment prevents the patient from holding the utensil with the tightly flexed grasp that is usually required when using a fork, comb, or pencil without a built-up grip. Subsequently the patient avoids a position of deformity by maintaining the smaller joints of the fingers and thumb in a less flexed position during gross grasp.

ENERGY CONSERVATION

Energy conservation, like joint protection, is taught to the patient to facilitate a more active patient role in the choice of equipment and to provide a rationale for use of the equipment (Exhibit 15–2). The incorporation of energy conservation and adaptive equipment be-

Exhibit 15–1 Joint Protection Principles

1. Avoid position of deformity.
2. Use stronger, larger joints that can perform the job, rather than smaller joints.
3. Avoid holding joints in one position for a long time.
4. Maintain correct anatomical planes of movement.
5. Respect pain by knowing when to stop an activity.
6. Protect against further injury (Watkins & Robinson, 1974).

comes a necessary adjunct to treating the patient with RA more effectively. The goal of energy conservation is to minimize steps and reduce energy required in ADLs, mobility, and ambulation.

COMPENSATORY TREATMENT APPROACH

Decisions about equipment selection are facilitated by formal assessment and the discharge planning process. These procedures provide information to the therapist and the patient about abilities and limitations in the areas of range of motion (ROM), muscle strength, coordination, endurance, ADL status, mobility, and ambulation. In situations where problem areas are not conducive to remediation, equipment is considered as one approach to compensate for limitations present in areas that have an impact on ADLs, mobility, and ambulation. Through the use of selective, adaptive equipment individuals have the ability to master elements of daily activities, fulfill needs, and achieve feelings of satisfaction with themselves. Gans (1987) reports that people with arthritis and similar disorders were found to be dysfunctional for two major reasons: (1) pain that resulted in decreased motor skills and (2) an inability to perform daily living tasks.

Gans (1987) states:

> With the appropriate use of technology, disabled people can achieve mastery over their environments. Several major strategies are used to this end: adaption of a patient's physical technique of doing an activity, use of an adaptive aid, adapting a specific environment to the needs of the patient, or providing a complete substitute technology to allow accomplishment of an activity without body work being performed.

The importance of adaptive equipment is observed with the postoperative hip replacement patient who must limit ROM at the hip in accord with surgical precautions for 6 to 8 weeks (Fisher & Seeger, 1982). The limitations significantly complicate lower extremity tasks. Through the use of extended equipment such as a long-handled shoehorn, dressing stick, reacher, and bath sponge, as well as sock aids, shoe-tying aids, and bathroom and toileting equipment, a patient can master these lower extremity dressing and bathing skills during recovery. This allows patients to return home and care for themselves. It has also been reported by Fisher and Seeger (1982) that a large majority of patients who used compensatory adaptive equipment or technique in occupational therapy were independent in ADLs upon discharge, thus achieving a major patient and occupational therapy goal.

Exhibit 15–2 Energy Conservation Principles

1. Avoid unnecessary motions by
   - minimizing steps in all tasks
   - sitting whenever possible
   - using labor-saving devices such as microwave ovens, food processors, utility carts, and electric appliances
   - creating an easy flow of work such as an assembly line for preparing food
   - avoiding overreaching by arranging items at easy-to reach heights
2. Avoid last minute hurrying by
   - planning ahead to allow time for rest breaks
   - performing more difficult tasks such as window washing and vacuuming the carpet earlier in the day
   - distributing heavier physical tasks throughout the week
3. Establish a proper work environment including good lighting, ventilation, and proper work heights.
4. Analyze which activities are essential parts of a daily work schedule and eliminate nonessential activities (Watkins & Robinson, 1974).

OTHER CONSIDERATIONS IN EQUIPMENT SELECTION

Other special factors that need to be considered in the selection of adaptive equipment and assistive devices are the following:

- The cost of most equipment is not covered by insurance companies (Riggs & Gall, 1984). Often only wheelchairs, bedside commodes, hospital beds, and lift chairs are partially covered by insurance. Therapists should encourage and assist the patient in exploring resources such as equipment catalogs and discount stores for other options before purchasing equipment.
- The patient's acceptance of equipment or gadgets will have an influence on overall compliance.
- The stresses of equipment on hand and wrist joints must be considered. For example, while using a trigger-handled reacher to compensate for limited hip ROM, small joints of the hand may be affected. It is also important to consider the impact on hand and wrist joints when the patient grasps standard mobility equipment (wheelchair, walker, cane).
- Medical implications and the safety of certain equipment need to be considered. Cardiovascular considerations are inherent in ambulatory devices and adaptive aids that require a constant isometric grasp. Patients need to be informed about risks involved in equipment misuse and possible faulty equipment fabrication.
- The effect of new mobility equipment on self-care, home management, work, and leisure pursuits must be considered. For example, meal-preparation evaluation would be required if the patient is responsible for cooking after discharge and has been issued a new ambulatory device (ie, a walker). In this situation, special equipment is needed to assist in transporting items because the hands are needed to maneuver the ambulatory aid and are not available to pick up or carry objects.
- The durability of the equipment becomes a factor when the patient uses the device on a regular basis. The patient may choose a more expensive model if he or she foresees constant use. The patient also needs to know where to get replacements.

Thus many factors need to be considered in the selection of appropriate equipment for the patient with RA. Ease of selection varies with the variety of abilities, limitations, and emotions inherent in each individual case. For example, the postsurgical hip replacement patient may accept equipment readily, knowing that it is only for short-term use, but a patient with end-stage rheumatoid arthritis who will need to use the equipment indefinitely may not. Therapists' use of discretion is important when equipment is issued. Both need and probable compliance should be assessed.

MOBILITY EQUIPMENT

The principles of joint protection and energy conservation should also be applied when using assistive devices to improve mobility skills and facilitate pain relief during gait. Mobility, particularly the activities of sit to stand and ambulation, becomes impaired with involvement of the hip and knee joints. Weakness of supporting musculature, in particular the quadriceps and gluteal muscle group, is likely to cause impairment in position changes such as sit-to-stand activities and in ambulation on level surfaces, slopes, or stairs (Ehrlich, 1986). Pain and weakness may result in gait deviations, such as decreased stride, decreased step length, or uneven cadence. Range of motion limitations also result in postural changes and gait deviations requiring increased energy expenditure, lowering efficiency and further lowering endurance. Limitation of ROM at the knee during gait has been found to correlate with pain. Instability of the knee, joint effusion, and synovial thickening or bony hypertrophy are found in patients with rheumatoid arthritis.

The assistive devices are used to improve the patient's level of independence during mobility and ambulation by unloading the painful joints that, in part, have created gait deviations. After a careful assessment an assistive device is selected and properly fitted to the patient. The patient should also be instructed in the proper use of the device. The determining factors to be considered include the following:

- Safety factors
- Stability at other joints
- Joint protection: use of an ambulatory aid should not cause stress or increase the load on the small joints of the upper extremity or on the unaffected lower extremity
- Weight-bearing classification
- Patient stability in terms of balance
- Energy expenditure required of the patient
- Sensation in weight-bearing extremities
- Cardiac status

Various assistive devices are available for the patient with RA whose mobility skills and ambulation are impaired.

Canes

A cane is used on the contralateral side (ie, the side opposite the affected joint). The force applied to the cane should not exceed 20% to 25% of the body's weight because of instability (Edwards, 1986). Two canes are required for safety or joint protection if the force applied exceeds 25% of body weight. In considering joint protection of the wrist and hand, a flattened or T-shaped cane handle is preferable to a C-shaped cane handle.

Optimally, the cane is advanced with the affected lower extremity to allow for reciprocal arm and leg movement during ambulation on a level surface. An alternative method of sequencing is to advance the cane first, then the affected lower extremity, and then the unaffected lower extremity. When ascending stairs, the patient should lead with the unaffected leg, followed by the affected leg, and then the cane; when descending stairs the cane, followed by the affected leg, and then the unaffected leg.

Crutches

Crutches may be used by the patient with good balance when the force applied to the assistive device is required to exceed 25% of body weight. The same sequencing pattern used for ambulation with a cane may be used. The use of a two-handed device is required if the force applied to the device exceeds 25% and the weight-bearing category/classification is no weight bearing, partial weight bearing, or full weight bearing (guarded). One or two crutches may be used when the patient's status is full weight bearing if there is instability, swelling, or pain in a lower extremity weight-bearing joint (Riggs & Gall, 1984).

If the patient has RA involvement of the wrist and/or hands the use of platform crutches is preferable. The platform crutches have a padded arm board with Velcro closures and a vertical hand grip instead of an axillary pad and horizontal hand grip. Weight-bearing forces are applied to the forearm when the elbow is flexed to 90° and placed on the arm board rather than through the joint of the wrist and hand.

Walkers

A walker should be used if only 50% of the body weight is on the affected extremity (partial weight bearing; Riggs & Gall, 1984). A standard pickup walker should be advanced with the patient remaining in an erect posture, followed by the affected lower extremity and the unaffected lower extremity. Energy expenditure, hand and wrist involvement, and safety are to be considered in selecting the appropriate walker. Platform attachments are available to adapt the walker when there is upper extremity involvement. Additionally, roller attachments are available and may be substituted for the front legs of the walker if the patient is unable to advance the walker without exceeding the weight-bearing restrictions and/or loss of balance. The reciprocating walker also provides another alternative under these circumstances.

Elevated Surfaces

Elevated surfaces are to be considered for the patient with hip and knee involvement who is impaired in position changes (ie, sit to stand). The use of raised toilet seats, bath chairs or benches, and elevated (high) chairs reduces the force on the hip and knee during sit to stand (Burdett, Habasevick, Pisciotta, & Simon, 1985).

Stairs

For the patient with impaired stair-climbing ability, elevators, lifts, and stair-glide devices are available. However, cost becomes an issue because this equipment is expensive and requires maintenance.

Wheelchairs

Patients severely limited by contractures may require the use of a wheelchair when ambulation is unrealistic. Wheelchairs are used on a temporary basis by those limited by joint pain or swelling. The wheelchair should be properly fitted to the width and height of the patient. Removable armrests and legrests are available to facilitate easier transfers to level and unlevel surfaces. Lightweight chairs made with an alloy frame facilitate an easier push and decrease energy expenditure. Electric wheelchairs and other transportation machines such as the Amigo are available to the patient with multiple joint involvement.

EQUIPMENT SUGGESTIONS

Equipment suggestions are summarized in Tables 15–1 to 15–10. They are not all-inclusive because of the wide variety of equipment that can be purchased or customized. Equipment vendors provide catalogs that describe adaptive equipment and assistive devices in more detail. Vendors of equipment and adaptive clothing are given in Appendix 15–A, along with patient self-help education resources.

Table 15–1 ADL Equipment: Feeding Equipment

Problem	*Equipment*
1. Poor hand grasp	1. Built-up handles on eating utensils, cylindrical foam padding placed on handles (Figure 15–1) 2. Utensil cuff, a cuff that fits over the palm of the hand into which utensils are inserted; used when a patient is unable to grasp utensils 3. Sandwich holder, a plastic holder that grips a sandwich
2. Decreased upper extremity ROM	1. Bent-up utensils; angle of utensil handle is adjusted to facilitate hand-to-mouth patterns 2. Long-handled utensils 3. Long straws (18 inches), clear plastic straws (Figure 15–1) 4. Straw holder placed on cup; holds long straw at appropriate angle (Figure 15–1)
3. Decreased upper extremity strength	1. Rocker knife, a knife with a long, curved blade; used to cut food with a rocking motion 2. Meat cutter, a cuff-type utensil that slips over the palm of the hand; used when the patient is unable to grasp utensil 3. Special knives with handles of various shapes and sizes; used to decrease ulnar deviation
4. Decreased upper extremity coordination	1. Nonslip padding (Dycem), a rubber pad placed under a plate to prevent slipping 2. Plate guard, a metal or plastic piece placed on the perimeter of a plate to prevent spilling; aids in getting food onto utensil

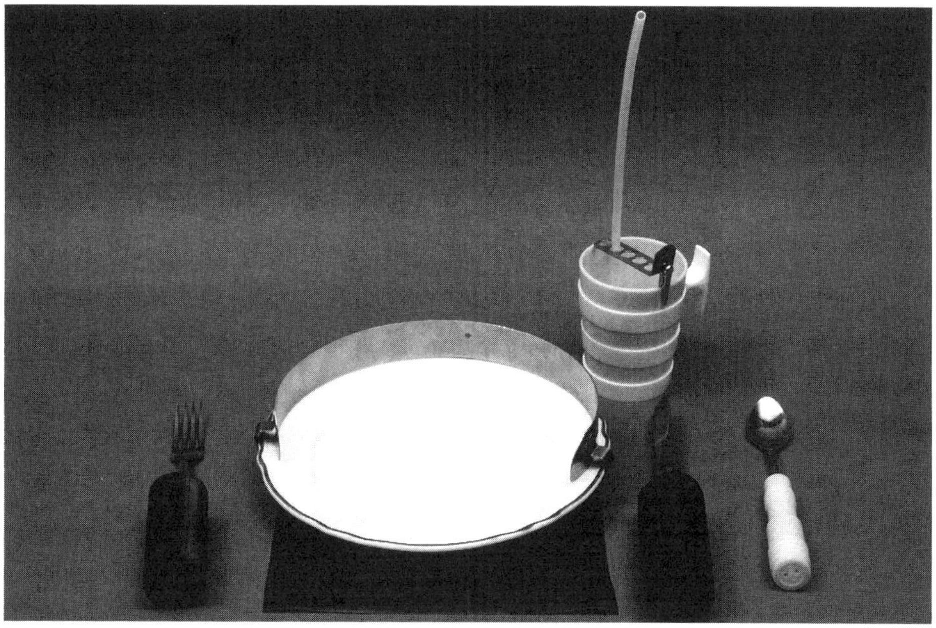

Figure 15–1 Feeding setup with nonslip (Dycem) plate guard, built-up utensils, long straw, and straw holder.

Table 15–2 ADL Equipment: Grooming Equipment

Problem	*Equipment*
1. Decreased upper extremity ROM	1. Extended handles on comb, hairbrush, and toothbrush 2. Extended faucet handles
2. Decreased upper extremity strength	1. Universal cuff (a cuff that slips over the palm of the hand where utensils are inserted) 2. Built-up handle, cylindrical foam padding placed on handles of combs, hairbrushes, toothbrushes, makeup, and razors (Figure 15–2) 3. Dental floss holder, a device used to hold dental floss 4. Wash mitt with Velcro closure
3. Decreased upper extremity coordination	1. Emery board glued to a wood base 2. Nonslip padding, a rubber pad placed under bottles 3. Suction nail and denture brush, a brush with suction cups that attach to a table 4. Electric shaver

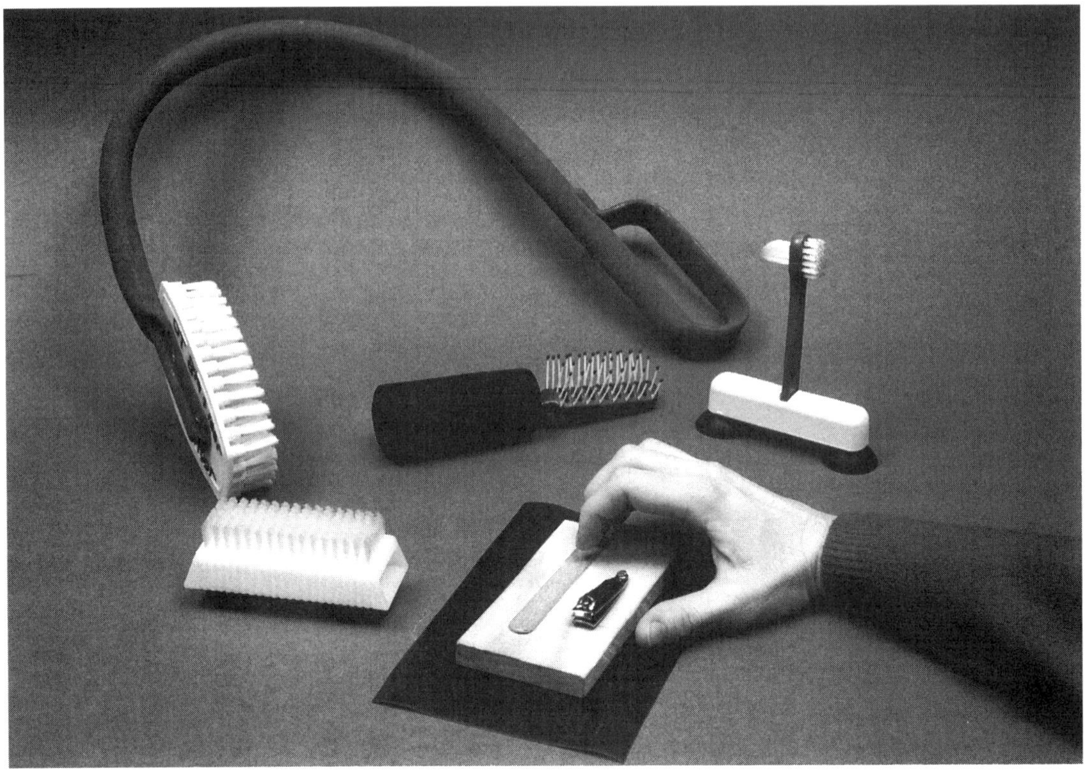

Figure 15–2 Grooming setup with built-up grip on hairbrush, toothbrush, and comb; emery boards on wood stabilizer with nonslip padding (Dycem); nail and denture suction brushes; and extended-handle bath brush.

Table 15–3 ADL Equipment: Dressing Equipment

Problem	*Equipment*
1. Decreased upper extremity and lower extremity ROM	1. Long-reach zipper pull, cord with ring attached 2. Long-handled dressing stick, reacher, and shoehorn (Figure 15–3) 3. Sock-donning aid; a sock or stocking is pulled over a rigid plastic piece, the foot is inserted, and sock and aid are pulled up 4. Shoe insert aid, a plastic piece that fits over the heel of a shoe so that the heel of the shoe does not bend over 5. Elastic shoe laces that do not require tying
2. Decreased upper extremity strength and coordination	1. Adapted Velcro fasteners, to replace buttons and zippers 2. Built-up handles on button aid and zipper pull 3. Zipper ring, a ring placed on zipper tab 4. Loose-fitting clothing with a minimal number of fasteners

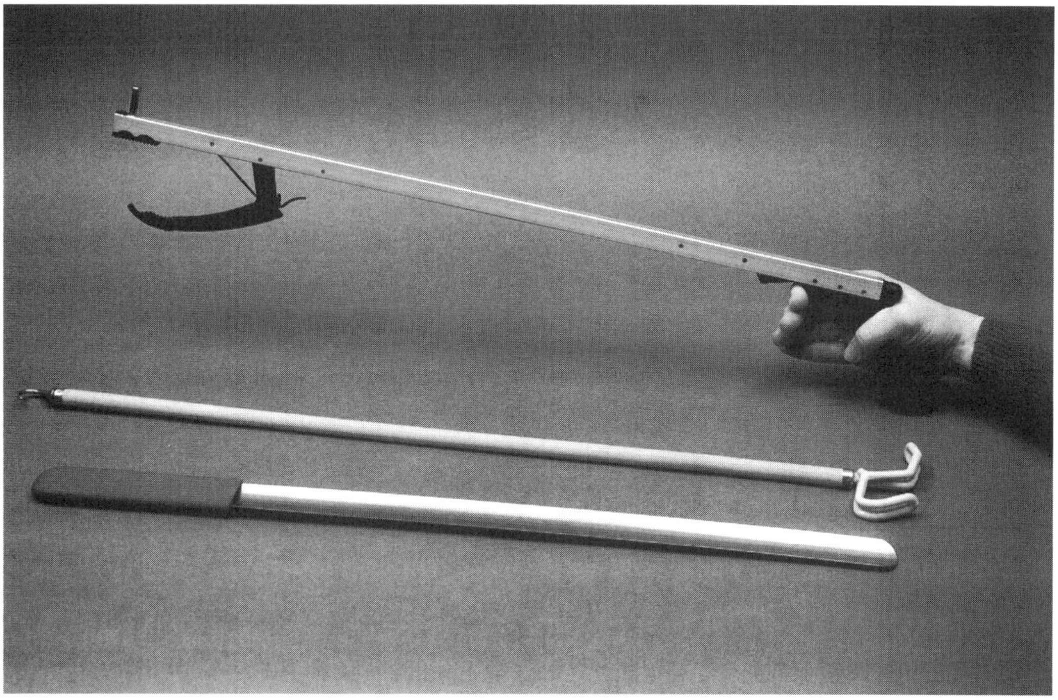

Figure 15-3 Dressing equipment, including a long-handled shoehorn, dressing stick, and reacher.

Table 15–4 ADL Equipment: Toileting Equipment

Problem	*Equipment*
1. Decreased ability to sit and stand	1. Raised toilet seat (Figure 15–4) 2. Safety rails (Figure 15–4)
2. Decreased lower extremity ROM	1. Raised toilet seat with right/left cut out
3. Decreased upper extremity ROM	1. Toilet hygiene aid, a plastic or metal aid with a clamp that holds toilet paper in place

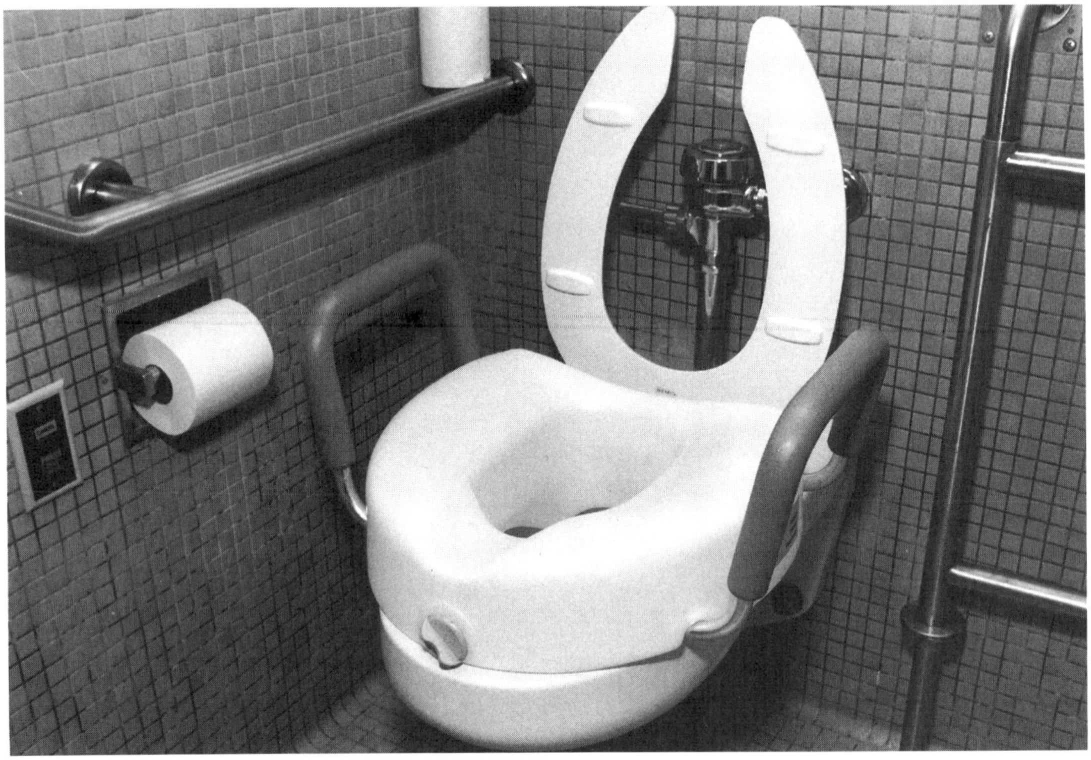

Figure 15–4 Toileting equipment with raised toilet and toilet rails.

Table 15–5 ADL Equipment: Bathing Equipment

Problem	*Equipment*
1. Decreased upper extremity and lower extremity ROM	1. Long-handled sponge 2. Hand-held shower hose
2. Decreased upper extremity strength and coordination	1. Wash mitt with Velcro closure 2. Suction rubber soap holder; holds down soap 3. Soap attached to a rope
3. Safety	1. Grab bar (Figure 15–5) 2. Safety treads on floor of shower or bath 3. Bath bench 4. Shower chair (Figure 15–5)

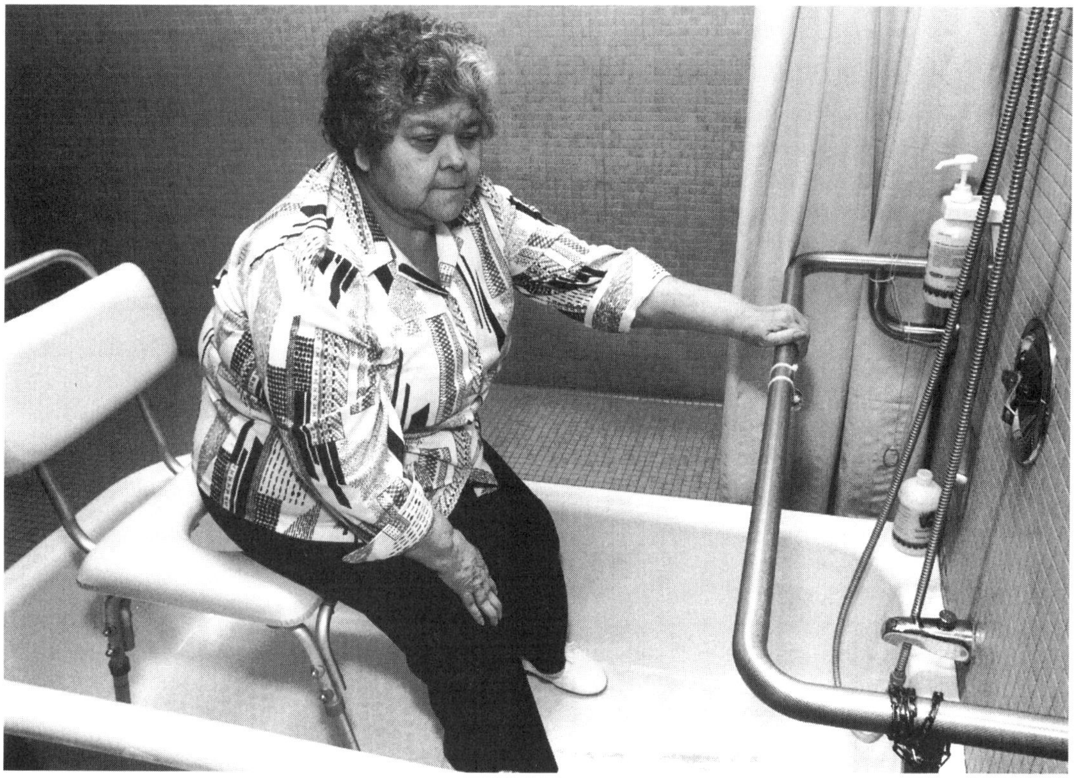

Figure 15–5 Bathing equipment with shower chair and safety rail.

Table 15–6 ADL Equipment: Communication Equipment

Problem	*Equipment*
1. Decreased upper extremity strength and coordination	1. Gooseneck phone holder, a flexible chrome tube that attaches to a table and holds the receiver in place (Figure 15–6) 2. Speaker phone, an electronic device that amplifies sound 3. Phone holder, a handle on the phone receiver that slips onto the palm of the hand 4. Book holder, a device that sits on a table and holds books 5. Built-up grips on pens and pencils, cylindrical foam padding placed on writing utensils

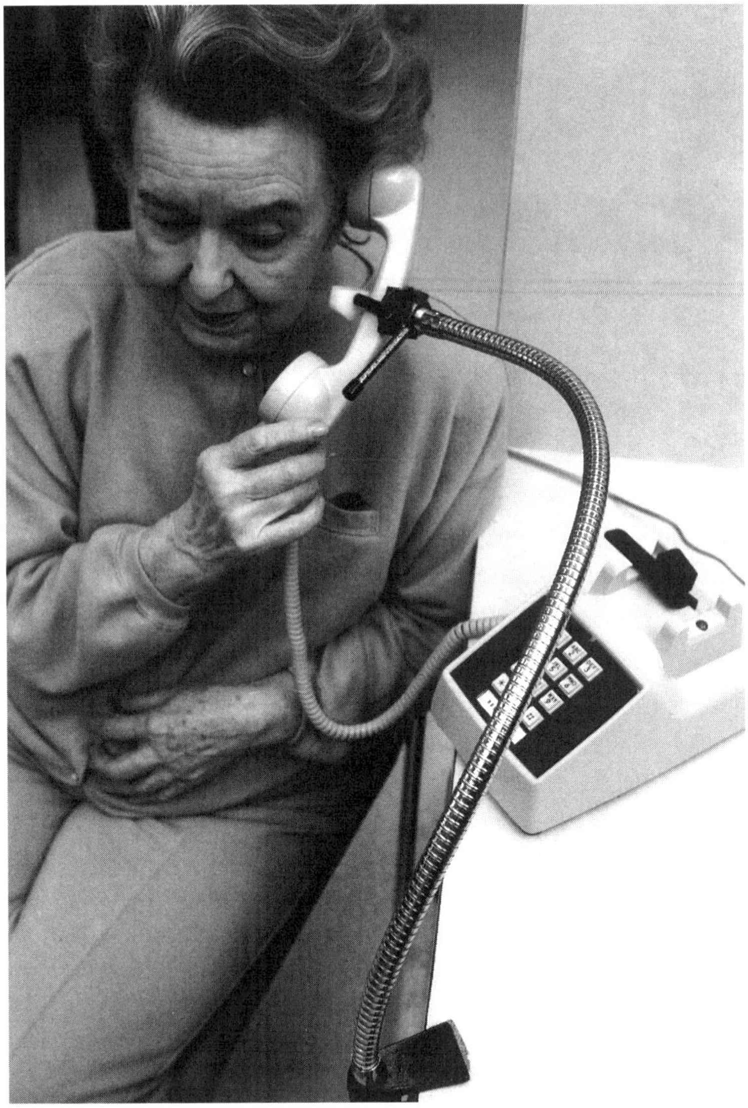

Figure 15–6 Communication equipment setup with gooseneck phone holder.

Table 15–7 ADL Equipment: Meal Preparation Equipment

Problem	*Equipment*
1. Decreased upper extremity ROM	1. Oven shove (an extended reacher) 2. Long-handled reacher with rubber grips
2. Decreased upper extremity strength	1. Loop scissors, spring loaded, self-opening handle 2. Vegetable peeler with a circular handle that fits in the palm of the hand 3. Bowl holder, a plastic or metal frame holds the bowl in place while mixing 4. Adaptive jar openers 5. Built-up handles on cooking utensils, cylindrical foam padding placed on handles (Figure 15–7) 6. Nonslip padding (Dycem), a rubber pad placed under bowls to keep them in place
3. Decreased endurance	1. Stool, kept in kitchen for conservation of energy 2. Lightweight cookware; avoid heavy iron cookware 3. Labor-saving devices such as microwave ovens, food processors, and electrical appliances; appliances with push buttons or levers 4. Convenience foods, such as frozen foods
4. Decreased mobility	1. Utility carts, rolling carts used to transport items 2. Walker bags and baskets; attach to walker to transport items (Figure 15–8)

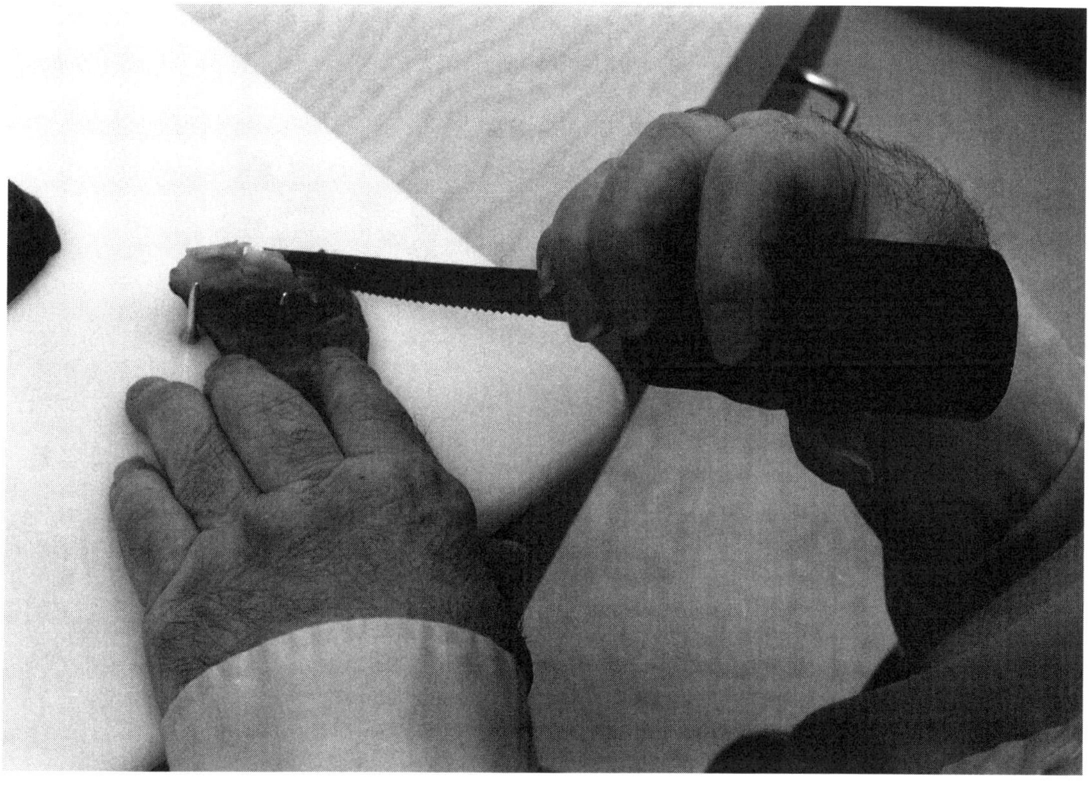

Figure 15–7 Meal preparation with built-up grip on knife and cutting board with suction feet and nail stabilizer.

Table 15–8 ADL Equipment: Home Maintenance Accessories

Problem	*Equipment*
1. Decreased upper extremity and lower extremity ROM	1. Long-handled dustpan (Figure 15–9) 2. Mop with easy-to-reach squeeze handle
2. Decreased upper extremity strength, coordination, and endurance	1. Doorknob and faucet turners, devices to increase leverage; aid in turning rotating knobs 2. Built-up grip on key holder 3. Rolling dolly for mop bucket 4. Lightweight appliances 5. Alternative electrical switches for easier environmental control
3. Decreased mobility	1. Utility cart, a rolling cart used to transport items 2. Walker bags and baskets; attach to walker to transport items 3. Chair with extended legs

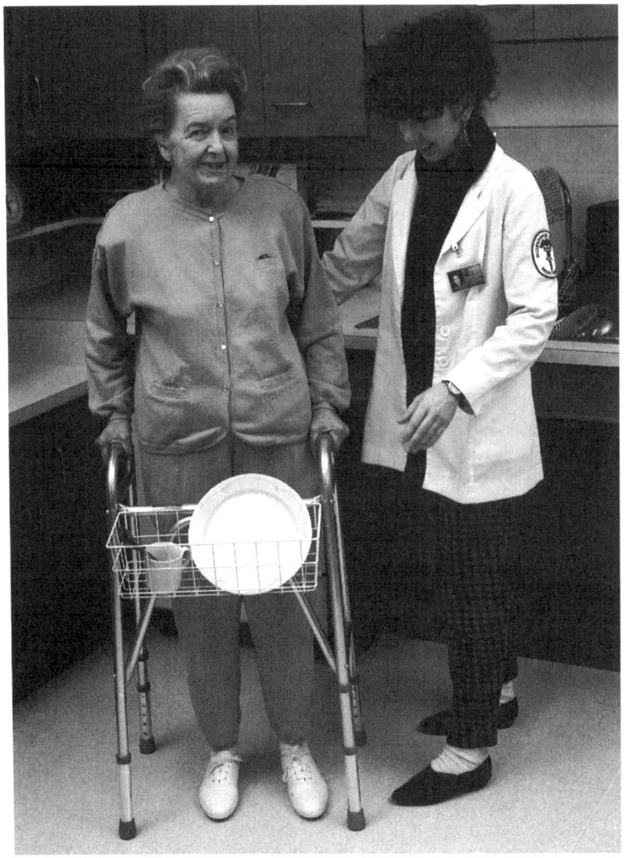

Figure 15–8 Using a walker with attached walker basket to transport items in the kitchen.

Table 15–9 ADL Equipment: Automobile Accessories

Problem	*Equipment*
1. Decreased upper extremity strength	1. Car door opener, a device to increase leverage 2. Built-up grip on keyholder; plastic frame holds keys (Figure 15–10) 3. Electric garage door opener

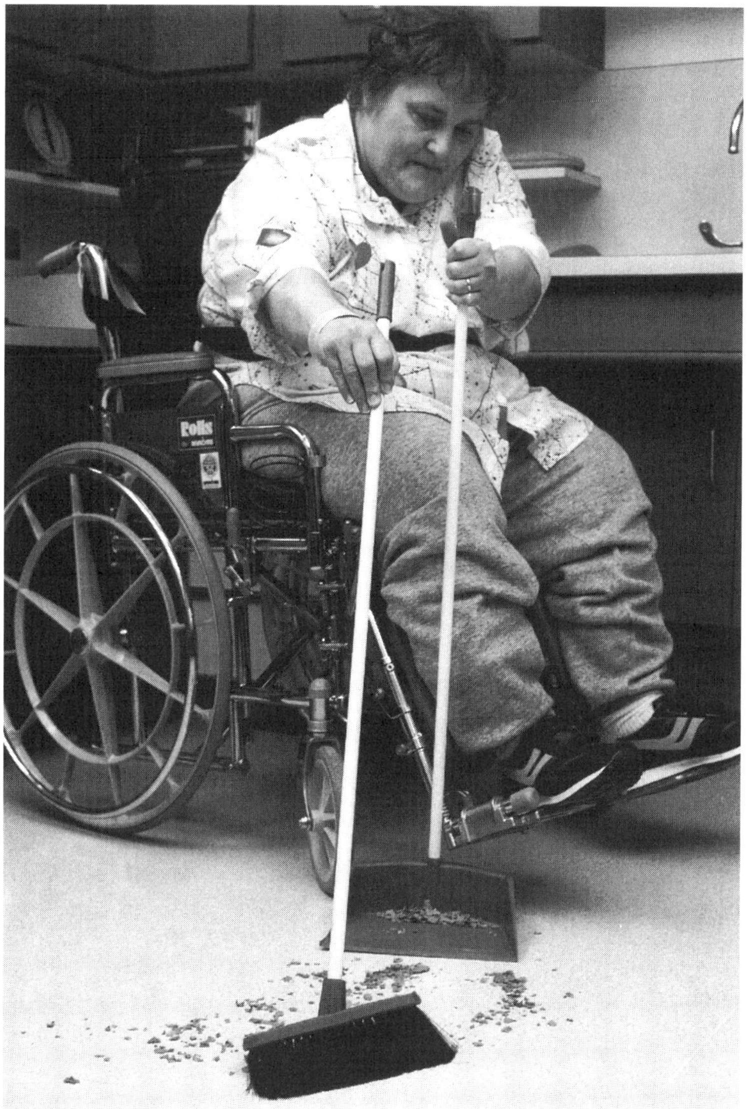

Figure 15–9 Using a long-handled dustpan and broom to increase upper extremity range of reach required in cleaning floors.

Table 15–10 Mobility Equipment: Ambulation Aids

Problem	*Equipment*
1. Decreased stride, step length, and cadence secondary to ROM limitations, pain, and/or muscle spasm	1. Cane, if force applied is less than 25% of body weight 2. Walker or crutches, if force applied is 50% of body weight
2. Decreased velocity	
3. Decreased balance	1. Walker (Figure 15–11)
4. Involvement of hand or wrist	1. Cane with flattened or T-shaped handle 2. Platform crutches 3. Platform walker
5. Poor endurance secondary to increased energy expenditure	1. Roller walker with or without platform attachment

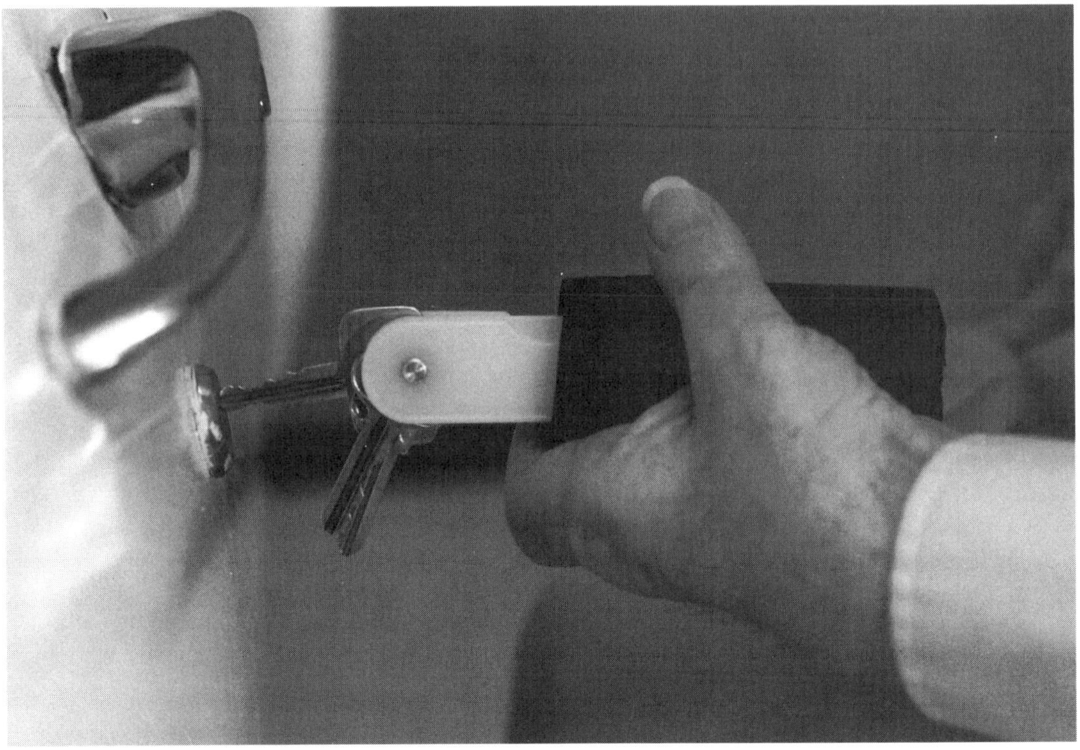

Figure 15–10 Using a built-up grip on key holder to open a car door.

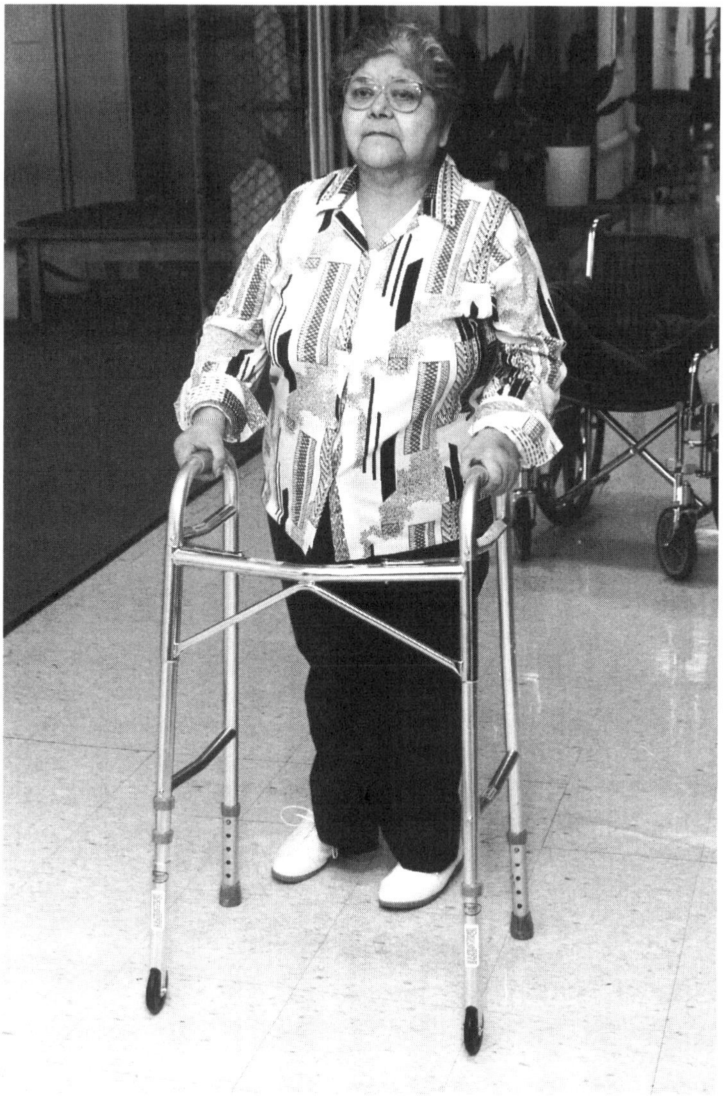

Figure 15–11 Using a walker to maintain balance.

CONCLUSION

Most adaptive equipment and assistive devices are readily available through manufacturers and suppliers. On occasion, specially designed equipment may be required to meet a patient's needs. The rehabilitation engineer then works in conjunction with the patient, occupational therapist, and physical therapist to customize the adaptive aid, mobility device, or environmental control setup.

Equipment can range from simple devices easily purchased from a hardware store to state-of-the-art technology. Gans (1987) reviewed current technological advances relevant to the needs of the arthritic patient. His review includes water faucets with "proximity detectors" that start and stop the flow of water, faster speed motors for wheelchairs that are quieter than older systems, and environmental control systems. As an example, Radio Shack's Home Control System is a remote-control system that can facilitate turning appliances on or off, thereby eliminating the need to do this by hand.

REFERENCES

Burdett, R.G., Habasevick, R., Pisciotta, J., & Simon, S.R. (1985). Biomechanical comparison of rising from two types of chairs. *Physical Therapy, 65*, 1177–1183.

Edwards, B.G. (1986). Contralateral and ipsilateral cane usage by patients with total knee or hip replacement. *Archives of Physical Medicine and Rehabilitation, 67*, 734–740.

Ehrlich, G.E. (1986). *Rehabilitation management of rheumatoid conditions*. Baltimore: Williams & Wilkins.

Fisher, L.A., & Seeger, M.S. (1982). Adaptive equipment used in the rehabilitation of hip arthroplasty. *American Journal of Occupational Therapy, 36*, 503– 508.

Gans, B.M. (1987). Rehabilitation engineering technology and the arthritis patient. *Journal of Rheumatology, 14*, 68–71.

Melvin, J. (1982). *Rheumatic disease: Occupational therapy and rehabilitation*. Philadelphia: F.A. Davis.

Riggs, G., & Gall, E.P. (1984). *Rheumatic diseases rehabilitation and management*. Boston: Butterworth.

Watkins, R., & Robinson, D. (1974). *Joint protection techniques for patients with rheumatoid arthritis*. Chicago: Rehabilitation Institute of Chicago.

SUGGESTED READING

Brinkman, J.R., & Perry, J. (1985). Rate and range of knee motion during ambulation in healthy and arthritic subjects. *Physical Therapy, 65*, 1056–1060.

Denham, R.A. (1959). Hip mechanics. *Journal of Bone and Joint Surgery [Br], 41*, 550–557.

Dimonte, P., & Light, H. (1982). Pathomechanics, gait deviations, and treatment of the rheumatoid foot. *Physical Therapy. 62*, 1148–1156.

Leek, J.L., Gershwin, E.M., & Fawell, W.M. (1986). *Principles of physical medicine and rehabilitation in the musculoskeletal diseases*. Orlando, FL: Grune & Stratton.

Reisman, M., Burdett, R.G., Simon, S.R., & Norkin, C. (1985). Elbow movement and forces at the hands during swing through axillary crutch gait. *Physical Therapy, 65*, 601–605.

Richards, R.L., Wessel, J., & Malowin, F. (1985). Muscle activation patterns in gait of rheumatoid arthritis patients. *Physiotherapy Canada, 37*, 220–228.

Swezey, R.L. (1978). Arthritis: *Rational therapy and rehabilitation*. Philadelphia: Saunders.

Trombly, C.A. (1983). *Occupational therapy for physical dysfunction*. Baltimore: Williams & Wilkins.

Van der Loos, H.F.M., Michalowski, S.J., & Leifer, L.J. (1986). Design of an omnidirectional mobile robot as a manipulation aid for the severely disabled. In *Proceedings of the Rehabilitation Engineering Society of North America 9th Annual Conference* (p. 247). Minneapolis: Rehabilitation Engineering Society of North America.

Appendix 15–A

Resources

EQUIPMENT SOURCES

Aamed, Inc., 1215 South Harlem, Forest Park, IL 60130

Abbey Medical, 6833 West Roosevelt, Berwyn, IL 60402

Accent on Living's Buyer's Guide, Box 700, Bloomington, IL 61701

Be OK! Fred Sammons, Inc., Box 32, Brookfield, IL 61513

Denson, 609 South Carlton Street, Wheaton, IL 60189

Designs for Independent Living, Whirlpool Corporation Administration Center, Benton Harbor, MI 49022

Ekco Housewares Co., 9234 West Belmont, Franklin Park, IL 60131

Enrichments, Bissell Healthcare Companies, P.O. Box 579, 145 Tower Drive, Hinsdale, IL 60521

Help Yourself Aids, P.O. Box 192, Hinsdale, IL 60521

Home Care Catalog, Smith and Davis Manufacturing Co., 1180 Central Industrial Avenue, St. Louis, MO 63110

Independent Living from Maddock, Inc., Ableware: Maddock Inc., Pequannock, NJ 07440-1993

Miles-Kimball, 41 West 8th Avenue, Kimball Building, Oshkosh, WI 54901

Resource: Help at Your Fingertips, Sears Home Health Care, Sears, Roebuck and Co., 925 South Homan Avenue, Chicago, IL 60607

The Capability Collection, Ways and Means, 28001 Citrin Drive, Romulus, MI 48174

The Independence Factory, P.O. Box 597, Middletown, OH 45042

Tru Trac Therapy Products, Diaz Road, Tenecula, CA 92390

ADAPTIVE CLOTHING SOURCES

Accessible Fashions, National Access Center, 1419 27th Street, N.W., Washington, DC 20007

Claypool Classics, 586 North Bank Lane, Lake Forest, IL 60045

Contour Fabrications, Inc., P.O. Box 56, Grand Blanc, MI 48439

Easewear, 44 Wexford Drive, Mendham, NJ 07945

Fashion Able for Better Living, 5 Crescent Avenue, Box 5, Rocky Hill, NJ 08553

PATIENT SELF-HELP EDUCATION RESOURCES

Abledata Information System, Marion Hall, National Director, P.O. Box 3368, University State, Charlottesville, VA 22903

Access Living, 310 South Peoria, Chicago, IL 60607

Arthritis Foundation, Arthritis Health Profession's Associates, 1314 Spring Street, N.W., Atlanta, GA 30309

Blair J., Gevin, C., and Schater, M.K. (1983). *Adapted equipment/rehabilitation engineering*. Rockville, MD: American Occupational Therapy Association.

Available from the American Occupational Therapy Association, 1383 Piccard Drive, Suite 300, Rockville, MD 20850. Comprehensive resources for adaptive equipment needs.

Davis, W.M. (1981). *Aids to make you able: Self-help devices and ideas for the disabled*. New York: Beaufort Books. Available from the publisher: 9 East 4th Street, New York, NY 10016. An occupational therapist compiled this book to assist in making appropriate selections of adaptive equipment.

Grainger, S.E. (1982). *Making aids for disabled living*. London: B.T. Batsford, Ltd. Publisher's address: 4 Fitzhardinge Street, London, England, WIHOAH. Provides patterns and photos for fabricating aids.

Hoffman, M.A., and Morris, W.W. (1979). *Clothing for the handicapped, the aged and other people with special needs*. Springfield, IL: Charles C Thomas Publishers. Publisher's address: Bannerstone House, 301–327 Cast Lawrence Avenue, Springfield, IL. A resource for selection and adaption of clothing.

Klinger, J.L. (1980). *Self-help manual for patients with arthritis*. Atlanta: Arthritis Foundation. Available from Arthritis Health Professions Associates, Arthritis Foundation, 1314 Spring Street, N.W., Atlanta, GA 30309. Excellent source for adaptive equipment and assistive devices.

Klinger, J.L., Frieden, F.H., and Sullivan, R.A. (1970). *Mealtime manual for the aged and handicapped*. New York: Essandress Special Editions, a division of Simon and Schuster, Inc. Publisher's address: 630 Fifth Avenue, New York, NY 10020

Lorig, K., and Fries, J.F. (1980). *The arthritis helpbook: What you can do for your arthritis*. Reading, MA: Addison-Wesley. A guidebook written for the arthritis patient that gives information on disease process, surgeries, medications, diet, exercise, and equipment needs.

Lowman, E., and Klinger, J.L. (1969). *Aids to independent living: Self-help for the handicapped*. New York: McGraw-Hill Publishing Co. Provides hundreds of photos and descriptions of adaptive equipment and assistive devices.

Thabault, G., and Ocone, L. (1984). *Tools and techniques for easier gardening*. Burlington, VT: Gardens for All. Publisher's address: 180 Flynn Avenue, Burlington, VT 05401

CHAPTER 16

Insights from Problem-Solving Theory for Arthritis Patient Education

Karen J. Connell

There is a growing and substantial interest in the potential benefit of education as an adjunct to medical and surgical interventions for persons with arthritis. Daltroy and Liang (1993) have observed that prior to 1980 there were fewer than 20 published research articles concerning arthritis patient education; by the end of the decade, there were more than 200. Clearly, there is growing and substantial interest in the potential benefit of education as an adjunct to medical and surgical interventions for persons with arthritis.

Early studies focused on increasing patients' knowledge about their disease and their compliance with treatment regimens. Research confirmed that most such programs *did* substantially increase patients' knowledge; increases in knowledge, however, typically did not lead to changes in behavior or ability to cope with arthritis-related problems (Haynes, Taylor, & Sackett, 1979; Lorig, Konkol, & Gonzalez, 1987; Mazzuca, 1982; Potts & Brandt, 1983). Focus then shifted to the development of interventions aimed at influencing *behaviors* thought to be beneficial, such as exercise and relaxation. The assumption was that positive changes in health behaviors would lead to improved health status, particularly reductions in pain, disability, and depression. Research did not support this assumption either. Lorig, Laurin, and Gines (1984), for example, found that increases in the use of exercise and relaxation techniques by patients who had participated in their arthritis self-management courses were not associated with improvements in pain, disability, and depression, although some patients did realize benefits in these areas. Lorig & Laurin (1985) then conducted a literature review, which suggested that lack of association between changes in health behaviors and health status is found in several other chronic diseases as well.

The EDUCIZE work referenced in this chapter was conducted while the author was Director, Education Component, Arthritis Division, Northwestern University Medical School, Chicago. EDUCIZE research was supported by the Division's National Institutes of Health Multipurpose Arthritis Center Grant No. P60 AR30692.

For further information about the application of Deweyan theory to patient and/or health professions education, contact the author at the Department of Family Medicine, University of Illinois at Chicago, 1919 W. Taylor (M/C 663), Chicago, IL 60612.

The author expresses her sincere gratitude to, and respect and affection for, Maureen R. Gecht, OTR/L, MPH, and Patricia Conlon-Grosso, OTR/L, MA. Their enthusiastic, thoughtful, persistent, and tireless work over many years to develop and test Dewey-based patient education strategies have made it possible for many allied health professionals and people with arthritis to benefit from the ideas discussed in this chapter. The author's own understanding has been significantly enhanced by their efforts and colleagueship.

More recently, investigators have turned to cognitive-behavioral theories to help them develop more refined interventions in the hope of improving outcomes. Lorig and her colleagues, for example, have based their investigations of the possible mediating role of self-efficacy in program outcomes on the social learning theory of Bandura (1977, 1986). Self-efficacy refers to one's confidence or belief that he or she can achieve a specific behavior or cognitive state. Lorig and her colleagues have found that self-efficacy predicts future health status and that interventions that affect self-efficacy often are associated with positive changes in health status (Lorig & Gonzalez, 1992; Lorig et al., 1989).

The arthritis self-management program (ASMP) now includes strategies to enhance participants' self-efficacy for pain management, physical functioning, and controlling other arthritis symptoms such as fatigue and depression. Similarly, Allegrante, Kovar, MacKenzie, Peterson, and Gutin (1993) used self-efficacy theory to guide development of some of the interventions in an 8-week walking education program for patients with knee osteoarthritis. At program end, participants had improved significantly on two functional measures, compared with control subjects, and one self-efficacy measure—ability to manage arthritis-related symptoms other than pain.

Research by other investigators suggests support for cognitive-behavioral approaches, particularly to pain management in rheumatoid arthritis (Keefe & Van Horn, 1993; Perker, Iverson, Smarr, & Stucky-Ropp, 1993). These approaches typically include such strategies as relaxation training, goal setting with self-reinforcement, communications training, problem solving, and/or assertiveness training. Whatever their particulars, such programs typically contain an educational phase, a skills-acquisition phase, and a maintenance phase that emphasizes ways to apply new knowledge and skills to problems in everyday life.

Still other researchers are pursuing investigations of the relationship between specific coping strategies used to deal with illness-related stressors and illness outcomes such as psychological well-being, disability, and pain (Parker et al., 1988; Schiaffino, Revenson, & Gibofsky, 1991). There is evidence for the effectiveness of problem-focused coping strategies as well as for the use of multiple rather than single coping strategies (Affleck, Urrows, Tennen, & Higgins, 1992; Blalock, DeVellis, Holt, & Hahn, 1993).

Clearly, research over the last 15 years has afforded us many useful insights into variables that are related to effective patient education for persons with arthritis. It is now clear that interventions that focus primarily on ensuring that participants acquire information about their disease and ways to manage it are not likely to influence behavior or health status. It also appears that we cannot assume that teaching patients behaviors generally accepted as desirable will ensure improvements in health status. Factors such as self-efficacy and problem-focused coping strategies appear to mediate improvements in health status and must be considered both when planning programs and when studying their effects.

Despite our progress, treatment gains, whatever the approach used, more often than not either are not maintained or diminish significantly over time (Bradley, Young, & Anderson, 1987; O'Leary, Shoor, Lorig, & Holman, 1988). Although the 4-year follow-up study by Lorig, Mazonson, and Holman (1993) of primarily patients with osteoarthritis who had participated in the ASMP found that the program resulted in significant reductions in pain ratings and arthritis-related physician visits, functional gains that had initially been realized were not retained. Keefe and Van Horn (1993) conclude their review on cognitive-behavioral treatment of rheumatoid arthritis pain by suggesting that two of the most important directions for future research are improving our understanding of the relapse process and evaluating methods for enhancing maintenance. In addition, as DeVellis and Blalock (1993) have noted, the mechanisms through which beneficial effects are obtained in patient education programs remain largely unknown.

The remainder of this chapter explores the possibility that the problem-solving theory of the American educational philosopher John Dewey can be used to enhance the effectiveness of arthritis patient education. Dewey developed his theory of reflective thinking or problem solving (he uses the terms largely interchangeably) in writings that spanned the 56-year period between 1882 and 1938. His work is widely regarded as the most comprehensive set of statements made to date about the nature of teaching and learning. Dewey's theory has formed the conceptual and philosophical basis for much curriculum research and development in elementary, secondary, and higher education. Some medical education researchers, including the author, have applied the theory in health professions education. Except for the efforts of the author and her colleagues (Connell, 1992; Connell, Gecht, & Conlon-Grosso, 1993; Connell & Sinacore, 1996; Perlman et al., 1990), Dewey's ideas have not been systematically applied to patient education.

Discussed are five central and interrelated educational concepts from Dewey's theory. The story of Marjorie, a middle-aged woman with severe American Rheumatism Association Functional Class III rheumatoid arthritis, is used to illustrate these concepts. Quotes from Dewey's work that have been integrated into the text are from *Democracy and Education* (1916) and *How We Think* (1933).

MARJORIE'S STORY

Marjorie was a participant in EDUCIZE, a combined aerobic exercise and problem-solving education program that was developed by the author and her colleagues, initially for people with rheumatoid arthritis (Perlman et al., 1990). Although EDUCIZE has been refined over the past dozen years as it has been used with varied audiences, its core philosophy has remained unchanged. EDUCIZE is designed to enhance the problem-solving skills of persons with arthritis concerning arthritis-related movement limitations.

Marjorie wanted to be able to travel again, with sufficient mobility to enable her to do the things that were especially important to her, including attending musical events and visiting art museums. She identified her deconditioned state, and particularly her limited strength and endurance, as problems she would need to address. In her EDUCIZE class, which met twice weekly, she came to the idea that a personal walking program that could be done every day at home would help with her strength and endurance problems. She measured some distances and identified a space at home in which she could carry out her program. She planned the time of day she would walk, as well as the music she would listen to while walking. She anticipated possible interruptions (e.g., phone calls) and made plans to control them. She considered and discussed with her EDUCIZE instructors, who were allied health professionals, different movements that might be particularly beneficial for her as well as those she would need to take care to avoid, given her rheumatoid arthritis. She projected the number of "laps" she would have to do to achieve a conditioning effect as well as how long it might take before she would be able to complete that number of laps. In advance of initiating her program, she discussed at length and actually tested her walking program in class with the other members of her EDUCIZE group. That process helped her identify possible problems in her plan that she had not anticipated. She created and tried out modifications of her plan in the group, a process which helped her feel more confident that she could carry out her program successfully.

Marjorie did initiate her walking program and did succeed in increasing her strength and endurance. Early in her work, she suffered an unexpected setback. She experienced a bad flare that interrupted her program for 3 weeks and, in effect, necessitated her starting again. But her determination persisted, she did resume, and she was able to achieve some of the things she once thought impossible, including a trip to Europe.

LESSONS FROM MARJORIE

Principles 1 and 2. The first two Deweyan principles illustrated by Marjorie's story are these: (1) "Learning *is* problem solving . . . and problem solving leads to 'intelligent learning'"; and (2) "The impetus for problem solving is a personally experienced problem."

Marjorie's recognition that her deconditioned state was a major obstacle to being able to achieve an important personal goal—the ability to travel once again—illustrates the role that a *personally experienced problem* plays in learning. That recognition set in motion a *problem-solving process*, a process that was self-propelled and led her to find a satisfactory solution to her problem. As she addressed her problem, she searched, she created, she used others as resources, she experimented, she made mistakes, she corrected her mistakes, she tried again, she found ways to overcome unexpected obstacles, and she kept on going until she resolved the situation to her satisfaction. This problem is, according to Dewey, learning, and learning is problem solving. "Only by wrestling with the conditions of [an experienced] problem first hand, seeking and finding his way out, does [the learner] think. . . . If he cannot devise his own solution . . . he will not learn . . . ."

A central premise of Dewey's theory is that all of us have a natural inclination to seek challenging experiences and find ways to work our way through them, to learn by solving problems. Unfortunately, formal education too often interferes. The tendency in education is to neglect direct experience in favor of *acquisition*, to organize learning around questions posed by the teacher or the textbook, to furnish answers and make judgments about whether learning has occurred based on the accuracy with which they are reproduced—these Dewey calls the "evils of education." "We can and do supply ready-made 'ideas' by the thousand; we do not usually take much pains to see that the one learning engages in significant situations where his own activities generate, support, and clinch ideas. . . ." Marjorie's instructors could have provided her with a good, packaged set of information about how to plan, implement, and evaluate a walking program. It is not likely, however, as research in patient education has demonstrated, that it would have prompted her to use it, even if she could, as Dewey says, "recite it with one hundred percent accuracy." It was the problem-solving process, stimulated by not being able to achieve an important personal goal because of her deconditioned state and the deliberate work by her instructors to facilitate that process, that produced for Marjorie "intelligent learning," learning that enabled her to resolve her problem.

What role, then, does information play in learning? When and how should educators provide information that they believe is important? A third Deweyan principle speaks to this issue.

Principle 3. Teachers should, Dewey says, give information or suggestions when ". . . curiosity has created an appetite that seeks to be fed . . . and . . . abstain from giving information when, because of a lack of a questioning attitude, it would burden and dull the sharp edge of the inquiring spirit."

Another look at Marjorie's story illustrates the importance of this idea. Marjorie *did* acquire a lot of information in the course of addressing her problem. She used the knowledge and skills of her group leaders to help her decide what movements would be safe and beneficial for her in her at-home walking program; she used her fellow group members to help her develop her plan, test it, and modify it. What is important to recognize is that she sought and acquired information as she needed it to proceed with her problem-solving process. Her instructors actively supported and guided her efforts by pushing her thinking and challenging her ideas until they were well thought out and ready to test. Her process would have been sidetracked or perhaps even squelched if her instructors had decided at various points to provide information or instruction they thought important before Marjorie perceived she needed it. Learning is inhibited, Dewey says, whenever information is given for its own sake rather than to help the learner along with the process of addressing a personally important problem. *Acquiring* is always secondary to *inquiring*.

Related to the question of when to provide information is the question of what ensures that learners acquire good information and make *good* judgments. Our fourth principle speaks to this issue.

Principle 4. It is important to distinguish between an "educative" and a "non-educative" experience. Both experiences tend to begin with the generation of rough ideas in response to a general problem, e.g., Marjorie's idea to develop a walking program. Teachers who let learners stop there and encourage them to "give their ideas a try" without refining them are promoting a "non-educative" or "mis-educative" experience. For an experience to be "educative," learners must be pushed to develop and refine their thoughts by actively looking into and taking account of ideas and facts that are pertinent to the problem on which they are working. Reading, discussing, observing, and any other methods to ensure that the learner moves toward the development of an informed, well-reasoned idea that is specific enough to test are appropriate. Ideas that are ready for testing, in this sense, have inherent in them questions or hypotheses that will cause the learner to notice what happens when the test is implemented, thus increasing the likelihood that the reasons for failed experiments will be understood well enough to help the learner devise a new strategy. Further, when one's strategy works, one can identify the reasons why, thus resulting in increased power and growth, in learning how to face and meet new experiences with some sense of mastery.

Had Marjorie's instructors simply encouraged her to go ahead and "give her walking program a try," they would have been promoting a "non-educative" experience, an experience that might have been momentarily fun or even exciting but one that would not have led to genuine insight or learning. What made Marjorie's experience an "educative" one was that she was pushed in the group to refine her thoughts, take into account known information about safe and unsafe movements for persons with rheumatoid arthritis, anticipate possible problems or distractions that might interfere with her program, pilot test her plans, notice the results, and refine her plans further. As part of her thorough preparation, she had been helped by her instructors to anticipate the possibility of a flare and learned that if it occurred, it was not likely to be related to her program. When it did occur, her program was interrupted only temporarily. Had she not been helped to prepare thoroughly and anticipate, she might have drawn the erroneous conclusion that her flare was associated with her program, abandoned it, and never realized the gains from her efforts that she eventually did.

It is the deliberate organization and facilitation by teachers of repeated educative experiences that are diverse in nature and complexity that ensures students' acquisition and use of the best available knowledge and skills, and of good judgments along the way.

A final principle concerns the kinds of attitudes Dewey says teachers must exhibit in order to promote genuine learning.

Principle 5. The teacher must model certain attitudes in order to foster genuine learning. In *Democracy and Education*, Dewey writes:

> The alternative to furnishing ready-made subject matter and listening to the accuracy with which it is reproduced is . . . participation, sharing, in an activity. In such shared activity, the teacher is a learner, and the learner is, without knowing it, a teacher . . . and upon the whole, the less consciousness there is, on either side, of either giving or receiving instruction, the better.

In addition, teachers must be "students of education," that is, like their learners, they too must be active problem solvers who develop and test well-reasoned strategies to address the educational problems or challenges they face. Finally, teachers must themselves possess and cultivate in their students certain attitudes: open-mindedness, intellectual self-confidence, willingness to postpone judgment, willingness to test one's beliefs, valuation of knowledge and thinking, demand for closure, and desire for intellectual consistency.

THE POTENTIAL OF DEWEYAN THEORY FOR ARTHRITIS PATIENT EDUCATION

It would be presumptuous to suggest that the ideas discussed above constitute a thorough representation of Dewey's educational ideas. They do reflect five central and interrelated Deweyan concepts, however, and hence can be considered a coherent set of theory-based guidelines for educational programs.

There are compelling reasons to investigate further the efficacy of Deweyan theory for arthritis patient education. It is the most developed theory that speaks directly to the goal that most arthritis patient educators would identify as their overriding goal, regardless of the specific focus of a particular program. Most of us would agree that we *intend* that our patients leave our programs as better problem solvers who are both more committed and able to address their arthritis-related problems in reasoned, informed ways. Dewey provides specific direction concerning both facilitative and nonfacilitative educational strategies for development of a learner's problem-solving skills.

Further, there is both anecdotal and empirical evidence that suggests the power of Dewey's ideas for arthritis patient education. Marjorie's story is not an isolated example. Others have achieved seemingly near-impossible feats in their EDUCIZE programs. An elderly (70s) man with severely limited neck, shoulder, and hip mobility due to his Class III rheumatoid arthritis was able to resume swimming, a lifelong passion, after many months of developing and testing various ways to manage his movement limitations in the water.

A woman in her 30s with rheumatoid arthritis who had not been able to skate for more than 5 years figured out safe and effective ways to do so. An elderly woman severely limited by her rheumatoid arthritis had wanted for years to find a way to clean the lower shelves and drawers of her refrigerator and did so. A woman in her 60s with osteoarthritis who had not been able even to go shopping for several years found a way to take a trip abroad. A woman with rheumatoid arthritis who had been unable to work at all or to travel even short distances returned to a job that involved international travel. A middle-aged woman with rheumatoid arthritis that seriously affected her wrists, hands, ankles, and feet was able to repeat an event that had had great meaning to her earlier in life—a climb up the falls at Ocho Rios in Jamaica.

Empirically, the initial EDUCIZE study (Perlman, et al., 1990) showed significant effects on disease status as well as physical and psychologic function. While certainly the vigorous exercise component of the program was a centrally important factor, there were some results not typical of exercise programs that make it reasonable to infer that the problem-solving emphasis enhanced program effects. For example, a subset of the study sample reported significant improvement on four of five quality of life indices that one would expect particularly the problem-solving focus to effect. Subjects said they were doing better overall, were less hampered by their arthritis, and were both better able and more determined to carry on activities important to them despite the fact that their arthritis discomfort, while lessened, did not change significantly. Also, though other research has indicated that older adults tend to experience physiologic but not psychologic benefits from exercise (Blumenthal, Schocken, Needels, & Hindle, 1982), older adults in this study experienced both. Additionally, only 19 percent of those who began the four-month, 32-session program withdrew, in sharp contrast to the 50 percent that would be more typical of exercise programs (Oldridge, 1984; Shephard, Berridge, & Montelpare, 1987). Finally, attendance, which tends to be sporadic in exercise programs, was excellent for this program. Seventy-seven percent of those who completed the program attended at least 75 percent of the 32 two-hour sessions. A later, controlled study involving 117 experimental subjects representing various types of arthritis and 105 volunteer control subjects showed results similar to those found in the first EDUCIZE study (Connell & Sinacore, in preparation).

It is interesting to consider other effective patient education programs from the standpoint of Deweyan theory. Lorig's revised ASMP, for example, which includes specific strategies to enhance participants' self-efficacy for pain management, physical functioning, and controlling other arthritis symptoms such as fatigue and depression, produced greater increases in health status than did the original ASMP (Lorig & Gonzales, 1992). If one examines the self-efficacy training reported by Lorig, it is clear that key elements of it are consistent with Deweyan theory. Skills mastery, for example, occurs by having participants contract to pursue self-management behaviors *they* want to accomplish, *not* behaviors suggested by others. To the extent that the self-management behaviors on which participants choose to work are chosen as a means of addressing a problem they consider important to resolve, this strategy is consistent with Dewey's ideas; it is facilitating participants' involvement in testing ways to address a problem important to them. Similarly, having patients establish success criteria for themselves so that they can monitor their own progress and make adjustments in their efforts is compatible with Dewey's ideas.

A program developed by Maisiak, Koplon, and Heck (1990) found that education and skills training by telephone improved patients' health status. Although the program almost certainly was not designed with Deweyan principles in mind, it nevertheless was based on Dewey's foundational principle. Users of the telephone service initiated the educational process; they called because they felt they needed some information or help. From a Deweyan perspective, this fact would explain the positive impact of the program. Following Dewey's ideas, program effects would likely have been even greater if those who provided information to the callers had been trained to facilitate deliberately a problem-solving process that would help callers develop ways to test and evaluate the potential usefulness of information they received.

The work of theorists and researchers in higher and medical education also has supported the Deweyan principles discussed in this chapter. Dillon (1968) and Ward and Tikunoff (1976), for example, suggest that teachers are likely to *inhibit* student thought if they ask questions designed to "lead" a student to see a point that the teacher believes is important. Instead, they should tune in to problems with which the student is struggling and ask questions that will help the student find his or her own answers. There has been considerable attention given to whether organizing instruction to enable learners to work on problems important to them influences both retention and effective use of information. Coppola and Gonnella (1968) found that the clinical clerks on a surgical rotation relied too heavily on routine and habit in dealing with medical problems and lacked any sense of the tentativeness of medical decisions. Determined to make learning an active process, they organized groups of students to explore problems they had experienced on the ward. They provided, in advance of the meetings, a host of resources (often conflicting, and including patients) and then participated as colleagues in the group. They found that students struggled with all sorts of ideas and views and increased their store of information (as well as their critical thinking skills) *because* they needed the information in order to resolve their problems. Gruber and Weitman (1962) conducted a number of studies of self-directed learning. They found, in a variety of subject areas, that students who faced real problems (e.g., engineering students facing engineering problems) struggled with them after brief instruction on some basic principles, received information from tutors only when they were stumped and could not proceed without it, and acquired more information and retained it longer than students who received traditional instruction. Inui (1976) worked with physicians on specific patient compliance problems and found that individualized tutoring that helped physicians "experiment" to enhance compliance was successful. Griffen (1983) improved the competencies of primary care physicians in rheumatology using tutorials and small group work that concentrated on individual physician problems in diagnosis. He concluded that significant changes in behavior occur when "teaching and learning . . . are aimed directly at areas in which learners recognize and work on their own difficulties or needs."

Connell and Alberti (1973), Connell, Alberti and Piotrowski (1977), and Monahan and Connell (1982) demonstrated the efficacy of Deweyan theory in health professions and higher education. They were able to train faculty to increase teaching behaviors compatible with Dewey's ideas and reduce incompatible behaviors. They found that as faculty behavior became more compatible with Deweyan principles, students' inquiry behavior increased. Recent work by Irby (1992) on the instructional reasoning and actions of distinguished clinical teachers in internal medicine confirms the role of experimentation (improvisation) and reflection in effective teaching, both key Deweyan ideas.

The use of a well-developed theory as a framework for planning, implementing, and evaluating patient education interventions offers important advantages. Prospectively, as illustrated by EDUCIZE, sound theory can help program planners ensure that decisions concerning program components and processes are logically connected and compatible with program goals. It also can provide a template against which those who implement programs can make reasoned rather than random instructional judgments as they pursue achievement of program goals. Retrospectively, theory can help program evaluators understand and interpret program effects, both expected and unexpected. If a program is intentionally organized to reflect the essential principles of a particular theory and it produces some or all of what is intended, the program developers can rationally explain their outcomes and develop systematic refinements to move forward with exploring further the potential application of their theoretical notions. If a theory-based program fails to produce expected effects, it can be reviewed systematically for ways in which it may have failed to reflect the theory adequately, or the value of the theory for the program's purposes can be reconsidered.

It is the author's hope that this chapter has stimulated interest in further testing Dewey's ideas in arthritis patient education. The guidelines offered can be used by individual professionals who work one-on-one with their patients as well as by those who plan programs having multiple components to help ensure that their efforts are directed toward better developing patients who are active problem solvers. Long-term study of the effectiveness of such efforts should contribute importantly to our understanding of what it takes for arthritis patient education to produce clinically meaningful and sustainable effects.

REFERENCES

Affleck, G., Urrows, S., Tennen, H., & Higgins, P. (1992). Daily coping with pain from rheumatoid arthritis: Patterns and correlates. *Pain*, *51*, 221–229.

Allegrante, J.P., Kovar, P.A., MacKenzie, C.R., Peterson, M.G.E., & Gutin, B. (1993). A walking education program for patients with osteoarthritis of the knee: Theory and intervention strategies. *Health Education Quarterly*, *20*, 63–81.

Bandura, A. (1977). *Social learning theory*. Englewood Cliffs, NJ: Prentice-Hall.

Bandura, A. (1986). *Social foundations of thought and action: A social cognitive theory*. Englewood Cliffs, NJ: Prentice-Hall.

Blalock, S.J., DeVellis, B.M., Holt, K., & Hahn, P.M. (1993). Coping with rheumatoid arthritis: Is one problem the same as another? *Health Education Quarterly*, *20*, 119–132.

Blumenthal, J.A., Schocken, D.D., Needels, T.L., & Hindle, P. (1982). Psychological and physiological effects of physical conditioning on the elderly. *Journal of Psychosomatic Research*, *26*, 505–510.

Bradley, L.A., Young, L.D., & Anderson, K.O. (1987). Effects of psychological therapy on pain behavior of rheumatoid arthritis patients: Treatment outcome and six-month followup. *Arthritis and Rheumatism*, *30*, 1105–1114.

Connell, K.J. (1992). Arthritis: The aerobics advantage. In *1992 medical and health annual* (pp. 391–394). Chicago: Encyclopedia Britannica, Inc.

Connell, K.J., & Alberti, J.M. (1973). Systematic inquiry and the education of health sciences faculty. In *Report to the faculty from the Center for Educational Development*. Chicago: University of Illinois College of Medicine.

Connell, K.J., Alberti, J.M., & Piotrowski, Z. (1977). What does it take for faculty development to make a difference? *Educational Horizons*, *55*, 138–145.

Connell, K.J., Gecht, M.R., & Conlon-Grosso, P. (1993). Multimedia dissemination of EDUCIZE for arthritis. *Arthritis Care and Research*, *6* (4), S22, S71.

Connell, K.J., & Sinacore, J.M. (1996). Training allied health professionals to conduct EDUCIZE: A controlled study of effects on people with arthritis. In preparation.

Coppola, E.D., & Gonnella, J.S. (1968). A non-directive approach to clinical instruction in medical school. *Journal of the American Medical Association*, *205* (7), 75–79.

Daltroy, L.H., & Liang, M.H. (1993). Arthritis education: Opportunities and state of the art. *Health Education Quarterly*, *20*, 3–16.

DeVellis, R.F., & Blalock, S.J. (1993). Psychological and educational interventions to reduce arthritis disability. *Bailliere's Clinical Rheumatology*, *7*, 397–416.

Dewey, J. (1916). *Democracy and education*. New York: Macmillan.

Dewey, J. (1933). *How we think: A restatement of the relation of reflective thinking to the educative process*. Lexington, MA: DC Heath.

Dillon, J.T. (1968). Using questions to depress student thought. *School Review*, *86*, 50–62.

Griffen, G.A. (1983). Rheumatic disorders: Training for improved care. *Practitioner*, *227*, 1149–1153.

Gruber, H.E., & Weitman, M. (1962). Self-directed study: Experiments in higher education. University of Colorado Behavior Research Laboratory Report #19.

Haynes, R.B., Taylor, D.W., & Sackett, D.L. (1979). *Compliance in health care*. Baltimore: Johns Hopkins University Press.

Inui, T.S. (1976). Improved outcomes in hypertension after physician tutorials: A controlled study. *Annals of Internal Medicine*, *84*, 646–651.

Irby, D. (1992). How attending physicians make instructional decisions when conducting teaching rounds. *Academic Medicine*, *67*, 630–638.

Keefe, F.J., & Van Horn, Y. (1993). Cognitive-behavioral treatment of rheumatoid arthritis pain: Maintaining treatment gains. *Arthritis Care and Research*, *6*, 213–222.

Lorig, K., & Gonzalez, V. (1992). The integration of theory with practice: A 12-year case study. *Health Education Quarterly*, *19*, 355–368.

Lorig, K., Konkol, L., & Gonzalez, V. (1987). Arthritis patient education: A review of the literature. *Patient Education and Counselling*, *10*, 207–252.

Lorig, K., & Laurin, J. (1985). Some notions about the assumptions underlying health education. *Health Education Quarterly*, *12*, 231–243.

Lorig, K., Laurin, J., & Gines, G. (1984). Arthritis self-management: A five-year history of a patient education program. *Nursing Clinics of North America*, *19*, 637–645.

Lorig, K.R., Mazonson, P.D., & Holman, H.R. (1993). Evidence suggesting that health education for self-management in patients with chronic arthritis has sustained health benefits while reducing health care costs. *Arthritis and Rheumatism*, *36*, 439–446.

Lorig, K., Seleznick, M., Lubeck, D., Ung, E., Chastain, R., & Holman, H.R. (1989). The beneficial outcomes of the arthritis self-management course are inadequately explained by behavior change. *Arthritis and Rheumatism*, *32*, 91–95.

Maisiak, R., Koplon, S., & Heck, L.W. (1990). Subsequent behavior of users of an arthritis information telephone service. *Arthritis and Rheumatism*, *33*, 212–218.

Mazzuca, S.A. (1982). Does patient education in chronic disease have therapeutic value? *Journal of Chronic Diseases*, *35*, 521–529.

Monahan, J., & Connell, K.J. (1982). Toward an inquiry atmosphere: An evaluation of the tutor experiment project. In *Report to the Council of West Suburban College Deans*. Chicago: Institute for Inquiry in Education, Inc.

Oldridge, N.B. (1984). Adherence to adult exercise fitness programs. In Matarazzo, J.D., Miller, N.E., Weiss, S.M., & Herd, J.A. (Eds.), *Behavioral health: A handbook of health enhancement and disease prevention*. New York: John Wiley & Sons.

O'Leary, A., Shoor, S., Lorig, K., & Holman, H.R. (1988). A cognitive-behavioral treatment for rheumatoid arthritis. *Health Psychology*, *7*, 527–544.

Parker, J., McRae, C., Smarr, K., Beck, N., Frank, R., Anderson, S., & Walker, S. (1988). Coping strategies in rheumatoid arthritis. *Journal of Rheumatology*, *15*, 1376–1383.

Perlman, S.G., Connell, K.J., Clark, A., Robinson, M.S., Conlon, P., Gecht, M., Caldron, P., & Sinacore, J.M. (1990). Dance-based aerobic exercise for rheumatoid arthritis. *Arthritis Care and Research*, *3*, 29–35.

Potts, M., & Brandt, K.D. (1983). Analysis of education support groups for patients with rheumatoid arthritis. *Patient Counselling and Health Education*, *4*, 161–166.

Schiaffino, K.M., Revenson, T.A., & Gibofsky, A. (1991). Assessing the impact of self-efficacy beliefs on adaptation to rheumatoid arthritis. *Arthritis Care and Research*, *4*, 150–157.

Shephard, R.J., Berridge, M., & Montelpare, W. (1987). Exercise compliance of elderly volunteers. *Journal of Sports Medicine*, *27*, 410–418.

Ward, B.A., & Tikunoff, W.J. (1976). The effective teacher education problem: Applications of selected research results and methodology to teaching. *Journal of Teacher Education*, *27*, 48–52.

CHAPTER 17

Vocational Rehabilitation for Persons with Rheumatoid Arthritis

Lynn Westerman Kirkbride, MS, and Caroline Ross, ScD

The vocational rehabilitation needs of persons with rheumatoid arthritis (RA) are overlooked in many treatment programs. One reason may be the subtle nature of work limitation and loss for such persons. Because the onset of RA usually occurs well into adulthood, many persons who suffer from this disease are diagnosed after career choices have been made, so the need for vocational services may not be apparent. Although the immediate effect of diagnosis on the individual's employment may be limited, the course of arthritis is slow and insidious and, over time, may impose subtle but pervasive limitations on the individual's ability to perform job tasks, work the necessary hours, or even get to work on time. Ultimately, these effects may limit promotions or earnings on the job or cause the individual to leave the work force. Nonetheless, many individuals are dependent on work emotionally and psychologically as well as to provide for their material well-being. Vocational services can play an integral part in the rehabilitation of persons with RA.

Formal vocational rehabilitation services may include the initial assessment interview, vocational evaluation testing, creation of an individualized written plan, job placement services (job development or job modification), and follow-up services after the individual is employed.

VOCATIONAL EXPERIENCE OF PERSONS WITH RHEUMATOID ARTHRITIS

Early and continuing attention to the vocational rehabilitation needs of the person with arthritis is critical because of RA's extensive impacts on economic and vocational potential. Since 1971 a number of studies have been published that examine the extent of work disability associated with arthritis (Haber, 1971), the cost of arthritis (Burkhauser, Butler, Mitchell, & Pincus, 1986), RA specifically (Stone, 1984), the nature of work disability and work loss associated with arthritis in general (Kramer, Yelin, & Epstein, 1983; Yelin, Henke, & Epstein, 1986), and RA in particular (Meenan, Yelin, Nevitt, & Epstein, 1981; Robinson & Walters, 1979; Yelin, Henke, & Epstein, 1987; Yelin, Meenan, Nevitt, & Epstein, 1980; Yelin, Nevitt, & Epstein, 1980). These studies base their findings on data from several sources: the 1966 and 1978 Social Security Administration, Survey of Disability and Work; the 1976 National Health Interview Survey; and several community samples.

According to Haber (1971), musculoskeletal conditions accounted for 30% of the 17.5 million noninstitutionalized persons aged 18 to 64 who had been disabled (defined as a limitation in the kind or amount of work for more than 6 months). With a disability rate of 53 persons per 1,000, this is the single largest cause of work limitation, followed by cardiovascular and respiratory conditions (43 and 19 per 1,000, respectively).

Musculoskeletal conditions are costly in terms of loss of wages. Burkhauser et al. (1986) estimated that $10.8 billion of lost earnings (in 1978 dollars) were associated with musculoskeletal disease each year. This figure reflects loss due only to arthritis and not due to other premorbid conditions, age, or race. On average, men with arthritis earned 21% less than men without arthritis and women with arthritis earned 15.4% less than women without arthritis. Stone (1984) used an incidence-based approach to estimate the direct and indirect costs of RA. Direct costs included medical care and costs for medication and adaptive equipment. Indirect costs were calculated to reflect the earnings lost during a lifetime for persons with onset of disease during a particular year. Indirect costs or lost earnings were dominant in the total lifetime costs of RA, nearly four times greater than the direct costs.

Several studies have described the nature of work limitation or loss among persons with rheumatoid arthritis. Using a community sample, Yelin, Henke, and Epstein (1987) found that 51% of persons who were working at the time of RA diagnosis were no longer employed 5 years later. Meenan et al. (1981) also estimated that the financial contribution of working individuals with RA to family income decreased from 69% to 32% between the date of disease onset and the study year, on the average a period of 8 years. The basis for this estimate is reduced earning capacity below what would have been expected given onset-year income. Reduced earning capacity may be due to lower earning opportunity on the job as well as wages lost as a result of leaving the work force.

A few factors may contribute either to ability to remain on the job or to work disability—the inability to remain on the job. In general, studies have examined disease, sociodemographic factors, and occupational and workplace factors to understand the reasons why people with arthritis do or do not continue working.

Work disability, defined as cessation of work, is associated with more severe arthritis of longer duration, older age, poor functional status, married status (presence of another wage earner), a lack of commitment to continue work, and characteristics of the job such as physical demands or fewer discretionary activities (Meenan et al, 1981; Yelin, Henke, & Epstein, 1986, 1987; Yelin, Meenan, Nevitt, & Epstein, 1980; Yelin, Nevitt, & Epstein, 1980). While the studies suggest that disease factors such as disease duration influence work disability, their influence is less than might be expected. Contradictory findings between studies on the relationship between the presence of other co-morbidities and work disability can be explained by sample differences: the community samples exclude patients with other major co-morbidities and report little relationship between existing factors and work disability. The Social Security Administration samples also included those persons reporting a positive relationship. The presence of other major diseases probably does influence work disability, although that influence may be less than expected. Sociodemographic factors such as sex, education, and race appear to have no, or sometimes only slight, relationship to work disability.

The most striking agreement across studies is found in the description of factors that are associated with continued employment. Consistent with the findings mentioned, characteristics of the job such as work autonomy, working hours, or the activities of work were consistently associated with continued employment. Self-employment was consistently associated with continued employment (Meenan et al., 1981; Yelin, Henke, & Epstein, 1986, 1987; Yelin, Meenan, Nevitt, & Epstein, 1980; Yelin, Nevitt, & Epstein, 1980). From the perspective of vocational rehabilitation, the most important finding is the relationship between ability to alter the activities of the job and disability. Yelin, Meenan, Nevitt, and Epstein (1980) and Yelin, Nevitt, and Epstein (1980) found that two thirds of those persons whose job activities could not be altered to increase autonomy and flexibility were work disabled. Less than half of those whose job could be altered were work disabled. This relationship was strongest for persons with the more severe forms of RA. Yelin, Meenan, Nevitt, and Epstein (1980) and Yelin, Nevitt, and Epstein (1980) suggested that the nature of RA (and other types of arthritis) with periodic flares and remissions and daily variation in symptoms is particularly incompatible with inflexible work situations.

A study by Robinson and Walters (1979) provides useful insight into the work experience of persons with RA. Interviews were conducted with 50 employed RA patients (unemployed persons were excluded) about their problems with RA and the coping methods they used to continue working. The need for extra time in the morning for medication to reduce morning stiffness or for dressing was commonly described. Major problems were encountered in using public transportation (eg, distance to bus stops, presence of stairs, and difficulty using private cars alone). The need to rest during the workday was commonly reported. Respondents indicated a need for assistance from co-workers or for scheduling more strenuous work early in the day. They expressed interest in their work and concern that they would become more physically disabled if they stopped working.

Based on the literature review, several suggestions can be made to guide the vocational rehabilitation process for persons with RA. First, most adults will have made their career choice before the onset of disease. The role of vocational rehabilitation is to assess whether individuals, with appropriate assistance, can remain in their present jobs or whether new positions in a related field are needed. Vocational intervention will evaluate job restructuring, transferability of skills, education of employers about the needs of the person with musculoskeletal disease, and job accommodation to increase flexibility and autonomy.

The increase in work limitation that leads to job loss may be quite gradual. The person with RA may be overlooked for promotion or salary increase or may need to reduce the number of hours worked. When the individual is employed, however, the need for vocational rehabilitation may not be recognized. Nonetheless, vocational counseling before these negative effects occur may be appropriate and beneficial for the person with RA.

VOCATIONAL REHABILITATION SERVICES AVAILABLE

Role of the Vocational Rehabilitation Professional

Vocational rehabilitation professionals are often called vocational rehabilitation counselors or vocational rehabilitation case managers, or vocational rehabilitation specialists. They are trained to consider the whole person and can lend considerable expertise to the team and to an individual's successful rehabilitation outcome, whether it be a return to a former employer with some modifications, a job with a new employer, or exploration of other options.

Vocational rehabilitation (VR) promotes independence through economic self-sufficiency. Across all impairment groups, the benefit-cost ratio for VR services is estimated at 8:1; for every one dollar spent for vocational services eight dollars are returned in increased lifetime earnings (Bitter, 1979). This significant statistic justifies the need for vocational services for people with RA.

State Vocational Rehabilitation Services

As a result of the progressive legislation started in the early 1900s, a state-federal system of VR exists in each state for the benefit of disabled individuals. These programs have certain uniform mandates such as eligibility criteria for services. The law states that an individual is eligible for service if (1) the individual has a physical or mental disability that constitutes or results in a substantial barrier to employment and (2) the services may be reasonably expected to benefit the individual's employability. Severity of disability does not preclude the rendering of services.

Despite uniform mandates, services do vary from state to state. State-level flexibility occurs because programs are financed by a federal-state matching monies system; through a formula, federal dollars are provided based on state contributions. Therefore, state programs are supported only partially by federal funds and within broad federal mandates states can set specific policies. Federal law mandates that those persons most severely disabled be granted services.

Although state VR systems are unable, by law, to refuse evaluation services to any person with a disabling condition, the financial resources that can be used to provide services beyond evaluation depend on state-level funding of the VR agency. Therefore, the amount of total dollars will determine the quantity of services.

The professional who makes a referral to the local state VR department must understand the services available and give the person with RA a clear idea of what to expect from the state VR agency. This is especially important for the person who may be well into a career and have an income that precludes state services beyond evaluation.

The state VR program can be viewed as a resource for evaluation services regardless of the specific state provisions regarding individual income and eligibility. State programs cannot deny evaluation services. Therefore, if the need for vocational interventions must be assessed and there are no qualified team members available to make the assessment, the state VR agency can do the assessment and make recommendations. The team members then can use the recommendations to assist them in interventions, even if further services are not available.

The state VR process may not be as expedient as one would like. State VR programs have carefully detailed protocols for evaluation, development of vocational plans, and provision of services. The individual must be prepared to cooperate to benefit from the agency's expertise. Coaching about what the state VR program can do for the individual and what to expect during the process will avoid disillusionment. Optimally, the VR specialist or someone from the medical team should become familiar with the system and then act as a liaison between the team and the state agency.

Private Vocational Rehabilitation Services

There is an alternative to the federal-state VR services—the private, for-profit VR vendor. Most often individuals who use these services are involved in workers' compensation cases or have comprehensive private medical insurance policies. Often a comprehensive medical policy can provide financial assistance for returning to work or can provide help determining appropriate job modifications that will accommodate an individual's functional limitations. Insurance carriers have a vested interest in returning a person to employment, finding that claimants stay healthier if they are productive and have substituted the role of "employee" for that of "patient."

EVALUATING VOCATIONAL REHABILITATION POTENTIAL

This section describes the process of evaluating the client and assisting in the identification of career alternatives and goals. The development of a vocational plan for the accomplishment of career goals can take place as a result of the initial assessment or following more formal evaluation. General vocational options are described. This section describes the crucial tasks of working with employers to accomplish vocational goals. These tasks include job analysis, job modification, and job placement.

Initial Assessment

The initial assessment interview begins the VR process. If a VR specialist is not available, these guidelines can be used by any member of the team who possesses skills in interviewing, such as a social worker or a psychologist. The initial assessment lasts from 1 hour to 2 hours and gives the professional the opportunity to get to know the client. During the initial assessment the VR specialist evaluates the following areas: age, sociodemographics, means of transportation, family support, educational background, work history, physical capacity, and adjustment to disability. Some agencies and organizations have established assessment interview protocols or formats. One major goal is to determine whether vocational testing would be useful.

At the beginning of the interview, the person's age is recorded. Since many persons with arthritis are older and have made career decisions and worked for years, their age will be a factor in locating new employment. Advanced age will limit opportunities in some respects, and the client and VR specialist should be realistic about this. The VR client will need adequate and dependable transportation for counseling appointments, job interviews, and eventually commuting to a job. Transportation options should be discussed during the interview. When reviewing the individual's financial status, a thorough examination of entitlement should be conducted. For many, the receipt of monthly Social Security Disability or even Supplemental Security Income (SSI) payments and Medicare/Medicaid can be a large disincentive to becoming employed. Individuals may be uncertain of their ability to maintain employment that will provide them with, at minimum, their present level of income and medical coverage.

Another important element in the success of VR intervention is the degree of the client's family support. The vocational rehabilitation specialist will need a sense of the family dynamics that might hinder or facilitate vocational goals. The supportive, encouraging family or spouse can contribute greatly to successful outcome (G.N.Wright, 1980). Close coordination with the team social worker should give the VR specialist insight into potential family-derived incentives or disincentives. An effort should be made to involve the patient's significant others in the planning process, and to gain cooperation and support. Vocational rehabilitation goals are often long-term and will take determination and drive to accomplish.

A crucial factor in determining VR potential is the individual's level of education. The highest level of formal education should be determined. Involvement in vocational training programs, adult education classes, or on-the-job training is also assessed. Clients' attitude toward school, their degree of success in school, the types of courses they enjoyed, and their interest in pursuing further education, if required, to obtain employment are explored. A patient with a strong educational background will have greater options in employability because often knowledge can compensate for physical limitations. The plan for a client with a fifth-grade education will probably require greater creativity than the plan for a client with a higher education level. Also, more motivation may be required to achieve a successful outcome than is needed for a successful plan for a high school graduate. On the other hand, a less educated individual might be content with entry-level employment and lower wages.

Next, a detailed list of previous positions and employers should be compiled. As part of the process, the skills that have been developed and could be applied to other positions are highlighted. Transferability of skills refers to "the process by which similar or related jobs are selected for a worker based upon the transference of previously demonstrated vocational skills" (Sink & Field, 1981, p. 100). An example of transferable skills would be those of an individual who worked in the construction trade as a laborer. He had worked in this capacity for 15 years. With the onset of arthritis, he is unable to meet the physical demands of the former job. A skill that might transfer well would be the ability to read blueprints and determine architectural specifications. This type of skill would transfer to other jobs, such as draftsperson, cost estimator, or technician.

In assessing a work history, patterns can be discerned in an individual's employment. This information can be used to determine the importance of work to clients and their potential behavior. How ingrained is their sense of work ethic? Did they hold jobs for long periods of time? Are there gaps in their history characterized by long stretches of unemployment? Were they often fired or did they mention terminating employment on several occasions because they were unable to get along with supervisors or co-workers? Did they change jobs frequently, stating that they were easily bored? Maybe they held the same position for 25 years. Why? What motivates an individual to work is a crucial question in determining future employment. Clients should be encouraged to formulate a vocational goal and to assist in planning further VR services.

For VR purposes, the physical capacity of the client should be assessed in functional rather than medical or diagnostic terms. The MD, PT, and OT should assist, but the individual's self-perception is crucial when employment is involved. Athelstan and Crewe (1984) recognize the need for this type of functional assessment to assist in determining whether clients can meet the physical demands of a specific job. Observations are useful, but questions should be asked, such as: What is their physical capacity to function in the home environment? How long can they sit, stand, walk? Can they bend, stoop, and perform fine finger movements? How much can they lift? Which are their most affected joints or limbs? How do they experience and perceive pain and thus cope with the variability of their disease? When is their most-reduced level of functioning? For example, do they experience daily morning stiffness or are they most affected by severe heat, humidity, or cold?

Much has been written about the individual's adjustment to disability. Theories such as those proposed by B.A. Wright (1960) can be useful to clinicians assisting persons with RA. The patient's personal response to disability should be explored. This response can vary from denial of the disability's existence to the exaggeration of its consequences, depending on the environmental and social variables and the psychological characteristics of the respondent. Information from the family, social worker, and team psychologist should be able to provide additional information.

Comments that will give clues about the person's level of adjustment should be noted. These attitudes will have an impact on the individual's ability to benefit from VR services. If much of a person's premorbid self-identity was derived from work, motivation to pursue vocational goals should be high.

Once the assessment is completed, a decision needs to be made about the need for further vocational services. The decision is based upon two questions: (1) Does the individual have vocational potential? and (2) Can the individual benefit from further vocational services? When making the decision, the severity of the disease and the client's functional status should be considered. The issue of vocational potential, however, will probably be determined by the individual's interests and motivation and the support available from the family. Patients with a high desire to work might be provided with further services even when there may be doubts about the chances of success.

Vocational Testing

Based on the initial assessment, vocational testing may be required to help in the planning process. If so, the individual's basic achievement levels, aptitudes, and interests as they relate to achieving vocational goals are specially tested. Further assessment of physical capacity may also be included.

Not all individuals will need vocational testing. Data on the nature of work loss in persons with musculoskeletal disease suggest that many persons will be employed in stable positions that they wish to retain and may need limited testing, if any. Candidates for formal testing will be those whose past educational and employment history cannot accommodate their changing physical condition, for example, a dental assistant with RA that has severely affected fine finger dexterity.

There is an extensive variety of assessment instruments on the market. Rather than describing these instruments, the purpose here is to describe the types of information that can be obtained through the assessment of achievement levels, aptitudes, and interests and suggest how this information can be used in the vocational planning process.

Achievement Levels

The assessment of an individual's intelligence (IQ) and general learning ability can be addressed by the team psychologist. Also important is the academic achievement level of a client with arthritis because it will relate to the types of basic skills necessary for employment. The client's reading (both vocabulary and comprehension), math, spelling, and language usage should be assessed.

Aptitudes

Once achievement levels have been analyzed, the VR specialist can determine other appropriate tests. Assessment of aptitudes refers to evaluating an individual's "potential" for performance in the future. It should be distinguished from skills that are actual "demonstrated proficiencies in performance resulting from training or practice" (Schwertzer & Linden 1979, p. 237). Differentiating among intelligence, aptitude, and achievement tests is not easy, and Schwertzer and Linden (1979) point out that people often naively assume that aptitude tests measure innate capacity. Instead, aptitude test data are thought to "predict subsequent performance; they are employed to estimate the extent to which individuals will profit from training or to forecast the level or quality of their achievement in a new situation" (p. 237). Aptitude tests can be helpful predictors of future performance on a job and a useful tool in the assessment process.

One of the most widely accepted and used systems of classification for aptitudes was developed by the United States Department of Labor. The Department of Labor developed a system of classification that has identified nine basic aptitudes essential to work performance. Consequently the General Aptitude Test Battery (GATB) was developed to evaluate these crucial areas. These recognized aptitudes are as follows:

1. General learning ability
2. Verbal aptitude
3. Numerical aptitude
4. Spatial aptitude
5. Form perception
6. Clerical aptitude
7. Motor coordination
8. Finger dexterity
9. Manual dexterity

When more specific information is desired about a person's aptitude in a task (ie, bookkeeping, drafting, filing), a work sample will be more useful. Work samples generally refer to real and simulated samples of work. Pruitt (1977) states that "work sample methods tend to incorporate the realistic aspect of actual work with the time-tested principles of test construction, i.e., standardized procedures for administration and scoring, use of appropriate norm groups, and statistical rigor in estimating validity and reliability" (p. 61). This type of instrument can also give information about the individual's physical tolerance of a particular job task. Some options for job modifications that will accommodate a person's physical limitations and can outline examples of commercial work sample systems include the McCarron and Dial, JEVS, JAP, Tower, and the Valpar systems.

Situation and Simulated Work Assessment

Other helpful evaluation techniques that a VR specialist might use are those of situational or simulated work assessment. Situational assessment can take place in a number of settings, but it is real work and takes place in a legitimate work setting. This could mean that the client's current employer allows the VR specialist to observe, in a systematic way, the patient's ability to perform while actually working on the job. It could also apply to a situation in which an individual works at a workstation located within a sheltered employment setting. Simulated work, on the other hand, "refers to a work setting that has the following characteristics: replication of the tasks and other aspects of a job or work process, control by the evaluator and location within an evaluation facility" (G.N. Wright, 1980, p. 346).

Assessment of Transferable Skills

A formal approach to determine whether a client possesses skills that might transfer to other occupations is a system named the Vocational Diagnosis and Assessment of Residual Employability (VDARE). The job classifications used in this system are based upon the US Government's Department of Labor publication, the *Dictionary of Occupational Titles* (*DOT*). The *DOT* is a compilation of thousands of job titles and short definitions. Alternate titles are described, and titles are cross-referenced (Hoppock, 1976). The VDARE system does not include all occupations listed in the *DOT*. The Department of Labor has classified each job title by educational levels, aptitudes, working conditions, physical capacities, and other categories. The VDARE uses this same classification system and can be a helpful tool in determining alternative employment options.

Assessment of Interests

Finally, an individual's interests should be assessed. Job satisfaction highly correlates with a person's interest in the tasks being performed. Consider, for example, an individual with limited mobility who is interested in law enforcement and desires to become a police officer. Given this individual's physical restrictions and low average of intellectual functioning, this goal is unreasonable. Nevertheless, this interest in law enforcement might be redirected into a more suitable position, such as an emergency dispatcher. This job would capitalize on the client's stated interest while considering the physical and cognitive level of functioning.

While a number of different systems have been developed for classifying jobs by interest (Holland, 1973; Super, 1957), one widely used approach is the data/people/things system upon which the *DOT* is based (Pierce, Cohen, Anthony, Cohen, & Friel, 1980). This system is useful because several of the tests described earlier are also based upon the *DOT*, and the information about achievement and aptitude can be related directly to job choices in the client's area of interest.

Each of the three categories (data, people, and things) is clearly defined. All of the 27,000 jobs included in the *DOT* are coded for their level of involvement with data, people, or things. By using the *DOT* and the data/people/things system the client can explore his or her interest in each category by looking at the definition or by reviewing the types of jobs in categories comparable to his or her interests. Once categories have been identified that reflect the client's interests, then the *DOT* can be used to expand the list of job possibilities.

Formulation of a Vocational Rehabilitation Plan

After the initial assessment and special testing, a formal written plan may be indicated. In the state-federal VR system, this is referred to as the Individualized Written Rehabilitation Plan (IWRP). It summarizes information from vocational assessment, states a vocational goal, and outlines steps to accomplish that goal. The client's input in the creation of a plan gives the individual a sense of ownership. Support for the VR plan from family members is also crucial to help with goal attainment. Examining the whole person is important. Goals and objectives set early are subject to change.

A comprehensive plan will encourage the cooperation of the rest of the rehabilitation team as well. Expertise from other members can enhance this process and safeguard against subjective judgments from the VR specialist. Both long- and short-term goals are key features of a good VR plan. Since the VR process is often lengthy, the patient's efforts and accomplishments should be commended regularly.

Most often the short-term plan will aim toward one of these six long-term goals: (1) continuation with current employer or return to former employer, (2) location of new employment, (3) training options, (4) supported employment, (5) location of suitable volunteer work, or (6) engagement in sheltered employment.

Continuation with Current Employer or Return to Former Employer

A continuation with or return to a current or former employer is always desirable because it will achieve the ultimate VR goal expediently. The employer knows and has formed an established relationship with the employee. Given a past good work record, an employer often has an interest in maintaining the original investment in the development of the employee. They will have a returned "tried and true" employee who is a cost-effective investment for them.

Approaching the employer to discuss the individual's illness and limitations or to seek re-employment should be done carefully using detailed knowledge about the individual's situation. The client's job performance, length of employment, and problem areas should be assessed carefully before the employer is faced. Depending on the circumstances, the client might prefer to negotiate with the employer without the help of the VR specialist. The VR specialist then assumes the role of counselor and discusses with the client how to approach the employer and the possible outcomes.

Often those with arthritis can maintain their present job if a few simple job modifications are made. A job modification is simply a revision or change of the work structure of a given job to make the existing work suitable for the disabled person's functional limitations. Because the clients know their own limitations they often can offer the best solutions. It is important to keep them involved in this process of job modification. The fears and questions the employer has must be addressed to save confusion, misunderstanding, and disillusionment later.

Location of New Employment

Many clients will have skills and a solid work history. Often they are eager to become employed, but still require assistance. Many are unsure about how to present their disease to an employer or how to go about searching for suitable positions. A job placement specialist can be contacted to assist the client and offer leads and coaching throughout the search. A job placement specialist is a VR professional who places individuals in competitive employment. This person has knowledge of the current employment trends and types of positions available in the marketplace.

Before a job placement specialist can begin working with someone, he or she should be considered "job ready." That means that the individual is ready at any time to begin employment. Transportation options have been determined, the individual has marketable skills, and he or she has decided on an appropriate job goal. This person should also be prepared with résumé in hand and possess adequate interviewing skills.

Training Options

Some individuals may not possess any marketable employment skills. Or they might have skills for types of employment that they do not desire or can no longer perform. These reasons might lead someone to choose to enter training or retraining. Training, as referred to here, ranges from the acquisition of a general equivalency diploma (equivalent to a high school diploma) to the completion of graduate studies. In between, there are short-term training programs, on-the-job training options, and junior college programs. Before training, it should be determined that, when training is completed, the client's functional limitations can be reasonably accommodated and he or she will be truly employable afterward. Furthermore, labor market information should be analyzed to ensure that jobs are available in the new area.

Supported Employment

A fairly new movement (1984) in vocational rehabilitation is supported employment (Rusch & Hughes, 1989), which could also work well with individuals with RA. Supported employment places a person in a competitive job in the community and then provides support services that will ensure success on the job. Supports are individualized but usually include job coaching (to help the employee learn the job or to find ways to accommodate for his or her disability) and follow-up services (weekly or monthly contacts by the VR specialist to the employer to help in the transition). The law recently changed to include part-time employment, which many RA individuals need to be able to work and manage their disease. Supported employment, as written by the federal VR system, requires that support for this type of individual be long term. With the ever-changing nature of RA this approach could be very helpful. A job coach could be called in at necessary intervals by the employer when new job tasks are added to the position or if a person's disease is progressing and is limiting in new ways. This is a new and more optimal option than sheltered employment.

Location of Suitable Volunteer Work

One goal of the VR plan might be volunteer work. Someone who has a tenuous medical status and fears loss of financial and medical benefits might find this type of "work" situation appealing. Many have a need to be involved outside the home, and volunteer work can offer this therapeutic outlet as well as the flexibility that many competitive employment positions do not offer.

Engagement in Sheltered Employment

Sheltered or noncompetitive work experiences are the least optimal of vocational goals. The client works in a sheltered workshop facility, usually performing tasks that are paid on a piece-rate basis. The nature of this work is primarily assembly-type tasks; it is geared toward those who are not competitively employable or those who need to develop the necessary work habits for competitive employment. For some with severe RA, this type of goal may be appropriate.

Job Placement Considerations

The VR specialist typically will request the assistance of a job placement specialist, who has a working knowledge of current labor market trends and has established employer relationships. There are different philosophies to the job placement process. The client-centered approach teaches the client how to conduct his or her own job searches with some assistance and guidance. This makes clients independent so that in future searches they can seek their own employment.

A selective placement approach has been suggested by Usdane (1976). A client is preselected for a given job. It involves knowing the worker and the job and matching them. Often those with arthritis need the intervention of a counselor to be successful in the job market. Both of these approaches can work, but the key is knowing the individual's needs and using the most effective method.

Employer attitudes can be the greatest barrier to securing employment. Myths that disabled workers are more likely to be absent or cause medical insurance rates to rise still exist. The placement specialist can help the employer to overcome these misconceptions and fears. With the passage of rehabilitation legislation, specifically the Americans with Disabilities Act (ADA), sections 501 and 503, which set affirmative action guidelines (US Equal Employment Opportunity Commission, 1991) and the hiring of disabled persons by those who work under federal contracts, many employers are requesting assistance for their hiring practices to ensure compliance. The effective placement specialist can prescreen qualified disabled applicants, which will assist in a good job match. When approaching an employer, the placement specialist can also offer the incentive of a tax shelter through the Targeted-Jobs-Tax Credit Programs or in making architectural changes or "reasonable accommodations." There is a federally run Job Accommodations Network (JAN), which is free to employers, to assist with individualized job accommodations. Thus, the involvement of a job placement specialist has clear advantages.

Strategies for assisting the individual to find employment are summarized below.

Job Analysis

Whether returning clients to previous employment or placing them in new employment, a job analysis often will be required. This analysis is done to determine whether the position is appropriate to an individual's level of physical functioning. Job analysis is the systematic examination of what a worker does, why it is done, how it is done, and the skill level needed to perform the task. For an individual with RA, the level of stress, cognitive skills, and the working hours also should be assessed. Because a high amount of stress and fatigue can aggravate RA, these are important considerations.

Although a job analysis does not guarantee successful placement, it can eliminate speculation regarding the client's ability to perform the job. For example, the requirements for a drill press operator of one employer might vary considerably from those of another employer.

Job Modifications

Often, the results of a job analysis will reveal that with "job modifications" a position can be manageable for the client. Job modification alters the workplace or a function of the employee's responsibility to accommodate his or her physical or cognitive limitations. Examples would be lowering shelves for the individual confined to a wheelchair, or possibly purchasing a specialized office chair that provides good back support and the ability to alter one's position to help prevent unnecessary stiffness.

Job restructuring is another approach. Wright states that this involves "examining the relationships among a number of the employers' jobs and rearranging tasks performed to create a position that is suitable" (G.N. Wright, 1980, p. 618). Job restructuring may be simply an understanding between the employer and the employee as to the tasks assigned or the order in which they are completed. If an understanding is reached on these kinds of issues, the employer will know that the employee is not malingering, nor will the employee be viewed as a chronic complainer. Another accommodation is to allow the client to work flexible hours. This is commonly referred to as flex time. Flex time would allow a period of rest during the day that is needed because of fatigue or to cope with morning stiffness associated with RA. Job sharing (making two part-time positions out of one full-time job) might also be considered.

Job restructuring might involve the identification and exchange of a specific task that cannot be performed for one that can be performed. For example, the individual with limited mobility would have difficulty delivering packages to the mailroom; this task could be exchanged for filing with a more mobile employee.

Job carving is the newest approach that might also be beneficial to individuals with RA. Job carving entails approaching the employer with the tasks your client can do, "carving," in a sense, the job to meet his or her capabilities. Often these tasks can be tasks other employees have little time to do, such as filing, typing, or paper shredding. This approach can free up the time of other employees while creating an ideal job for an individual with RA.

Follow-Up Services

Once a client has secured employment, follow-up services are important to ensure job retention. For many who suffer from arthritis, the transition and adjustment to employment can be problematic. For example, it may take someone with RA time to build up the necessary stamina to work the hours the job requires. Having someone to discuss problems with often makes the difference between losing or maintaining the job.

Follow-up services are also important because the functional status of an employee with arthritis changes periodically. The changes are usually gradual, but if the VR specialist or job placement specialist is aware of the situation, longer job retention can be expected. There may be direct contact with the employer at specified intervals or on an as-needed basis.

The Americans with Disabilities Act

July 26, 1990, saw the passage of monumental legislation affecting people with disabilities: The Americans with Disabilities Act, or the ADA. This Act applies to private employers, as well as state and local governments, labor unions, and employment agencies. July 25, 1994, saw the inclusion of employers with 15 or more employees. (The original legislation covered employers with 25 or more employees.)

The ADA basically prohibits discrimination based on disability in all employment practices and covers all "qualified people with disabilities." In keeping with past rehabilitation legislation, an individual with a disability is a person "who has a physical or mental impairment that substantially limits one or more major life activities." A "qualified" person refers to a potential employee "who meets legitimate skill, experience, education, or other requirements of an employment position that he or she holds or seeks, and who can perform the 'essential functions' of the position with or without reasonable accommodation." An employer does not have to give preference to a qualified applicant with a disability over other applicants, but must consider them. A reasonable accommodation is any modification made to the work environment or to assist in the application process that will allow a person with a disability to perform essential job functions.

In the past, there have been many barriers to employment for people with disabilities. The ADA provides civil rights protection to those with disabilities and tries to break down barriers that have imposed staggering costs to society. In the past, society has not received the full benefit from the talents and skills of people with disabilities. The ADA will help overcome these barriers so that rehabilitation can be successful for individuals and society as a whole.

CONCLUSION

Vocational rehabilitation should be an integral part of the rehabilitation of those with arthritis, but it is often overlooked. Many suffering from RA have vocational needs. Attending to these needs will facilitate their rehabilitation program because they will be independent and feel that life still holds meaning and value. People that are fulfilled often stay healthier.

As health care professionals it is imperative to confront our own attitudes toward the vocational potential of this population and use the resources available. If a VR specialist does not exist on staff, a VR specialist consultant should be hired to do this work. Alternatively, resources such as the state VR system and the private, for-profit VR specialist should be used. Other staff professionals can also be involved in the VR process.

Rheumatoid arthritis is challenging to the client and the VR specialist due to its variability. The prognosis that usually accompanies this disease is complicated by uncertainty and ambiguity. However, people with RA who feel productive and worthwhile often have greater success in managing their disease.

REFERENCES

Athelstan, G.T., & Crewe, N.M. (1984). Vocational assessment and management. In *Functional assessment inventory manual* (pp. 163–189). Materials Development Center, Stout Vocational Rehabilitation Institute: University of Wisconsin-Stout.

Bitter, J.A. (1979). *Introduction to rehabilitation*. Saint Louis: Mosby.

Burkhauser, R.V., Butler, J.S., Mitchell, J.M., & Pincus, T. (1986). Effects of arthritis on wage earnings. *Journal of Gerontology*, *41*, 277–281.

Haber, L.D. (1971). Disabling effects of chronic disease and impairment. *Journal of Chronic Diseases*, *24*, 469–487.

Holland, J.L. (1973). *Making vocational choices*. Englewood Cliffs, NJ: Prentice Hall.

Hoppock, R. (1976). *Occupational information* (4th ed.). New York: McGraw-Hill.

Kramer, J.S., Yelin, E.H., & Epstein, W.V. (1983). Social and economic impacts of four musculoskeletal conditions. *Arthritis and Rheumatism*, *26*, 901.

Meenan, R.F., Yelin, E.H., Nevitt, M., & Epstein, W.V. (1981). The impact of chronic disease: A sociomedical profile of rheumatoid arthritis. *Arthritis and Rheumatism*, *24*, 544–549.

Pierce, R.M., Cohen, M.R., Anthony, W.A., Cohen, B.F., & Friel, S.T. (1980). *The skills of career counseling*. Psychiatric Rehabilitation Practice Series, Book 4, Baltimore: University Park Press.

Pruitt, W.A. (1977). *Vocational work evaluation*. Menomonie, WI: Walter Pruitt Associates.

Robinson, H.S., & Walters, K. (1979). Patterns of work—Rheumatoid arthritis. *International Rehabilitation Medicine*, *1*, 121–125.

Rusch, F., & Hughes, C. (1989). Overview of supported employment. *Journal of Applied Behavioral Analysis*, *22*, 351–363.

Schwertzer, B., & Linden, J.D. (1979). *Fundamentals of individual appraisal: Assessment techniques for counselors*. Boston: Houghton Mifflin.

Sink, J.M., & Field, T.F. (1981). Vocational assessment planning and jobs. Athens, GA: VDARE Service Bureau.

Stone, C.E. (1984). The lifetime economic costs of rheumatoid arthritis. *Journal of Rheumatology, 11*, 819–827.

Super, D.E. (1957). *The psychology of careers*. New York: Harper & Row.

US Equal Employment Opportunity Commission & US Department of Justice Civil Rights Division. (1991). The *Americans With Disabilities Act Questions and Answers*. Washington, DC: National Institute on Disability and Rehabilitation Research.

Usdane, W.M. (1976). The placement process in the rehabilitation of severely handicapped. *Rehabilitation Literature, 37*, 162–167.

Wright, B.A. (1960). *Physical disability: A pychological approach*. New York: Harper & Row.

Wright, G.N. (1980). *Total rehabilitation*. New York: Little, Brown.

Yelin, E.H., Henke, C., & Epstein, W.V. (1986). Work disability among persons with musculoskeletal conditions. *Arthritis and Rheumatism, 29*, 1322–1333.

Yelin, E.H., Henke, C., & Epstein, W.V. (1987). The work dynamics of the person with rheumatoid arthritis. *Arthritis and Rheumatism, 30*, 507–512.

Yelin, E.H., Meenan, R.F., Nevitt, M., & Epstein, W.V. (1980). Work disability in rheumatoid arthritis: Effects of disease, social, and work factors. *Annals of Internal Medicine, 93*, 551–556.

Yelin, E.H., Nevitt, M., & Epstein, W.V. (1980). Toward an epidemiology of work disability. *Milbank Memorial Fund Quarterly, 58*, 387–415.

SUGGESTED READING

Jacobs, R.P. (1982). *Psychosocial factors that limit the rehabilitation of patients with chronic arthritis*. Final report, Project #R-561982. Washington, DC: National Institute of Handicapped Research, Department of Education.

Leek, J.D., Gershwin, M.E., & Fowler, W.M., Jr. (1986). *Principles of physical medicine and rehabilitation in the musculoskeletal diseases*. Orlando, FL: Grune & Stratton.

McCarty, D.J. (1985). *Arthritis and allied conditions: A textbook of rheumatology* (10th ed.). Philadelphia: Lea & Febiger.

Miller, J.J., Spitz, P.W., Simpson, U., & Williams, G.F. (1982). The social function of young adults who had arthritis in childhood. *Journal of Pediatrics, 100*, 378–382.

Nagy, S.Z. (1976). An epidemiology of disability among adults in the United States. *Milbank Memorial Fund Quarterly, 54*, 439–468.

Tolbert, E.L. (1980). *Counseling for career development* (2nd ed.). Boston: Houghton Mifflin.

CHAPTER 18

Social Supports and Community Resources for Persons with Rheumatoid Arthritis

Mary C. Kozy, LCSW, ACSW

The goal of this chapter is to view the person with rheumatoid arthritis within the context of a social system that includes the individual, family, support systems, and the community. Social supports as well as federal, state, and local community resources can aid the individual and family in coping effectively with the consequences of this chronic disease.

Resources and eligibility requirements vary from place to place and among subgroups within a community. This chapter is an overview of the types of social supports and resources that may be helpful in optimizing the functioning of the person with rheumatoid arthritis. Some barriers to locating and utilizing resources are also identified.

For the purpose of this chapter, working definitions of social supports and community resources are employed. Social supports are those people within the individual's environment who provide emotional or concrete help. They may include family, neighbors, coworkers, peers, friends, or any other significant relationships. Community resources are those formalized or institutionalized agencies and programs that provide services or assistance to a specified clientele.

Although many government, public, and private programs exist, a variety of factors influence securing these resources. Knowledge, attitudes, skills in negotiating systems, and eligibility criteria must be considered.

AN ECOLOGICAL-SOCIAL SYSTEM PERSPECTIVE

A model that synthesizes information from ecology and social systems theory is a helpful framework for understanding the individual within the context of the family and the community (Grief, 1986). A system is made up of component parts, each related to the whole. A change in one part of the system causes change in other parts (Anderson & Carter, 1978). This holistic view identifies the individual as the smallest unit. As the individual relates to other systems (eg, family, church, health care, and school), each component affects and is affected by the complex transactions. A system, whether it is a family or an institution, strives to maintain a steady state. However, because of the constant interaction between systems and parts of systems, this steady state is, in reality, dynamic. Ecology lends the view that there is a delicate balance between living things and their environment (Hartman, 1978). Furthermore, all living things require nurturance and sustenance from the environment and are interdependent.

A case example illustrates the interdependence and interrelatedness of the social system as it attempts to maintain its steady state. A 30-year-old wife and mother of three young children is newly diagnosed with rheumatoid arthritis. Prior to onset of the illness she held a part-time job, contributing to the family income. At home, she fulfilled roles of homemaker, caregiver, nurturer, lover, listener, social planner, and joint decision maker. The system ran smoothly and fairly independently, although there were connections to outside systems such as work, church, and extended family. With the onset of the rheumatoid arthritis, the family system's functioning was thrown into a crisis state. Roles were disturbed. Additionally, the family was forced to look outside the nuclear family for assistance from parents, child care and health care agencies, and counseling services. These outside supports brought additional energy and aid into the system, helping it reestablish its equilibrium. However, since rheumatoid arthritis is a chronic condition and because the family changes and goes through transitions over time, it must continually readapt.

THE FAMILY

The family is the basic social unit of society and can be the best resource to aid the person with arthritis. The family is a natural social system with roles, rules, power structure, and communication patterns (Goldenberg & Goldenberg, 1991). Everyone belongs to at least one family. From a functional standpoint, the family socializes its members. Values are instilled and norms transmitted across generations (Bradshaw, 1993). It provides a mutual-aid network that includes help during time of illness (Leslie, 1967).

For the person with rheumatoid arthritis, the family may supply emotional as well as concrete support. Emotionally, the family listens, nurtures, spends time, and provides intimacy, sense of belonging, and acceptance. Concretely, the family escorts the person to physician appointments, assists with activities of daily living, and may be instrumental in procuring formal community resources. The family through its reciprocal interactions creates a positive dependency of its member. According to Power and Dell Orto (1980), positive dependency is a significant quality for the readaptive disabled person.

Traditionally, the nuclear family consists of two adults living in a socially sanctioned relationship with their minor children; yet, in the United States, only a small percentage of families fit this description (Walsh, 1982). Many alternative family styles are represented in our current culture. These include single-parent families, extended families or kin networks, and those related through marriage or former marriage (eg, in-laws, grandparents, and ex–in-laws). Other alternative family lifestyles include the blended family reconstituted through successive marriages, homosexual relationships, and other communal relationships. Because of these changing trends in family structure, a broader definition of the family as any two or more people who fulfill the functions (roles, rules, values, shared history, sense of belonging, and so forth) of a family is a more accurate definition.

Each family system is unique. In its attempt to establish a functioning system, each family develops distinct roles, relationships, and sets of behaviors. Every family has strengths and weaknesses. The family's ability and willingness to lend adequate aid to the person with arthritis depend on many variables. For example, willingness to provide support may depend on previous interpersonal relationships within the family. If the relationship was conflictual or weak, the commitment might not be strong enough to overcome previous negative feelings. If, on the other hand, prior to the onset of the arthritis, the family socialized frequently with extended family and held warm affectionate feelings toward the person who became ill, the basis for adequate support is already in place.

Family rules and styles of interaction must also be considered. Some families have an open-family system with the free flowing of energy in and out, and interact easily. Other families have a more closed-system perspective, with rules of not sharing personal problems with outsiders. This style may make acceptance of help difficult.

It is essential for the health care professional to consider the family's ability to provide support to its member. Ability to cope and interact with outside systems is influenced by such factors as educational level, learning style, and interpersonal skills. Other existing family problems must be evaluated in assessing the family's available energy for lending support.

Despite problems, the family is still the best resource for a chronically ill member (Bass, 1990). Families provide 80% to 90% of care in the United States (Briar & Kaplan, 1990). Bonds are strong and emotions deep seated. Through counseling and the linkages to concrete services, the family can be strengthened to provide effective support to its member with arthritis. Therefore, the resources that are identified to aid the person with arthritis are also resources that will help maximize family function.

UTILIZING RESOURCES

Use of resources is determined by the individual's attitudes, capacities, and the availability of appropriate resources. Psychological and socioeconomic needs must be met to achieve maximum adjustment (Fineblatt, Anderson, & Gordon, 1986). The person with rheumatoid arthritis may need accessible housing, information about the disease, family counseling, socialization opportunities, problem-solving skills, or help in learning to negotiate systems. Although the needs may be readily apparent to the health care professional, solutions to these problems cannot be imposed upon the individual. Most important are the client's view of the situation, needs identification, and his or her willingness to engage in change (Hollis, 1970).

Attitudes

The individual's and/or family's attitudes play a significant role in accepting help and utilizing resources. Motivation affects the person's acceptance of change or of using a resource. For example, the person experiencing severe pain will seek medical relief. The individual with no money for groceries may apply for food stamps. Attitudes are complex, however, and may not even be at a conscious level. For instance, although a motorized wheelchair may make the person with severely disabling rheumatoid arthritis independent at a community level, the person who views the chair as a symbol of disability and dependence will reject its use. This attitude may be especially prevalent among those with invisible disabilities who fear becoming stigmatized as disabled or sick. To identify resources that will be used by the person with rheumatoid arthritis, it is essential to understand the underlying feelings and attitudes that affect behavior. For example, it would seem logical that a person with severe mobility limitations caused by rheumatoid arthritis would eagerly move from a third-floor walk-up apartment to an accessible apartment specifically designed for persons with disabilities; but if that now-inaccessible apartment has been home to the individual for many years, the combination of familiar surroundings and support from caring neighbors may be too great a price to pay for accessibility.

Another misconception is that if a resource is available and has been found to be helpful for some people, it will be beneficial to all. For example, myriads of educational materials are distributed free by the Arthritis Foundation. This information may be used enthusiastically by someone whose style is to learn through reading, who is at a coping stage where such materials can be useful, and who is receptive to new information. However, for the person who has poor reading skills or who may not be at a level of adjustment to absorb this knowledge, such materials, although obtained, may never be used. Resistance is a major barrier to obtaining and using resources. Since people may not be consciously aware of the resistance factors, and, because they do not wish to appear uncooperative, they may seem to be accepting of the suggested resource or service yet never follow through in obtaining it. This is particularly true for resources for which a high degree of motivation is required or when a significant financial or emotional cost is involved. For instance, counseling is often indicated for the individual or family to enhance coping or to deal with the impact of the arthritis. Even though the client may recognize the need for counseling, these other factors may interfere with engaging in a therapeutic relationship.

The highly motivated person, on the other hand, is able to overcome seemingly impossible obstacles, such as completing lengthy applications for services and patiently dealing with frustrating bureaucracies to acquire the desired resource or service.

Capacities

Everyone has strengths and weaknesses (Cowger, 1994). Some people take an active, assertive approach to life. Others see themselves as victims of fate. People vary in their intelligence level, problem-solving skills, and coping resources. For some, their strengths are their flexibility and openness to change. For others, rigidity and resistance to change are prime characteristics. Families, too, as a social group possess variance in their skills, talents, and personal resources. These individual differences must be considered when attempting to make resource linkages. For example, would the individual be able to appeal a denied Social Security Disability Income decision? Because the ability to find and use resources varies, it is not sufficient to write a name and address of a resource on a piece of paper and expect the person to follow through automatically. Additional information, more explanation, repetition, or time to think and engage in decision making may be required. Some individuals may even need someone to accompany them physically or assist them in accessing the service. The person with rheumatoid arthritis may be more or less open to using help at various points in the disease process or stages of adjustment. During an exacerbation, the individual may be more accepting of intervention. On the other hand, the person in crisis may not have the energy to contact or use services.

Availability

Availability is a major factor in resource linkages. Most people have family, kin, or other significant relationships. Research indicates that if close kin are not available more distant kin or other supportive persons are substituted to provide social support (Goldberg, Cantrow, Kremen, & Lauter, 1986). Influences in our rapidly changing society, however, such as family mobility, higher divorce rates, increasing numbers of women in the work force, and smaller family size, may have negative impact on the availability, frequency, and depth of social support.

Variance in Services

Some resources are national in availability and scope (such as Social Security Disability Income). Others, although national, vary in local programming (such as resources of the Arthritis Foundation). Service delivery systems vary from state to state and community to community in eligibility criteria, population served, and extent and nature of service.

Multiple programs and organizations may be available in urban areas but absent in rural communities; yet rural communities may offer multiservice centers not found in the city. Besides location, transportation may be a major factor in resource access. A service located four blocks from the person's home will be as inaccessible as one 100 miles away if the individual cannot get to the facility because of mobility limitations or transportation barriers.

Eligibility requirements include or exclude identified populations from receiving services. These requirements may change as funding changes or the focus of the agency shifts. Limited funding or quotas often impose restrictions on the numbers of clients served by a given program. Demand for services frequently exceeds supply. For example, waiting lists for accessible subsidized housing in metropolitan areas may exceed 10 years. Increasing demand and scarcer resources are major concerns of social service providers in today's economic and political climate.

NATURAL HELPING NETWORKS

In addition to the nuclear family and extended family, informal support systems are most often turned to for aid. In a study by Burchardt (1985), perceived social support was found to be a contributing factor in quality-of-life ratings of 94 adults with arthritis. Social support networks have been measured in terms of size, density, and ability to provide affection, affirmation, and aid (Lambert & Lambert, 1985). Informal support systems are often turned to because they are familiar, less stigmatizing than seeking help from a formal organization, and more easily accessible. The self-help group has received attention in the literature with conflicting findings of efficacy (Briley, 1986; Shern & Fireman, 1985). Support groups and mutual aid networks offer opportunities to share common concerns with peers, give and receive help, observe role models, gain information, and engage in practical problem solving (Wells, Schacter, Little, Whylie, & Balogh, 1993). Although many of these groups are sponsored by formal agencies (such as the Arthritis Foundation), they tend to emphasize lay leadership and peer support.

Churches and other religious organizations are examples of natural support networks. The clergy is often the first turned to in times of need by those with existing connections to a denomination. Pastoral counseling offers emotional and spiritual help to members. Churches and synagogues may also offer social, recreational, and other support services. Ethnic organizations may provide services for those with strong cultural identification. These groups share common values and culture and are committed to taking care of their own. Some religious and ethnic organizations (such as Catholic Charities, Jewish Family Services, and Asian-American Services) have become formalized into organizations serving the community as a whole.

Neighbors, friends, colleagues, landlords, and other interpersonal connections are sources of informal social support. Because these relationships may not have the depth of commitment or shared history as family, these people may best be relied on for specific types of support. For example, the neighbor may run an errand for the homebound individual. The landlord may bring mail upstairs for the tenant with mobility limitations. The beautician can provide empathetic listening. Individuals may have these informal support networks already in place. If not, building such networks can provide valuable support for the person with arthritis.

GOVERNMENT-FUNDED RESOURCES AND ENTITLEMENTS

Federal, state, and local governments have enacted legislation and social welfare policies to meet the needs of their citizens. Several major programs that may be pertinent to people with rheumatoid arthritis and their families are outlined below.

Social Security

The federal Social Security Act of 1935 created a program to provide income to retired workers, their survivors, and their spouses. A worker may retire at age 62 and receive partial benefits, or wait until age 65 for full benefits. The widow of a worker may receive benefits at age 60.

Social Security Disability Income

Social Security Disability Income (SSDI) became effective nationwide in 1956, to provide income to workers who had paid into the program and became disabled. Eligibility is based on proof of disability and having accumulated a sufficient number of work credits to qualify. The term *disability* is a legal concept (Brown, 1986). The key words from the perspective of the Social Security Administration are that the person's physical or mental impairment prevents him or her from performing any substantial gainful activity and that the impairment is expected to last at least 12 months or result in death. Number of quarters of earned credit required depends on age at onset of the disability. For the person with rheumatoid arthritis the determination of disability is not always clear-cut and many claims initially may be denied. It is crucial that the physician treating the claimant provide adequate documentation, including physical findings and laboratory tests, to substantiate the claim.

Often the applicant must see another physician arranged for by the Social Security Administration for a consultation. If the claim is denied initially, the applicant may file for reconsideration and submit additional documentation. Many claims previously denied are approved at this level. If the claim is denied at reconsideration, an appeal may be filed.

For the eligible disabled worker, there is a 5-month waiting period, with benefits beginning on the sixth month after disability onset. The Social Security Administration has established a 9-month trial work period for SSDI recipients in an attempt to counteract the economic disincentives and psychological anxieties of successful reentry into the work force (Social Security Administration, 1992). Other work incentives include deductions for impairment-related expenses and extension of Medicare benefits.

Family members may draw Social Security benefits from a retired, deceased, or disabled worker. Frequent legislative changes are made to the Social Security Act. Up-to-date information can be obtained by contacting the Social Security Administration.

Although Social Security has been a major source of income for retired and disabled workers and their families, the intent of the program never was to provide a comprehensive pension plan to its recipients. Therefore, many who depend solely on Social Security income struggle because of a lack of adequate financial resources.

Medicare

Medicare is considered to be the most significant piece of federal social legislation for the elderly of the United States (Brody, 1977). Established in 1965, the intent of this federal health insurance program was to protect against the high cost of medical care rather than to provide comprehensive coverage. In fact, Medicare pays less than 50% of the medical costs for those covered under the program. The Social Security Administration encourages Medicare recipients to purchase supplementary insurance. Medicare recipients who have limited income may qualify for additional assistance through state Medicaid programs. Beneficiaries include those covered under the Social Security retirement program and individuals who have been receiving Social Security Disability Income for 2 years. Certain other family members, such as a developmentally disabled child, may receive Medicare benefits through an eligible retired, deceased, or disabled parent.

Medicare hospital insurance (Medicare Part A) is available at no cost for those eligible. A benefit period begins when a Medicare beneficiary enters a hospital. During the first 60 days of this benefit period, all hospital expenses are covered after a deductible is met. After those first 60 days the beneficiary is entitled to 30 co-insurance days. If the hospitalization continues longer, there are 60 lifetime reserve days that may be used once. A new benefit period begins after the individual has been out of the hospital for 60 days.

Although Medicare Part A is available at no cost, Medicare Part B, medical insurance, is a voluntary program in which the individual must enroll. Premiums are deducted from the individual's Social Security check. The medical insurance part of the program pays for a percentage of physician services and other medical expenses incurred outside a hospital. Medicare excludes many medical costs, such as eyeglasses, dental care, hearing aids, and prescription drugs.

Medicare offers limited coverage for skilled nursing facilities and for approved home health care services. The key word is *skilled* and there are strict guidelines for determination of skilled care. Although Medicare meets a proportion of the acute health care needs of its beneficiaries, it does not address the long-term care needs or maintenance health care needs of the elderly, disabled, or chronically ill.

Supplemental Security Income

Supplemental Security Income (SSI), established in 1972, became the first federally standardized, needs-based, income maintenance program for the aged, disabled, and blind in this country. Disability determination is made in the same way as for SSDI. Criteria for determining SSI eligibility are strict and look at income and assets. Supplemental Security Income benefits are not dependent on the person's previous work history. There is no waiting period to begin receiving SSI checks; therefore, it is critical for the potentially eligible recipient to apply as soon as he or she becomes eligible. Payments are modest, with the monthly benefit for an individual in 1994 being $446 and for a couple $669 per month; payments are less if the person is in a shared living situation. Recipients residing in institutions such as nursing homes currently receive a monthly check of $30. Some states supplement benefits to recipients. The SSI recipient is considered categorically needy and may qualify for other financial and social programs such as Medicaid.

Medicaid

Also known as Title XIX, Medicaid was established to fund medical costs for the medically needy. Medicaid is administered by the states, with funding responsibilities shared jointly between federal and state governments. Eligibility criteria and extent of coverage vary from state to state. In general, for those who qualify, coverage is fairly comprehensive. Medicaid usually covers hospitalization, physician charges, laboratory tests, X-rays, supplies, equipment, transportation to medical appointments, home health services, and nursing home care. Prior authorization is often required for hospitalization, equipment, and other medically necessary services. Letters of justification written by physicians are often essential in obtaining services or equipment.

Because of the health care situation in the United States, Medicaid is frequently becoming the first encounter with the public welfare system today for the working poor, the uninsured, persons on Medicare without supplementary insurance, and those whose insurance benefits become depleted.

Other Public Welfare Programs

Aid to Families with Dependent Children (AFDC) provides monthly income and medical benefits to families with minor children. Some states have work incentive or training programs for AFDC families in an attempt to break the welfare cycle and provide opportunities for achieving economic independence.

The food stamp program is a federal program providing monthly stamps specifically designated to be used for food items. A separate food stamp application is required.

General assistance and aid to the medically indigent are offered in some localities to provide minimal monthly subsistence or emergency medical assistance for those with no income or resources and who are ineligible for other programs. Emergency cash assistance may be available for some groups of recipients, but programs vary from state to state.

Applicants for these public welfare programs must have verification of identity (citizenship, age, and residency) as well as proof of financial need. These lengthy and time-consuming applications and procedures may be frustrating and discouraging for those already dealing with physical, emotional, and financial debilitation.

Veterans Administration

The Veterans Administration (VA) is a federal agency available to those who have served in the Armed Forces of the United States and who have an honorable or a general discharge. Proof of service is required to receive services. A regional network of VA Hospitals provides inpatient and outpatient care to those who are eligible. Eligibility criteria for other services, such as pensions, are dependent on the veteran's status (eg, service-connected illness or having served during wartime). Other benefits that may be available to an eligible veteran include limited funding for nursing home placement, home health care services, equipment, and assistance for modifying an automobile. Veterans Administration benefit counselors are available to apprise veterans of their rights. Consumer groups such as the Paralyzed Veterans of America, Disabled American Veterans, and the Blinded Veterans of America are also sources of information and advocacy.

Other State and Local Government Resources

States and local governments may fund a variety of other programs that can benefit the person with rheumatoid arthritis. These may fall under the jurisdiction of the state, county, township, or municipality and sometimes share responsibility across governmental levels. Some potential resources include state, county, or city hospitals that offer medical or psychiatric care; county chronic care facilities or nursing homes; public health departments that operate clinics or home nursing services through the county or city; housing authorities providing accessible or subsidized housing for elderly, disabled, or families; mental health and counseling services offered through local communities; transportation available through regional transportation authorities, townships, or local communities; public or special education schools available through the administration of state, districts, or local communities; and services to senior citizens, including case management, nutrition sites, home-delivered meals, recreational programs, chore housekeeper, or financial energy assistance. Local communities are instrumental in removing architectural barriers such as curbs and enforcing handicapped parking requirements. With the passage of the Americans with Disabilities Act in 1990, public awareness of the needs and rights of citizens with disabilities has increased.

MEDICAL AND HEALTH CARE RESOURCES

A continuum of resources to meet the health care needs of the person with rheumatoid arthritis must be considered. These include the primary care physician, rheumatologist, and other health care specialists found in acute care hospitals, rehabilitation programs, and ambulatory care facilities. Access to health care is a prime concern in the United States today.

Funding for hospital care comes from private insurance, health maintenance organizations, Medicare, Medicaid, and private pay. With the imposition of diagnosis-related groups (DRGs) in 1983 for those covered under Medicare came a heightened awareness of hospital costs. Many hospitals have arrangements with third-party payers such as preferred providers or managed care contracts that impose restrictions on types of service covered and length of stay. Hospital stays have decreased in length, and earlier discharges create new problems in resource acquisition for ensuring continuity of care (Patchner & Watenberg, 1985).

Trends in the insurance industry reflect rapid changes with far-reaching implications for the person with rheumatoid arthritis. Some of the current requirements include prior authorization for service, preadmission screening for hospitalization, mandatory second opinions, and the use of preferred providers. Case management is increasingly being used by insurance plans to oversee the available benefits and conserve resources in the case of catastrophic illness or chronic disease. Rheumatoid arthritis is considered a chronic disease eligible for case management services under many plans.

Obtaining affordable, adequate health insurance is often a problem for those with arthritis. Insurance companies frequently deny insurance to those they label as too great a risk. Legislation adopted in several states provides for comprehensive health insurance plans (CHIPs), enabling the person who has been rejected for insurance to purchase it through a shared risk pool.

Another approach to checking rising health care costs is the trend toward use of ambulatory care services. Patients are treated in outpatient facilities, satellite centers, immediate-care facilities, outpatient therapy centers, and day treatment programs.

The rehabilitation hospital specializes in a unique program of coordinated team care for the person with arthritis (Sculco & Sculco, 1976). The patient and family play an active role in treatment of the disease. The multidisciplinary team of professionals shares its expertise to find solutions that help the patient decrease pain and maximize physical, psychological, and social function (Brattstrom, 1975).

For some individuals whose medical care needs cannot be met in the community, the nursing home is a health care option. These facilities may be referred to as extended care facilities, convalescent homes, or rest homes. Regardless of what they are called, nursing home placement may be the only realistic care alternative for the person whose medical needs are too great or whose social supports are inadequate for management in the community. Nursing homes vary in size, ownership, medical support, and level of care. Level of care is determined by medical needs, cognitive status, and self-care independence. Nursing home stays may be short-term for the person who is recovering from an illness such as a flare-up of arthritis or who is in need of therapy after joint replacement surgery. For others, nursing home placement becomes the permanent living and care arrangement. Costs for long-term care are astronomical. Most families cannot bear this financial burden. Although some private health insurance companies or Medicare may cover the initial cost of a nursing home stay, long-term nursing home arrangements are ultimately financed by the individual or by Medicaid. Long-term care insurance is a new but limited option.

Families often experience great emotional distress around the decision-making process for nursing home placement. Such a decision may create a crisis for the family system's functioning, challenging values and causing guilt feelings to surface. Family financial resources are stressed. Additionally, major role changes occur as a result of the absence of the placed family member.

THE ARTHRITIS FOUNDATION

Founded in 1948, the Arthritis Foundation is a national agency working to find answers to the more than 100 arthritic conditions (Whiebell, 1983). It is a valuable resource for both the health care professional and the person with arthritis. Through the efforts of the Foundation, the public's level of knowledge about arthritis has been raised (Smyth, Freyberg, & McEwen, 1985). Although research is the focus of the organization, other programs are available throughout the chapters, including educational materials, self-help courses, support groups, exercise or aquatics programs, and advocacy. Pamphlets on specific forms of arthritis, management techniques, and coping strategies are available free in single-copy requests. Books are published and sold by the Foundation for both the professional and the lay person. The arthritis self-help course, developed at Stanford University, was adopted by the Foundation in 1981. The self-help course encourages the individual with arthritis to take an active role in his or her health care and arthritis management (Lorig & Fries, 1986).

Another venture of the Arthritis Foundation is to promote aquatics programs. Through cooperative efforts with the YMCA, a network of swim programs tailored to the specific needs of the person with arthritis are available. Certified instructors lead these programs, and pools are maintained at the recommended 83°F water temperature. It is well recognized that for those with severe arthritis, swimming is one of the best all-around exercises (Rodman & Schumacher, 1983). Social benefits occur through interaction with others and participation in an enjoyable activity.

Support groups are offered by many chapters of the Foundation. These provide opportunities for education, social contact, sharing of experiences, and group identification. Other programs and services vary among chapters. They may include physician referral, equipment, and information and referral services provided by trained volunteers. Becoming a volunteer with organizations such as the Arthritis Foundation may be a positive coping strategy for some individuals with arthritis. The Lupus Foundation of America and the Scleroderma Foundation are other agencies providing information and support for specific related rheumatic diseases. Voluntary health agencies play an important role in the provision of services to the chronically ill (Black, Dornan, & Allegrante, 1986).

SENIOR SERVICES

Case Management Units

Coordinated services may be offered through city or county departments on aging, township senior programs, church-affiliated service organizations, or other social service agencies. They provide information and referral as well as case management to ensure continuity of care.

Senior Centers

Senior centers may be operated by local communities, social service agencies, or churches. Many offer nutrition sites, providing a subsidized meal and socialization opportunities. Transportation may be furnished to the center or to medical appointments, shopping centers, and recreational events. Some senior clubs sponsor political caucuses, involving their members in legislative issues. Health promotion classes are often available. Also, social services such as counseling, assistance in locating housing, and help in completing complicated forms may be provided. A few centers also offer legal services. Involvement with the senior center additionally provides opportunities for exposure to other available resources.

Geriatric Assessment Services

Older-adult programs are becoming prevalent in hospitals and social service agencies. These services use a multidisciplinary holistic team approach to evaluating the needs of the elderly and their living situations. Programs recommend medical management or counseling or may coordinate services to optimize the functioning of the geriatric client. A few home health care agencies have developed such specialized programs as well.

Adult Day Care

Day care centers offer a viable alternative for the individual with arthritis who requires supervision or could benefit from increased socialization. Many are open 5 days a week and provide structured activities, meals, and personal care assistance. They may best serve the elderly person who lives with family and whose physical or cognitive impairments require supervision. They may also provide part-time respite care. Fees vary and may be waived for those with limited financial resources. Some centers offer transportation. Adult day care programs may be sponsored by churches, nursing homes, proprietary companies, or social agencies.

Resources for the Active Senior

For the senior whose arthritis does not impose major physical limitations, a wide range of resource options are available for active community participation. Park districts and community colleges are sources of recreation and education. Travel agencies, banks, and other commercial organizations offer seminars and travel opportunities for seniors. The elder hostel program is one example. Volunteer opportunities exist in many settings, such as the Retired Senior Volunteer Program (RSVP), local hospitals, schools, churches, and foster grandparent programs. Organizations created to inform and mobilize the growing senior population include the American Association of Retired Persons (AARP) and the Gray Panthers. Many discount services are available to senior citizens, including reduced fares on public transportation and discounts in restaurants, movies, and sightseeing attractions.

HOMEBOUND SERVICES

There is increased awareness in our society of the importance of providing supports to enable the homebound individual to maintain as much independence as possible within the home setting. Home health care services and home-delivered meals are probably the best known and most used.

Home Health Care Services

Home health care services are an alternative to an extended hospital stay. Their purpose is to assist the recently hospitalized patient in making a smooth transition to home. Comprehensive services may include nursing, physical therapy, occupational therapy, speech pathology, respiratory therapy, social work, and home health aid and laboratory services. For Medicare reimbursement, as well as for many private insurance companies, a person must recently have been discharged from a hospital, have a physician's order, be homebound, and be in need of skilled in-home health care services. Agencies providing this type of service include public health departments, community nursing services, proprietary home health care agencies, or hospital-based home care units. Funding comes from private insurance, health maintenance organizations, Medicare, Medicaid, self-pay, or free care offered by the local community. Third-party reimbursement for these services is limited. Care is viewed as intermittent and time limited. It will usually meet the needs of a person with arthritis who has experienced a temporary flare-up or who has undergone joint replacement surgery and will soon return to independence.

For the person with ongoing maintenance care needs or a chronic condition, costs for home health care may become prohibitive. Many agencies offer several levels of assistance on a private-pay basis. Most individuals choose to look for less expensive help or are forced to go without needed assistance. Some states offer home attendant care for those who physically and financially qualify. The intent of these programs is to keep the person with a severe disability or illness from becoming institutionalized. These alternative care programs are essential for the homebound person with ongoing needs who lives alone or has minimal family support.

Home-Delivered Meals

Home-delivered meals programs are becoming available across the country. They may be provided by a city, township, hospital, or community service organization. Some are subsidized and others are purchased for a fee. Meals are generally delivered 5 days per week, with the homebound person receiving one or two meals each day. Eligibility for this service assumes that the individual can make meal arrangements for other times. The meals may be subscribed to in a short-term arrangement (such as after joint replacement surgery) or a long-term arrangement. Home-delivered meals may be prepared by hospitals, nursing homes, catering services, restaurants, or volunteers. A variety of dietary restrictions can be accommodated. For the homebound isolated person, the contact with the meal deliverer can serve as some social connection and a "check-in" system.

Adjunctive Homebound Services

Some adjunctive medical services, such as dentistry, optometry, and podiatry, are offered as a courtesy by particular medical professions to the homebound. In certain localities formal groups have been formed by the governing medical societies to provide such services for the handicapped, elderly, or otherwise homebound.

Counseling may be offered by some family service agencies, geriatric assessment programs, or private practitioners who are trying to meet the needs of the stay-at-home society (Whitington, 1985). For the person with arthritis, homebound counseling may offer a solution to architectural, transportation, mobility, and fatigue barriers.

Emergency Response Systems

Several types of emergency call systems are being marketed. The individual carries or wears a device that can be depressed in an emergency. This activates a call for help. Some systems, such as Lifeline, are linked directly to a hospital, which can immediately dispatch help. Others automatically dial preprogrammed numbers of the individual's choice. Emergency response systems may be rented monthly or purchased outright.

Assistive Technology

Environmental control technology is expanding rapidly. Individuals with even the most severe mobility limitations can use this assistive technology to dial phones, operate computers, turn lights on and off, open doors, use tape recorders, and control televisions.

Some individuals with arthritis have recently benefited from acquiring service dogs. These trained animals assist with mobility needs such as pulling wheelchairs, picking up dropped items, and opening doors.

Telephone Reassurance and Friendly Visitor Programs

Care call programs may be operated by volunteers who telephone the homebound person. Frequency of contacts vary from daily to weekly. These calls provide social contact and empathy and may identify problems requiring intervention. For the person who lives alone and is isolated socially, this can be a very valuable resource. Some of these programs are run by church-affiliated outreach service organizations or by other volunteer agencies, such as the Red Cross. A growing trend is to make these services available on a fee-for-service basis. Telephone reassurance services can decrease anxiety for family members who are geographically separated from their homebound relative.

Friendly visitors are usually volunteers who come weekly to talk, run errands, write a letter, or just provide companionship. Many of these programs have become formalized and may be provided by church ministries, respite care services, settlement houses, or social service agencies. There is a growing peer-visitor movement, in which individuals with similar conditions provide support and share information. Centers for independent living and disease-specific organizations are resources for locating trained peer visitors.

Additional Homebound Services

An increasing number of services are now accessible through mail order and telephone. Mail-order businesses will deliver clothing, equipment, medication, furniture, or adaptive devices. The use of credit cards and toll-free telephone numbers makes this means of shopping convenient for the person who is homebound. Furthermore, the telephone is a useful tool for the mobility-limited person. Businesses such as grocery stores, pharmacies, dry cleaners, and department stores often accept telephone orders and deliver.

TRANSPORTATION

Transportation is probably the major barrier to accessing community resources for the person with arthritis. Options and their limitations are discussed below.

The Automobile

Many persons with arthritis are able to drive themselves. Some individuals may benefit from vehicle modifications or adaptive driving devices. Driver education specialists can evaluate and make recommendations. Additional mirrors, a built-up key, power locks, or hand controls may make the difference between driving oneself and depending on others. For those with severe disabilities, modified vans with wheelchair lifts may be best.

Handicapped parking placards or license plates are available for those who have difficulty walking long distances. Application is made to the state or local authority, and physician certification is required. Designated handicapped parking spaces are required by law.

With the enactment of the Americans with Disabilities Act (ADA) in 1990, public awareness is increasing regarding community access as it relates to public transportation and the removal of environmental barriers.

Public Transportation

If the person with arthritis can use mass transit, some communities offer reduced-fare cards to seniors or those with physical disabilities. The rider must be certified as a special user. Designated priority seating located near the front of many buses facilitates access. An increasing number of public transit systems are acquiring accessible lift buses. Pain, limited range of motion, joint deformities, or energy limitations of the person with arthritis may be obstacles in accessing mainstream public transportation.

Taxis as an Option

Taking taxicabs may be a viable transportation solution for some individuals with arthritis since standing and waiting for public conveyances are eliminated. If the person has difficulties transferring into or out of the vehicle, however, this may not be an option. Lending physical assistance is at the driver's discretion. Furthermore, the cost of taxi transportation may be prohibitive for many.

Dial-a-Ride and Para-Transit

The Americans with Disabilities Act of 1990 prohibits discrimination in any federally aided transportation program based on impairment (US Congress, 1990). Therefore, para-transit services are offered in some communities to comply with the provision of comparable transportation services to individuals who qualify. These services are often extremely limited and drastically inadequate to meet the transportation needs of individuals who are elderly or disabled. Some communities use a dial-a-ride system whereby the individual calls in to schedule a trip. People with arthritis who wish to use para-transit services must be certified by the transportation authority as functionally limited. Drawbacks to the system include complicated scheduling arrangements, limited geographic areas, and long waiting lists. Because service is only provided curb-to-curb, it does not meet the needs of those who require assistance on stairs at home or at their destination.

Medi-Cars

The use of the medi-car (also known as medi-van) is an expensive solution to the transportation problem. These for-profit businesses have accessible vans and drivers will assist persons up and down stairs. Costs vary but generally include a base rate and standard mile charge with extra charges for services such as assistance on stairs. This expensive alternative limits its use, for most individuals, to essential trips or medical appointments.

Other Carriers

Airplanes are an efficient way for persons with mobility limitations to travel. Individuals with arthritis usually find airline personnel accommodating in providing wheelchair assistance through terminals and early boarding. Amtrak offers some discounts for persons with disabilities. More accessible train cars are becoming available, but assistance at the station is at the discretion of railroad personnel. Greyhound offers a "helping hands" service, allowing a companion of a person with a disability to ride at no charge. Other bus companies offer similar discounts.

It is important to recognize that transportation barriers are attitudinal as well as architectural (Boblitz, 1986). Response to these transportation barriers is highly individual. The person may find the application process too complicated or scheduling too cumbersome. The young person with arthritis may be self-conscious about using transportation designated primarily for the elderly. Acceptance of the use of special services may suggest the existence of a disability the person is not yet psychologically ready to acknowledge.

HOUSING

Locating suitable, affordable, accessible housing has become a major problem for many Americans today.

Federal Housing

The Federal Housing Act of 1956 was the first social legislation to provide public housing for the elderly (Mathiasen, 1977). It was expanded to include the disabled in 1964. Housing programs sponsored by the Department of Housing and Urban Development include public housing and rent-subsidy programs. To qualify for federal subsidized housing, the individual must meet certain income guidelines. Under rent subsidies (commonly referred to as Section 8), the renter pays one third of his or her income and the federal government contributes the remainder to yield the fair market price. Applications for Section 8 certificates are lengthy, and waiting lists are often extremely long.

Local Government Housing Programs

State and local governments may have housing programs for the elderly, disabled, or families. Assistance may be available for low-income or moderate-income households with income guidelines established by the housing authority. Various programs exist for new construction, rehabilitated housing, or other subsidies. In addition to income, other eligibility requirements such as age, family size, and physical status vary from program to program.

Housing for the Elderly

Many innovative programs are being developed for the elderly, some of whom may have special needs secondary to an arthritic condition. Creative alternatives are emerging due to the efforts of commercial developers, social service organizations, church groups, and housing coalitions. Options span the gamut from low-income apartments to luxurious condominiums. Along this continuum are retirement hotels, independent senior apartments, assisted-living arrangements, and home sharing. Living situations may be rental or for purchase. They may be aimed at healthy independent seniors or they may be life care facilities.

Other Alternatives

Architects with expertise in barrier-free design can build housing that will meet the needs of the person with arthritis by incorporating joint protection and energy-conservation features. Companies specializing in home modifications can adapt a living situation to the needs of the individual. For example, elevators, ramps, lowered cabinets, and adaptive doorknobs make the home more accessible. Special-interest groups have founded not-for-profit corporations to build housing that will accommodate special populations. These facilities may be apartments, condominiums, or group living situations or may reflect a transitional independent living philosophy.

Independent Living Centers

Centers for independent living (CIL) are unique programs that provide information and support to persons with disabilities. The creation of the CIL grew out of the 1978 amendments to the Rehabilitation Act of 1973. These amendments encouraged the formation of resource centers to empower persons with disabilities to acquire the information and resources to function independently in the community. There are more than 300 CIL in the United States today. Emphasis is on consumer control. A variety of services are provided to assist the individual. Independent living, peer support, advocacy, and information and referral are core components of all CIL. These centers have been instrumental in promoting the ADA and addressing disability awareness issues. Although impact of these centers on the individual and on the community must be researched further (Budden, Petty, Ray, Nelson, & Couch, 1986), these centers appear to be a valuable resource for the person with arthritis.

COUNSELING RESOURCES

Professional counseling may be an essential resource to aid in handling the emotional stresses or coping difficulties of the person with arthritis. In addition, counseling may be indicated to address issues extraneous to the arthritis, such as marital problems, depression, or loss issues. Substance abuse is an issue for many Americans. In fact, use of drugs or other medications may be more prevalent among persons who are exposed to polypharmacy approaches to treatment. Although more research on the disabled population must be conducted (Greer, 1986), the health care professional treating people with arthritis must be aware that other problems in addition to the arthritis may cause difficulties for them and their families.

Therapists in private practice may be psychiatrists, psychologists, clinical social workers, pastoral counselors, or family therapists. Charges are on a fee-for-service basis with reimbursement sometimes available through insurance. Many counseling agencies operate on a sliding-fee scale to make these services accessible for those with limited finances. Such agencies include community mental health centers and family service agencies. Hospital outpatient departments may also be a source for locating counselors.

OTHER COMMUNITY RESOURCES

Multiservice Agencies

Agencies providing a wide range of services to individuals and families are found in many communities. Some religious-affiliated social service agencies include Catholic Charities, Jewish Family Services, and Lutheran Social Services. They may offer case management, homemaker services, counseling, parenting classes, and outreach services to both children and adults. Multiservice agencies to assist those of certain ethnic backgrounds are often found in areas where there are high concentrations of persons of Spanish,

Greek, Asian, Native American, or African-American heritage. These agencies have the advantage of insight into cultural values and beliefs and may be more acceptable to the client as a source of help.

The Easter Seals Society is another multiservice agency found in many local communities. The center may offer therapy or loan equipment, or sponsor support groups. The American Red Cross is another national organization. Services may include transportation, telephone reassurance, volunteer opportunities, and counseling. Programs vary among local affiliates.

Hot Lines

Most communities have telephone information and referral service available to aid in locating resources. These may be operated by the United Way or sponsored by the city or county. Some 24-hour hot lines are staffed by professionals or trained volunteers to deal with crises or handle emergency situations.

Recreation and Leisure

For the person with arthritis, the use of leisure time presents unique issues. Because of the unpredictable nature of the disease, exacerbations may occur that complicate planning for activities. To overcome this obstacle, people must develop coping strategies of flexibility and contingency planning to compensate successfully for their fluctuating health status. Some communities have developed special outreach programs to meet the needs of the person with arthritis (Rusk, 1965).

Park districts offer a range of activities from crafts to exercise classes. Many persons with arthritis may be able to take advantage of these mainstream programs either with no modifications or with minor accommodations. Special recreation associations offer programs to meet the needs of special populations.

For those who must modify their leisure activities or develop new interests secondary to the limitations of arthritis, many special services exist. For example, the talking book program supplies recorded books to people who cannot read regular print because of a physical or visual disability. Books are distributed free through a nationwide network of cooperating libraries. This same group of print-handicapped persons may also take advantage of one of the 120 radio information services located across the country. Daily newspapers and other current materials are read over special receivers.

For the hobbyist, HandiHams promotes amateur radio for people with disabilities. *Expressions Magazine* encourages disabled writers. There are also organizations to foster interest in art, music, and theater.

Several travel agencies and tour planners specialize in developing tours for persons with mobility limitations. Some individuals with arthritis have found cruise ships especially accommodating to their individual needs. Specially designed outdoor adventure trips, such as those offered by Wilderness Inquiry II, provide a safe yet challenging canoe or dog-sled experience for the person with arthritis.

CONCLUSION

It is the person who has knowledge of community resources and is empowered to use social supports who does best in coping with life's challenges. The health care professional can be a vital source of information in assisting the individual with rheumatoid arthritis to locate and access these resources.

REFERENCES

Anderson, R.E., & Carter, I. (1978). *Human behavior and the social environment: The social systems approach.* New York: Aldine.

Bass, D. (1990). *Caring families: Supports and interventions.* Silver Spring, MD: National Association of Social Workers.

Black, R.B., Dornan, D.H., & Allegrante, J.P. (1986). Challenges in developing health promotion services for the chronically ill. *Social Work in Health Care, 31*, 287–293.

Boblitz, M. (1986). Transportation evaluation, counseling and training. In G.E. Ehrlich (Ed.), *Rehabilitation management of rheumatic conditions* (pp. 206–231). Baltimore: Williams & Wilkins.

Bradshaw, J. (1993). *Bradshaw on the family.* Deerfield Beach, FL: Health Communications.

Brattstrom, M. (1975). Teamwork in the rehabilitation of patients with chronic rheumatic disease. *Annals of Clinical Research, 7*, 230–236.

Briar, C., & Kaplan, C. (1990). *The family caregiving crisis*. Silver Spring, MD: National Association of Social Workers.

Briley, M. (1986). Taking command of your arthritis. *Modern Maturity*, *29*, 41–45.

Brody, E.M. (1977). Aging. In J.B. Turner (Ed.), *Encyclopedia of social work* (pp. 55–78). Washington, DC: National Association of Social Workers.

Brown, J.M. (1986). The role of the lawyer in the rehabilitation process and in disability coverage. In G.E. Ehrlich (Ed.), *Rehabilitation management of rheumatic conditions* (pp. 349–355). Baltimore: Williams & Wilkins.

Budden, J.F., Petty, F., Ray, C., Nelson, C., & Couch, R.W. (1986). Evaluating the impact of independent living centers on consumers and the community. *Journal of Rehabilitation*, *52*, 68–72.

Burchardt, C. (1985). The impact of arthritis on quality of life. *Nursing Research*, *43*, 11–16.

Cowger, C. (1994). Assessing client strengths: Clinical assessment of client empowerment. *Social Work in Health Care*, *39*, 262–268.

Fineblatt, A., Anderson, F.S., & Gordon, W. (1986). Psychosocial and vocational considerations. In J. Leek, E. Gershwin, & W. Fowler, Jr. (Eds.), *Principles of physical medicine and rehabilitation in the musculoskeletal diseases*. Orlando, FL: Grune & Stratton.

Goldberg, G., Cantrow, R., Kremen, E., & Lauter, L. (1986). Spouseless, childless elderly women and their social supports. *Social Work in Health Care*, *31*, 104–112.

Goldenberg, I., & Goldenberg, H. (1991). *Family therapy: An overview* (3rd ed.). Pacific Grove, CA: Brooks/Cole.

Greer, B. (1986). Substance abuse among people with disabilities: A problem of too much accessibility. *Journal of Rehabilitation*, *52*, 34–38.

Grief, J. (1986). Eco-systems perspective. *Social Work in Health Care*, *31*, 225–227.

Hartman, A. (1978, May). Presentation at Social Work Family Course at the Rehabilitation Institute of Chicago, Chicago, IL.

Hollis, F. (1970). The psychosocial approach to the practice of casework. In R.W. Roberts & R.H. Nee (Eds.), *Theories of social casework* (pp. 33–76). Chicago: University of Chicago Press.

Lambert, V., & Lambert, C., Jr. (1985). The relationship between social support and psychological well-being in rheumatoid arthritic women from two ethnic groups. *Health Care for Women International*, *6*, 405–414.

Leslie, G.R. (1967). *The family in social context.* New York: Oxford University Press.

Lorig, K., & Fries, J. (1986). *The arthritis help book.* Reading, MA: Addison-Wesley.

Mathiasen, G. (1977). Housing for special groups. In J.B. Turner (Ed.), *Encyclopedia of social work* (pp. 667–684). Washington, DC: National Association of Social Workers.

Patchner, M.A., & Watenberg, S.H. (1985). Impact of diagnosis related groups on hospital social service departments. *Social Work in Health Care*, *30*, 259–261.

Power, P., & Dell Orto, A. (1980). *Role of the family in the rehabilitation of the physically disabled.* Baltimore: University Park Press.

Rodman, G., & Schumacher, R. (1983). *Primer on the rheumatic diseases*. Atlanta: Arthritis Foundation.

Rusk, R. (1965). Public recreation and the arthritic patient. *American Journal of Occupational Therapy*, *19*, 303–305.

Sculco, C.D., & Sculco, T.P. (1976). Coordinated team approach to one health problem. *International Nursing Review*, *23*(3), 80–83.

Shern, M.A., & Fireman, B. (1985). Stress management and mutual support groups in rheumatoid arthritis. *American Journal of Medicine*, *78*, 771–775.

Smyth, C.J., Freyberg, R.H., & McEwen, C. (1985). *History of rheumatology*. Atlanta: Arthritis Foundation.

Social Security Administration. (1992). *Working while disabled*. Washington, DC: Department of Health and Human Services.

US Congress. (1990). *Public Law 101-346: Americans with Disabilities Act of 1990*. Washington, DC: Library of Congress.

Walsh, F. (1982). *Normal family process*. New York: Guilford Press.

Wells, L., Schacter, B., Little, S., Whylie, B., & Balogh, P. (1993). Enhancing rehabilitation through mutual aid: Outreach to people with recent amputations. *Health and Social Work*, *18*, 221–228.

Whiebell, B. (1983). *Taking charge: Learning to live with arthritis*. Atlanta: Arthritis Foundation.

Whitington, R. (1985). House calls in private practice. *Social Work in Health Care*, *30*, 261–264.

SUGGESTED READING

Blumefield, S. (1986). Psychological and social effects of rheumatoid disease during late life. *Clinical Rheumatology and Practice*, *4*, 5–10.

Booth, G., Goldklang, G., & Roth, H. (1971). Rehabilitation of indigent arthritis patients in the District of Columbia. *Medical Annals of the District of Columbia*, *40*, 304–308.

Brown, T.M., & Scammell, H. (1988). *The road back: Rheumatoid arthritis, its cause and its treatment*. New York: M. Evans.

Campbell, R., & Chenoweth, B. (1981). Health education as a basis for social support. *Gerontologist*, *21*, 619–627.

Fries, J.F. (1986). *Arthritis: A comprehensive guide* (rev. ed.). Reading, MA: Addison-Wesley.

Henkle, S. (1975). Social group work as a treatment modality for hospitalized people with rheumatoid arthritis. *Rehabilitation Literature*, *36*, 334–341.

Hill, R.H., Herstein, A., & Walters, K. (1976). Juvenile rheumatoid arthritis: Follow-up into adulthood—Medical, sexual, and social status. *Canadian Medical Association Journal*, *114*, 790–796.

Kushner, I. (1984). *Understanding arthritis*. New York: Charles Scribner's Sons.

APPENDIX A

Tools for Multidisciplinary Evaluation and Assessment

Exhibit A–1 Occupational Therapy Department Evaluation Plan: Short Form

☐ Initial ☐ Recheck ☐ Discharge

Period Covered From____________To____________ Number of Treatment Days____

Age_______ Sex________ Onset____________________________

Diagnosis ____

Reason for Referral ______________________________________

Patient Name

RIC Number

Physician

Date

☐ Inpatient ☐ Outpatient

Precautions

II PSYCHOLOGICAL A-Adequate for Treatment/Life Style
I-Interferes with Treatment/Life Style

☐ Social Interaction
☐ Knowledge of Disability
☐ Adjustment to Hospital/Home/Discharge Situation

III COGNITION Attention, Memory, Orientation, Safety, Problem Solving

☐ Not an identified deficit area

III SENSORY

☐ Not an identified deficit area
☐ Patient reports no change in status

	Left	Right
Sharp/Dull		
Proprioception		
2 Point/Steriognosis		

Key: N = No Apparent Deficit
P = Partial Deficit
S = Severe Deficit

III PERCEPTUAL—MOTOR Tactile, Motor, Visual

☐ Not an identified deficit area

IV POSTURE/BALANCE/MOBILITY Sitting/Standing

☐ Not an identified deficit area

TOLERANCE/ENDURANCE ☐ Not an identified deficit area

Tolerates _____ min./hour(s) of non-resistive activity in Sit/Stand with _____ rests

Tolerates _____min./hour(s) of resistive activity in Sit/Stand with _____ rests

2-013205-10

IV MOTOR SKILLS Upper Extremity Strength/Active/Passive Range of Motion

☐ Not an identified deficit area

	Clinical Status	Left PROM	Left AROM	Left Strength	Right PROM	Right AROM	Right Strength
SHOULDER	Scapular Elev (trapezius)	■	■		■	■	
	Flexion (ant delt) 0–180						
	Extension (post delt) 0–40						
	Abduction (mid delt)0–180						
	Horiz Abduction (post delt)	■	■		■	■	
	Horiz Abduction (pecs)	■	■		■	■	
	External Rotation 0–80						
	Internal Rotation 0–80						
ELBOW	Flexion 0–150						
	Extension	■	■		■	■	
	Supination 0–80						
	Pronation 0–80						
WRIST	Flexion 0–80						
	Extension 0–70						
FINGERS	Flexion (extrinsics)						
	Extension (extrinsics)						
	Intrinsics	■	■		■	■	

IV HAND FUNCTION ☐ Not an identified deficit area

	LEFT Current Measure	LEFT Previous Measure	LEFT Norm	RIGHT Current Measure	RIGHT Previous Measure	RIGHT Norm
Grasp						
Lateral Pinch						
3 Point Pinch						
Coord. (nine hole test)						

IV USE FUNCTION Quality of Movement, Tone, Pain, Functional Use

☐ Not an identified deficit area

ARM PLACEMENT

	Left	Right
Table Top		
Top of Hand		
Overhead		
Side Reach		
To Feet		
Behind Back		

Key: N = No Apparent Deficit
P = Partial Deficit
S = Severe Deficit

POSITIONING/EQUIPMENT

☐ None required

continues

Exhibit A–1 continued

IV SELF-CARE ACTIVITIES

Key 7 = Independent
6 = Independent with adaptive equipment/modified environment
5 = Independent with set-up/distant supervision
4 = Minimal assistance/intermitent supervision
3 = Moderate assistance/continuous supervision
2 = Maximal assistance
1 = Dependent
0 = Not applicable

ALL CORE ITEMS NOTED WITH BOLD LETTERING MUST BE RATED. If skills vary within component groups, an average rating is used for the core item functional level. If there is ***No goal***, or the patient is already at his/her expected level, rate the goal the same as the functional level. ***Meal preparation, Homemaking, Community Re-integration, and Work Skills*** may be deferred until they can be addressed. On discharge, the date the goal was set shall be noted in the date column.

A = ADMISSION STATUS G = DISCHARGE GOAL CIRCLE = DISCHARGE STATUS R = RECHECK STATUS

	1	2	3	4	5	6	7	
FEEDING								
UPPER EXTREMETY DRESSING								
LOWER EXTREMITY DRESSING								
TOILETING								
GROOMING								
BATHING								
COMMUNICATION								
MEAL PREPARATION DATE								
Basic								
Complex								
HOMEMAKING								
Light Homemaking								
Heavy Homemaking								
COMMUNITY INTEGRATION								

FAMILY INSTRUCTION HOME PROGRAM

Patient/Family Teaching Provided?
☐ Yes ☐ No ☐ NA

Fanily aware of ADL Status
☐ Yes ☐ No ☐ NA

Patient/Family able to safely and successfully assist with/perform:
ADL: ☐ Yes ☐ No ☐ NA
Home Programs: ☐ Yes ☐ No ☐ NA

Home Program/Teaching covered the following areas:

FOLLOW-UP

☐ Recheck in _________Wks/Mos
☐ Outpatient—Frequency _________
☐ RIC ☐ Other
☐ Home Health—Frequency _______ /Wk
☐ Not Indicated

VOC/LEISURE Present/Previous

GENERAL ASSESSMENT/DISCHARGE SUMMARY

XIV PATIENT/FAMILY GOALS:

Goal	Goals for OT Treatment (See ADL Goals Above)	Plan/Outcome

Key LTG = Long Term Goal
STG = Short Term Goal
GG = Group Goal

Therapist Date

Exhibit A–2 Physical Therapy Department Orthopaedic Evaluation Form

Patient Name

RIC Number

☐ Initial Evaluation ☐ Discharge Evaluation

Physician

Treatment Interval ________ to ________ No. of R_x ________

Date

Duration of Treatment ______ to ________ No. of R_x ________

Inpatient Floor ________

Diagnosis: ____________

Precaution: ____________

Reason for Referral: ____________

I. MEDICAL

____

Vitals: Rest Pulse ________ BP ________ Activity ________ Pulse ________ BP ________

Incision/Skin: ____________

IV. FUNCTIONAL SKILLS

LE ROM (Supine) (☐ AROM) (☐ PROM)

	Initial		Discharge	
	L	R	L	R
hip flex				
hip ext				
hip abd				
knee ext				
(sitting) knee flex				

LE Strength

	Initial		Discharge	
	L	R	L	R
hip flexors				
hip extensors				
hip abd				
quadriceps				
hamstrings				
PF/DF				

leg length: ____________

UE ROM: ____________

UE Strength: ____________

Bed Mobility: *Initial:* ____________

Discharge: ____________

Sit—Stand: *Initial:* ____________ *Discharge:* ____________

Transfers

	Assistive Device		Physical Assistance		Equipment Used	
	Initial	Discharge	Initial	Discharge	Initial	Discharge
bed						
toilet						
tub						
car						

Gait: *Initial:* ____________

Discharge: ____________

Sit—Stand: *Initial:* ____________ Ramp/ *Initial:* ____________

Discharge: ____________ Curbs/ *Discharge:* ____________

continues

Exhibit A–2 continued

Exercise Program Treatment Techniques used: ______

Equipment: ______

Additional Comments (e.g., social history, pain, sensation, etc.): ______

TREATMENT/PROGRESS OVER THIS TREATMENT INTERVAL (include classes, pool, modalities, home visit, family instruction):

Discharge: ______

INTERPRETATION/GENERAL ASSESSMENT:

Initial: ______

Discharge: ______

GOALS

GOAL—SET A DISCHARGE GOAL AT ADMISSION. If there is no goal, or the patient is already at his/her expected level, rate the goal the same as the functional level.

PLEASE DO NOT LEAVE BLANK.

Circle Functional Level		ADMISSION	Goal		DISCHARGE
Date ⇒					
Initials ⇒					
Bed Mobility		1 2 3 4 5 6 7			1 2 3 4 5 6 7
*W/C Propulsion	0	1 2 3 4 5 6 7		0	1 2 3 4 5 6 7
Bed Transfer		1 2 3 4 5 6 7			1 2 3 4 5 6 7
Toilet Transfer		1 2 3 4 5 6 7			1 2 3 4 5 6 7
Tub/Shower Transfer		1 2 3 4 5 6 7			1 2 3 4 5 6 7
Car Transfer		1 2 3 4 5 6 7			1 2 3 4 5 6 7
**Ambulation		1 2 3 4 5 6 7			1 2 3 4 5 6 7
***Stair Climbing		1 2 3 4 5 6 7			1 2 3 4 5 6 7

Patient/family (circle) has participated in goal setting? Yes____ No____

If no, why not? ______

Indicate by checkmark (√) if it is a short or long term goal

Long Term	Short Term	

PLAN (Treatment frequency, techniques, discharge follow-up care):

Initial: ______

Discharge: ______

Discharge Destination: ______

______ Initial Therapist Date

______ D/C Therapist Date

Exhibit A–3 Vocational Rehabilitation Department Administrative Policy

SUBJECT: Vocational Evaluation	DATE:
TITLE: Patient Initial Assessment	Dept. Head Approval:

It is the policy of the Department that the VRS will be responsible for patient intake. The purpose of the initial assessment is to determine the patient's readiness for the vocational rehabilitation services in the Department at the time of referral.

The initial assessment will consider the following areas: education history, employment history, medical/functional history, current status and tentative functional prognosis, financial status, and level of family support.

Specific areas to be addressed:

Education History:	level completed, current academic functioning, its relationship to work/training
Employment History:	degree of physical requirement at work; consistency of employment; skill level at work; relationships with co-workers, management, and unions
Medical/Functional:	time since onset and circumstances, current medical complications (if any), cognition, competence in managing affairs, memory, substance abuse, physical return potential
Financial:	status of benefits, financial resources available, degree of comfort with financial status
Behavior:	expressed motivation for vocational services, cooperation, past history with vocational rehabilitation services
Psychosocial:	family, peer support, physical, financial, emotional

The observation and interpretation sections of the Initial Plan have to support clearly the recommendations made regarding the patient's ability to benefit from vocational services at that time.

Exhibit A–4 Vocational Rehabilitation Department Initial Assessment Form

Name: ______________________________
RIC #: ______________________________
Physician: ___________________________
Inpatient _________Outpatient _________
Date: _______________________________

I. OBSERVATION V.O. Vocational Training

Gender: Male _________ Female _________

Birth Date: ____/____/____ Age: _________

Ethnic Background:

Black ____ Hispanic ____ White ____

Native American ____ Asian ____

Other __________

Diagnosis: ____

Referred by: ____

Reason for Referral:____

MEDICAL HISTORY:

Onset Date: ____/____/____

Circumstances:____

Past/Present Treatment:____

____

____

Future Treatment: ____

____

____

Medications: ____

Allergies: ____________________________________ Seizure: ___________________

Other Medical Conditions: Pain _____________ Coma _____________ Length _____________

High Blood Pressure _____________

Other:____

____

Medical Records Reviewed: ____

____

continues

Exhibit A–4 continued

CURRENT ACTIVITIES:

Arrived on time for Interview? Yes ____ No ____

Accompanied by Spouse/Family member/Friend? Yes ____ No ____

Persons in Attendance: ____________________

Relationship: ____________________

List Daily Activities: ____________________

____

____

EDUCATIONAL HISTORY:

Highest Grade Completed: ____________ G.E.D. Yes ___ No ____

Dates ____/____ to ____/____

High School: ____________________

College: ____________________ Dates ____/____ to ____/____

Major(s) ____________________

Trade / Tech: ____________________

Favorite Subjects: ____________________

Difficult Subjects: ____________________

Veteran: Yes ____ No ____ Branch (if yes) ____________________

Rank: ____________________ Type of Discharge: ____________________

Discharge Date ____/____/____

Military Training: ____________________

WORK HISTORY:

Job Title: ____________________Pay: ____________________

Employer: ____________________

Dates: ____/____/____ to ____/____/____

Job Duties: ____________________

____

____

Reason for Leaving: ____________________

Liked Job? Yes ____ No ____ Hours worked per week: _____

Other: ____________________

____

____

continues

Exhibit A–4 continued

Job Title: ______________________________ Pay: __________

Employer: ______________________________

Dates: ____/____/____ to ____/____/____

Job Duties: ______________________________

____

____

Reason for Leaving: ______________________________

Liked Job? Yes ____ No ____ Hours worked per week: _____

Other: ______________________________

____

____

PSYCHOSOCIAL INFORMATION:

Marital Status: Single ____ Married ____ Separated ____

Divorced ____ Widowed ____

Spouse Works? Yes ____ No ____

Number of Children: ____ Ages: ______________________________

Living Arrangements: ______________________________

Mobility: Walks Independently ____ Battery-Operated Cart ____

Crutches/Walker/Cane ____ Confined to Bed ____

Standard Wheelchair ____ Electric Wheelchair ____

Other: ______________________________

ADLs: Independent ____ Requires Assistance ____

Attendant Care: ______________________________

____

____

Hobbies: ______________________________

____

____

Smokes: Yes ____ No ____ Quantity ______________

Alcohol: Yes ____ No ____ History ____ Current Treatment ____

Drugs: Yes ____ No ____ History ____ Current Treatment ____

continues

Exhibit A–4 continued

Current Sources of Income and Support:

No Source of Income	____	Supplemental Security Inc.	____
Self-Employment Income	____	Veterans Benefits	____
Savings	____	Unemployment Comp	____
Workers' Comp Benefits	____	Pension / Retirement Fund	____
Litigation Settlement	____	Soc. Sec. Disability Ins.	____

Public Assistance or Aid to Families with Dependent Children ____

Other ____________________

Litigation: Yes ____ No ____ If Yes: W/C ____ PI ____ Victim ____

Arrest Record: Yes ____ No ____ If Yes: ____________________

____

Transportation:

Valid Driver's License:	Yes ____	No ____
Available Car:	Yes ____	No ____
Medically Released to Drive:	Yes ____	No ____
Public Transportation:	Yes ____	No ____
Special Transportation Services:	Yes ____	No ____

Patient's stated current vocational/educational goals: ____________________

____

____

____

Barriers to Vocational Activities Identified by Patient: ____________________

____

____

____

Strengths / Skills for Vocational Activities Identified by Patient: ____________________

____

____

____

INTERPRETATION:

Patient's Presentation/Communication Style during Interview:

____

____

____

____

continues

Exhibit A–4 continued

Motivation to Return to Work/School: ______________________________

____

____

____

____

Positive Indicators for Vocational Outcomes: ______________________________

____

____

____

Negative Indicators for Vocational Outcomes: ______________________________

____

____

____

____

Patient's Awareness of Deficits for Vocational Planning: ______________________________

____

____

____

____

Patient's Readiness to Engage in Vocational Rehabilitation Activities: ______________________________

____

____

____

Initial Impression of Vocational Potential: ______________________________

____

____

____

____

Long-Term Goal for Further Vocational Rehabilitation Training: ______________________________

____

PLAN:

1. ______________________________
2. ______________________________
3. ______________________________

______________________________ M.S., CRC ____/____/____

Vocational Rehabilitation Specialist (Date)

Exhibit A–5 Social Work Department Short Initial Evaluation Form

Patient Name ______________________

Date of Admission ______________ Date of Initial Contact ______________ RIC NO. ______________

PHYSICIAN ______________

INITIAL EVALUATION

I. Psychosocial Information:

A. Presenting Medical Information ______________

B. Family Involvement & Living Arrangements ______________

C. Patient/Family Understanding of Goals ______________

D. Patient/Family Coping/Adaption ______________

E. Education/Employment Background ______________

F. Financial Status ______________

G. Tentative Discharge Plan ______________

II. Psychosocial Assessment:

____

III. Treatment Plan:

1. ______________
2. ______________
3. ______________
4. ______________

Name & Title ______________ Date ______________

Exhibit A–6 Social Work Department Short Discharge Summary Form

Patient Name ____________________
RIC NO. ____________________
Physician ____________________
Admission Date __________ Discharge Date __________

I. Discharge Destination: ____________________

____

Primary Caregiver/Contact ____________________
Current Address ____________________ Zip Code __________
Phone Number (_____) ____________________

II. Social Work Intervention(s) During Stay:

A. Resource(s) (include status)

1. Financial Entitlements
   a. Social Security ____________________
   ____
   b. Insurance ____________________
   c. Other ____________________
2. Home Services
   a. Department of Rehab Services/Department of Aging ____________________
   Contact Person ____________________ Telephone Number (_____) __________
   ____
   ____
   b. Community Agency ____________________
3. Transportation ____________________
4. Home Health Agency ____________________
5. Outpatient Therapies ____________________
6. Other Referrals ____________________

B. Psychosocial Summary ____________________

____

____

____

____

____

____

____

____

____

____

____

____

____

Name & Title ____________________ Date __________

Exhibit A–7 Social Work Department Initial Evaluation Form

NAME ______________________

RIC NO. ______________________

ADMISSION DATE ______________________

INITIAL CONTACT/ DATE OF INTERVIEW ______________________

PHYSICIAN ______________________

I. IDENTIFYING INFORMATION

II. PSYCHOSOCIAL OBSERVATIONS

A. FAMILY CONSTELLATION AND INVOLVEMENT

B. FAMILY & PATIENT PERCEPTIONS—DIAGNOSIS, PROGNOSIS, GOALS

continues

Exhibit A–7 continued

C. FINANCIAL ENTITLEMENTS

SOCIAL SECURITY ____________________

MEDICARE ____________________

MEDICAID/PUBLIC AID ____________________

OTHER ____________________

D. COMMUNITY AGENCY(S) INVOLVEMENT

HEALTH CARE/SOCIAL SERVICE ____________________

EMPLOYMENT/SCHOOL ____________________

OTHER ____________________

E. TENTATIVE PLANNING

OWN HOME ____________________

WITH OTHERS ____________________

INSTITUTIONAL CARE ____________________

III. PSYCHOSOCIAL ASSESSMENT

IV. GOAL

V. PLAN

Exhibit A–8 Social Work Department Functional Assessment Scale

Patient Name ______________________
RIC Number ______________________
Date ______________________
Physician ______________________

(Please Circle) **ADMISSION** **DISCHARGE**

DEGREE OF PROBLEM
(Please Circle)

(See Department Key) FUNCTIONAL AREAS		**Severe 1**	**Mod-Sev 2**	**Moderate 3**	**Mild-Mod 4**	**Mild 5**	**Minimal 6**	**No Prob 7**	**GOAL***
FINANCIAL RESOURCES		1	2	3	4	5	6	7	
HOUSING		1	2	3	4	5	6	7	
TRANSPORTATION		1	2	3	4	5	6	7	
COMMUNITY PLACEMENT		1	2	3	4	5	6	7	
SUPPORT NETWORK		1	2	3	4	5	6	7	
GUARDIANSHIP/LEGAL	0 = NA	1	2	3	4	5	6	7	
FAM. UNDERSTANDING	0 = NA	1	2	3	4	5	6	7	
FAM. ADAPTATION	0 = NA	1	2	3	4	5	6	7	

GOAL = SET A DISCHARGE GOAL AT ADMISSION.** If there is no goal, or the patient is already at his/her expected level, rate the goal the same as the functional level. ***PLEASE DO NOT LEAVE BLANK.

____
Social Worker Signature and Title

FINANCIAL RESOURCES: Congruency between economic needs and the economic resources available to meet medical and basic living needs. Financial planning for medical care, daily living needs, and health maintenance (e.g., third–party payer coverage, Social Security Income, Social Security Disability Income, General Assistance).

HOUSING: Availability and accessibility of living arrangements with considerations of the physical and financial assistance required. At discharge, this rating should reflect the patient's vocational plan, medical and psychosocial needs.

TRANSPORTATION: Availability and accessibility of transportation resources such as private car or van, medicar, taxi, and public transportation systems. At discharge, this rating should reflect the patient's vocational plan, medical and psychosocial needs.

COMMUNITY PLACEMENT: Disposition at discharge within home or out of home. Problems regarding placement at home, in a nursing home, residential treatment facility, foster care, other institutions, and utilization of community resources regarding placement.

CONTINUITY OF CARE: Post-discharge planning for home health care, medical or psychosocial treatment, continuing hospitalization, planning for medical or psychiatric care (e.g., Department of Rehabilitation Services, Department of Aging, attendant care) for community reintegration.

SUPPORT NETWORK: Amount of assistance required by family to provide support for patient care needs.

GUARDIANSHIP/LEGAL ISSUES: Extent to which there is a need for consideration or involvement with a court as a result of disability that impacts on the individual's decision regarding person or estate (e.g., guardianship, commitment, protective services, power of attorney).

FAMILY UNDERSTANDING OF DISABILITY: Family's understanding of the nature and implications of illness/disability. Attitudes of significant others toward illness/disability. Family's perception of the future limiting aspects of the patient as a result of disability. Congruency or discrepancy experienced with the environments regarding information about disability, limitations, psychosocial reactions, and prognosis.

FAMILY ADAPTATION: Family's adjustment to disability, including coping resources, stage of family life cycle, effective and consistent communication, flexibility of family roles, tolerance of individuality, support, and self-esteem.

Exhibit A–9 Initial Medical Assessment Form

Name ______________________ Birth Date ____________ Sex ________
Address ______________________ Marital Status ______________________
City, State, Zip ______________________ Ethnic Origin ______________________
Phone: Home ______________________ Occupation ______________________
Work ______________________ Religion ______________________

Social Security Number ______________________

Referring Source:
Name ______________________ Address ______________________
Phone ______________________ ______________________
City, State, Zip ______________________

Patient's Local Physician: ______________________ Address ______________________
Name ______________________ ______________________
Phone ______________________ City, State, Zip ______________________

Medical Records ______________________ Address ______________________
Institution ______________________ ______________________
File Number ______________________ City, State, Zip ______________________

DATABASE

Chief Complaint: ______________________

History of Present Illness
Including JOINTS: Pain, heat, redness, swelling, total number involved, morning stiffness (hours), pattern, overall severity, course (cyclic, persistent, migratory), prior skeletal trauma, hypermobility, remissions (none, partial, total), plantar heel pain, Achilles heel pain, stress-aggravated pain, night-aggravated joint pain, rapidity of onset (insidious, abrupt, other), response to antirheumatic therapy (none, partial, total), response to other therapy (none, partial, total), ARA functional classification (normal, adequate, limited, incapacitated, other)

Date: ______________________ ______________________M.D./NUMS

continues

Exhibit A–9 continued

DATABASE

Past Medical History

Pediatric and Adults Illnesses	Date	Hospitalization Medication/Sequelae

Social History (daily routine, housing, job description, capabilities, etc.):

Habits (tobacco, alcohol, drug addiction, etc.):

Allergy (allergies, symptoms, dates):

continues

Exhibit A–9 continued

Current Medication (name, dose, frequency):

Family History (Circle positive and explain): Rheumatism, Arthritis, Lumbago, RA, Systemic Lupus Erythematosus, Spondylitis, Gout, Psoriasis, Tuberculosis, Scleroderma, Cancer, Diabetes, Peptic Ulcer, Renal Disease, Hypertension, etc.

Family Tree (Include age and health of parents, siblings, spouse, and children of propositus) Note: The symbols for the father and mother of the patient are already on the figure. Arrange the patient and siblings in the order of birth.

= Male

= Female

= Propositus

SYSTEMS REVIEW (Circle positive and explain)

General

Fatigability, fever, shaking chills, weight loss, recurrent infections, lymph node enlargement, photosensitivity, other (specify)

continues

Exhibit A–9 continued

Skin:

Malar rash, psoriasis, skin ulcers (digital), skin ulcers (other site), purpura, ecchymosis, other rash (specify), abnormal pigment, alopecia (disease or drug), Raynaud's phenomenon (# of phases), change in skin texture, urticaria, other (specify)

____

____

____

____

____

Head and Neck:

Temporary head pain, occipital head pain, other head pain, dry eyes, conjunctivitis, other ocular inflammation, nasal complaints, ear complaints, oral mucosal inflammation, sore throat, dry mouth, salivary gland enlargement, other (specify)

____

____

____

____

____

Cardiopulmonary:

Pleurisy, dyspnea on exertion, cough, wheezing, angina pectoris, other chest pain, orthopnea, paroxysmal nocturnal dyspnea, dependent edema, other edema, hemoptysis, other (specify)

____

____

____

____

____

Gastrointestinal:

Anorexia, dysphagia, abdominal pain, vomiting, hematemesis, melena, jaundice, diarrhea, constipation, other (specify)

____

____

____

____

continues

Exhibit A–9 continued

Genitourinary:

Dysuria, urethral discharge, renal stone, hematuria, menstrual abnormality, proteinuria, other (specify)

Hematological:

Anemia, lymph nodes, abnormal swelling, other (specify)

Neuromuscular:

Seizures, paresthesias, neuropathy, muscle pain, muscle weakness, altered sensorium, other (specify)

Psychiatric:

(specify)

Attending Physician

continues

Exhibit A–9 continued

Physical Examination (Circle positive findings and explain):

			Right Left		
Height	____________	BP/Sitting	________________	Temperature	____________
				Pulse	____________
Weight	____________	BP/Lying	________________	Respiration	____________

Skin:

Telangiectasia, erythematous knuckle pads, purpura, digital ulcer, digital scars, other ulcerations, sclerodactyly only, acroscleroderma, generalized scleroderma, dermal calcinosis, discoid rash, other rash, erythema nodosum, periungual erythema, heliotrope eyelids, malar rash, psoriasis, alopecia, keratodermia, blenorrhagica, nail pitting, abnormal pigmentation, urticaria, clubbing, erythema marginatum, rash of juvenile rheumatoid arthritis, other (specify)

____

____

____

____

____

Head and Neck:

Abnormal fundi, cataract, conjunctivitis, episcleral-scleral disease, chronic uveitis, acute iritis, ulcers, abnormal thyroid, pharyngitis, lymphadenopathy, abnormal pinnae, xerostomia, salivary gland enlargement, Schirmer test (mm ____), other (specify)

____

____

____

____

____

Lymph Nodes:

Enlargement; tenderness in cervical, axillary, epitrochlear, or inguinal; other (specify)

____

____

____

____

____

continues

Exhibit A–9 continued

Chest:

Moist rales, dry rales, wheezing, pleural effusion, pleural rub, other (specify)

Breast:

Nodules, symmetry, discharge, other (specify)

Cardiac:

Enlarged, systolic murmur (location), diastolic murmur (location), pericardial rue, edema, other edema, arrhythmia, abnormal P_2, other (specify)

Arteries:

Abnormal temporal arteries, Raynaud's phenomenon, absent pulses, other (specify)

continues

Exhibit A–9 continued

Abdomen:

Hepatomegaly, splenomegaly, pain, other (specify)

____

____

____

____

____

Genitalia:

Ulcerations, rashes, urethral discharge, rectal abnormality, pregnancy, other (specify)

____

____

____

____

____

Muscles:

Tenderness, proximal weakness, distal weakness, muscle atrophy, other (specify)

____

____

____

____

Neurological:

Cranial nerve palsy, peripheral motor neuropathy, entrapment neuropathy, peripheral sensory neuropathy, psychosis, other (specify)

____

____

____

____

____
Attending Physician

continues

Exhibit A–9 continued

Peripheral Joints

Axial Skeleton (neck, chest wall, lumbosacral spine; Schoeber, sacroiliac joints)

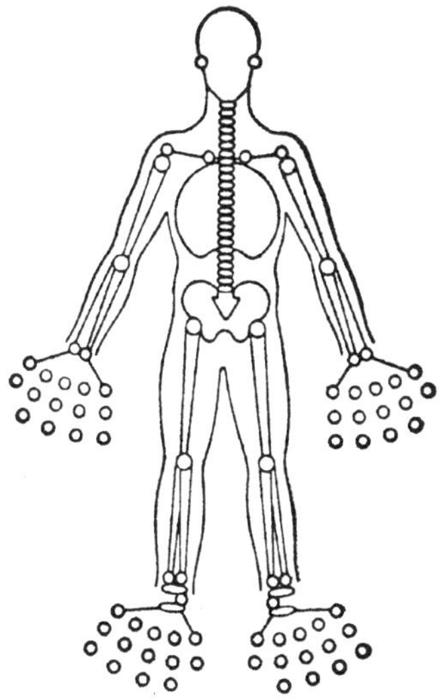

Soft Tissues (bursae, tendons, muscle spasm, nodules, tophi)

continues

Exhibit A–9 continued

SUMMARY BY INITIAL OBSERVER

Time

______________________ M.D.

______________________ Date

Reevaluation Summary #1

______________________ M.D.

______________________ Date

Reevaluation Summary #2

______________________ M.D.

______________________ Date

Index

L

M

N

O

P

T